Training and Conditioning Young Athletes

SECOND EDITION

Tudor O. Bompa, PhD
Sorin O. Sarandan, PhD

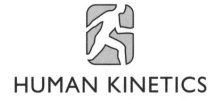

HUMAN KINETICS

Library of Congress Cataloging-in-Publication Data

Names: Bompa, Tudor O., author. | Sarandan, Sorin O., 1975- author.
Title: Training and conditioning young athletes / Tudor O. Bompa, PhD,
  Sorin O. Sarandan, PhD.
Other titles: Conditioning young athletes
Description: Second edition. | Champaign, IL : Human Kinetics, [2023] |
  "This book is a revised edition of Conditioning Young Athletes,
  published in 2015 by Human Kinetics, Inc." -- Title page verso. |
  Includes bibliographical references and index.
Identifiers: LCCN 2022028597 (print) | LCCN 2022028598 (ebook) | ISBN
  9781718216143 (paperback) | ISBN 9781718216150 (epub) | ISBN
  9781718216167 (pdf)
Subjects: LCSH: Physical fitness for children.
Classification: LCC GV443 .B619 2023 (print) | LCC GV443 (ebook) | DDC
  613.7/042--dc23
LC record available at https://lccn.loc.gov/2022028597

LC ebook record available at https://lccn.loc.gov/2022028598

ISBN: 978-1-7182-1614-3 (print)

The web addresses cited in this text were current as of June 2022, unless otherwise noted.

Senior Acquisitions Editor: Roger W. Earle; **Developmental Editor:** Amy Stahl; **Managing Editor:** Shawn Donnelly; **Copyeditor:** Joanna Hatzopoulos Portman; **Proofreader:** Erin Cler; **Indexer:** Rebecca L. McCorkle; **Permissions Manager:** Hannah Werner; **Senior Graphic Designer:** Joe Buck; **Cover Designer:** Keri Evans; **Cover Design Specialist:** Susan Rothermel Allen; **Photograph (cover):** Stevica Mrdja / EyeEm / Getty Images; **Photographs (interior):** part IV by Sorin Sarandan; all others by Human Kinetics, unless otherwise noted; **Photo Asset Manager:** Laura Fitch; **Photo Production Manager:** Jason Allen; **Senior Art Manager:** Kelly Hendren; **Illustrations:** © Human Kinetics, unless otherwise noted; **Printer:** Versa Press

Human Kinetics books are available at special discounts for bulk purchase. Special editions or book excerpts can also be created to specification. For details, contact the Special Sales Manager at Human Kinetics.

Printed in the United States of America

10 9 8 7 6 5 4 3 2 1

The paper in this book is certified under a sustainable forestry program.

Human Kinetics
1607 N. Market Street
Champaign, IL 61820
USA

United States and International
Website: **US.HumanKinetics.com**
Email: info@hkusa.com
Phone: 1-800-747-4457

Canada
Website: **Canada.HumanKinetics.com**
Email: info@hkcanada.com

E8818

Tell us what you think!
Human Kinetics would love to hear what we
can do to improve the customer experience.
Use this QR code to take our brief survey.

Training and Conditioning Young Athletes

SECOND EDITION

Contents

Part III Training Methods

Part IV Selected Exercises for Strength, Power, Agility, Speed, and Flexibility

Preface

Coaches and instructors of young athletes could noticeably improve their training methodology if they borrowed a concept used in home construction: Build from the ground up, from a strong foundation, and work your way up to the roof. The stronger the foundation, the more floors you can build. By analogy, the stronger the players' physical foundation, the higher their chances of growing up to be top athletes.

Unfortunately, this simple concept is rarely applied in youth sport. In their desire to quickly produce successful athletes, some sport enthusiasts are eager to start from the roof down. Others may not understand how to apply the concept unless they are exposed to readily available scientific and methodological information.

Without a long-term vision and guidelines, the development of young athletes will not improve as expected. In most current training programs for young athletes, the emphasis is mostly on acquiring technical and tactical skills. Although skills are determinants of achieving athletic goals, young athletes must also be exposed to progressive long-term training programs intended to improve athleticism, the ability to perform the fastest moves and actions with the highest power and agility possible and for the longest time needed in the selected sport.

The purpose of this book is to discuss and propose a long-term training methodology for young athletes. It aims to offer parents and coaches specific, long-term progressive training programs that will help young athletes realize their athletic dreams. This book shares the best modern methods and exercises to train athletes from under 12 (U12) to physical and technical maturation (U23).

Finally, this book is not just a theoretical forum. On the contrary, the information presented in each part is based on the science and best methodology available. Therefore, it is meant to be applied in each stage of athletic development.

Throughout the stages of athletic development—from under 12 (U12) through under 23 (U21-23)—we have proposed specific guidelines to follow with your athletes. Nutrition and methods of assessment of your athletes' improvements are also discussed, illustrating how we did it, and how to follow them. The largest part of the book is dedicated to what methods to use and how to apply them to develop sport-specific strength, power, maximum speed, agility, flexibility, and specific endurance. The final part of the book provides photos of selected exercises to develop these components in the training and conditioning of young athletes.

As you will expose your athletes to the best available training methodology, it is essential to follow proven scientific information because it works and it is good for you!

We sincerely wish you a successful application of the information we offer.

Tudor Olimpius Bompa, PhD, DHC

Sorin Octavian Sarandan, PhD

Acknowledgments

The 2022 date of publication of this book represents an anniversary for me: the 40th anniversary of my professional collaboration with Human Kinetics. These past 40 years have included many years of work on the publication of several books and the opportunity to meet many professionals from this company—professionals with incredible qualities. This is not flattery but rather a reality.

A book cannot be published without the contributions of these publishing professionals. Authors are recognized with their names on the book cover, but the behind-the-scenes contributors are not very visible. This is why it is our privilege to make their names known:

- Roger W. Earle, acquisitions editor. Roger and I have cooperated together on projects for some 25 years. Roger, sincere thanks for your outstanding leadership and guidance. To us, Roger was the captain of the Human Kinetics team because we worked together as a team.

- Amy Stahl, developmental editor. In my mind, I called Amy "my angel" because she took care of everything regarding the manuscript, correcting all my errors I made while working on this book. Amy, sincere thanks for everything you have done to pull the book through to the finish line.

- Shawn Donnelly, managing editor. Shawn, this is the second book we have worked on together. Thank you for your continued editorial contributions and diligent work.

- Sincere thanks for the work and contributions made by Joanna Hatzopoulos Portman, copyeditor; Hannah Werner, permissions editor; Joe Buck, graphic designer; Keri Evans, cover designer; Susan Rothermel Allen, cover design specialist; Laura Fitch, photo asset manager; Jason Allen, photo production manager; Kelly Hendren, art manager; and Matt Harshbarger, illustrator.

Tudor Olimpius Bompa

Sorin Octavian Sarandan

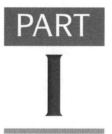

PART I

TRAINING CONSIDERATIONS

Train from early stages of development to maturation with careful progression.

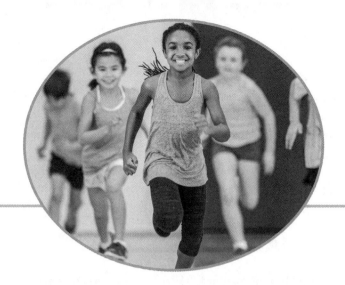

## chapter 1

Effects of Long-Term Training on Young Athletes

Parents, medical experts, social psychologists, and sport scientists generally agree that children enjoy sports and leisure and that athletic activities result in the healthy development of young people. Early years of a young athlete's involvement in sports are essential to a positive start in training and conditioning by following an organized training program and, as a result, to progress naturally in the development of specific skills and physical training attributes of the selected sport. For maximum benefits and enjoyment in any sporting activities, a training program organized according to the age, physical, and emotional potential specific to the young athletes is essential.

POSITIVE EFFECTS

Scientific literature provides substantial information regarding the benefits of children's participation in sports and leisure activities. Systematic physical activity that includes strength, flexibility, and cardiorespiratory endurance for a minimum of 60 minutes, two or three times a week, results in visible health benefits in school-aged children (Janssen and LeBlanc, 2010). In its 2018 study, Newport Academy concluded that young athletes experience benefits such as higher confidence, better concentration and alertness, reduction in the level of overall tension, improvement in cognitive function, enhancement in the ability to cope with stress, and increases in critical thinking (Nettle and Sprogis, 2018).

Furthermore, Richard Stead and Mary Neville (2010) claimed that many positive correlations exist between physical activity and mental health, cognitive functions (e.g., improved memory and concentration), enhanced academic achievements, school attendance, skill acquisition, improved personal development, positive social behavior, self-discipline, and teamwork.

Other authors have referred to the positive effects of sport and leisure activities on the development of youth, such as positive social climate, feeling of satisfaction, optimism, and positive influence on mental well-being. In addition, participation in sports has been shown to reduce stress, anxiety, and depression; improve relationships with adults and peers; improve social, emotional, and behavioral skills; improve self-esteem; lessen symptoms of depression; improve psychological health and nutrition; and decrease obesity (Holt and Neely, 2011; Passer, 2012; Eime et al., 2013; Peirce et al., 2018; Wiersma, 2020).

POTENTIAL CHALLENGES

Exposing children to high-intensity training has also resulted in some contradictory, sometimes even negative, repercussions. Pushing young athletes too hard and adopting a mindset of winning at all costs may cause significant emotional stress and mental disorders, such as depression, anxiety, social phobia, obsessive-compulsive disorder (OCD), and eating and sleep disorders. Unfortunately, self-worth is too often related to team performance. If the team is losing a game, criticism is directed to specific athletes, who often are sidelined. As a result, they become rudderless and experience mental health challenges. However, some parents and caregivers also bear the responsibility for children's reactions after losing a game or not making a team. Under such conditions, sports have more negative repercussions than the benefits outlined earlier.

MAKING POSITIVE CHANGES IN YOUTH SPORT

This chapter has explained that children benefit from practicing sports for enjoyment and for improving health and well-being. It has also identified some ways that participation could lead to serious mental health challenges. These conflicting results may lead you to wonder whether youth sports are worth the effort. However, a more important question may be how adults involved in youth sports can make efforts to effect positive change.

Youth participation in sports can have positive and negative physical, psychological, and social effects (Merkel 2013). Potential positive physical effects like increased physical activity, decreased risk of obesity and chronic disease, and improved fitness and motor skills must be considered alongside potential negative physical effects like increased risk of injury resulting from underdeveloped coaches, safety precautions, or institutional policies and practices. Similarly, positive psychological effects involving improved behavior and mental health must be weighed against the stresses and pressures caused by sport participation, as must positive social effects like opportunities for socializing, character building, and learning life skills against negative social effects like financial challenges and unequal access.

Positive changes for the future of youth sport culture must involve sport culture, parents, and coaches (Merkel 2013). In particular, more emphasis should be placed on sport safety, coach education and training, proper funding, and using positive reinforcement so that sport participants prioritize learning skills, desired social behaviors, and having fun over winning.

In his private sports psychology practice, Murray (2018) cautions about the 10 biggest issues seen in youth sports practice. These issues, along with ways to cope with them, are described as follows:

- *Competitive pressure.* Some children perform well during practice but not during games. Not all children are able to deal with the pressure of competition. Techniques such as guided imagery, relaxation, and goal setting can help.

- *Anxiety.* Some children overthink, become obsessed, or worry about the game and what people, parents, and coaches might think if they lose the game. Techniques to deal with anxiety include pregame treatment, relaxation, and guided imagery (e.g., "Imagine yourself as being relaxed and confident during the game"). Using imagery can often help control anxiety, resulting in improved training and conditioning.

- *Low self-esteem or lack of self-confidence.* Not all children are born with confidence. Often, past or present failure can abate any technique used to boost confidence. However, coaches and parents can help boost confidence by illustrating past achievements in training, offering modifications in self-talk, telling stories, giving examples, and showing videos recorded in previous training sessions.

- *Distraction.* People can easily be distracted. Use mental skills such as focusing and guided imagery with relaxation (imagining successful aspects of the game) to increase confidence, self-esteem, and self-talk. If needed use professional guidance.

- *Anger and frustration.* An upcoming contest may often exacerbate some athletes' behavior, such as eagerness to compete or, on the contrary, be doubtful about own success in a good performance. However, specific psychological treatment of anger and frustration made by a professional psychologist can be successful. Coaches and parents should also improve the pattern of communication with athletes during training and game preparation by rehearsing imagery during practice before the game. Encouraging children to focus on positive outcomes rather than dwell on negative thoughts can help diffuse feelings of anger before the game.

- *Poor relationships.* Negative emotions and actions among athletes, such as envy and lack of enthusiasm and confidence prior to and during the game, may negatively affect tactical communications and even athletic performance. Improve the relationships between athletes, different positions on the team (offensive and defensive players), and eventually between athletes and coaches and other staff members, to create a positive atmosphere that promotes collective confidence. Avoid favoritism and special treatment of some athletes. Children's feelings must be properly regarded. Be relaxed, assertive, fair, and perceptive. Fairness ensures a good team relationship.

- *Perfectionism.* Some children aim for always being technically perfect. However, perfection is difficult to achieve, and mistakes are a natural part of learning and practicing skills. Perfectionism can become a disorder. Encourage this type of athlete to strive for excellence while remembering that perfection is difficult. Ask athletes to aim for advancement rather than perfection.

- *Depression.* Depression is sometimes a mental disorder that can be best treated by specialists who use medication, talk therapy, or a combination of both. One can be stigmatized or labeled as a weak athlete. Keep an eye on the severity of athletes' depression and, if needed, refer them to a doctor for a medication evaluation or treatment.

- *Low motivation or wanting to quit.* Some athletes want to quit the sport with no explanation. Some athletes may lose passion for a sport for many reasons, including relationships, maturation, and simply having other interests. Use motivation techniques to refocus the love for sports. You may also refer the athlete to professional specialists to detect reasons and increase motivation.

- *Trauma, substance use, and addictive disorders.* Negative circumstances of the past (e.g., severe injuries, sexual abuse, domestic violence, drugs) can result in changing behaviors. In the case of appealing to drugs to improve performance, the reason can often be inappropriate training methods (poorly selected strength training methodology that does not result in improved performance as expected). Personal problems and change in status on the team can lead some athletes to drug use or eating and sleep disorders. Both parents and coaches should watch for signs of these conditions and disorders and seek professional help as needed for their athletes.

Courtesy of John F. Murray.

Sports, particularly team sports, are very complex activities. It takes more than just an athlete to enjoy sports participation. Coaches, staff members, parents, and medical and psychological professionals should work together to create a positive atmosphere and specific conditions to enjoy athletic satisfaction.

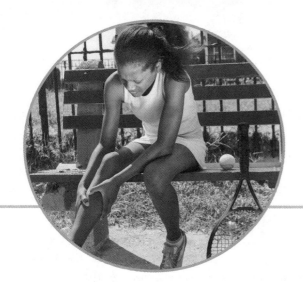

chapter 2

Injuries and Injury Prevention

In the United States alone, 30 to 40 million young people participate in sports. Unfortunately, that impressive number also comes with a high number of sport-related injuries. According to Stanford Children's Health (2022), each year, 3.5 million sport-related injuries occur; the attrition rate is 70 percent, and more than 775,000 children aged 14 and younger are treated in hospitals annually for sports-related injuries. The cost of sport injuries in high school athletics ranges from $5.4 billion to $19.2 billion per year (Fair, 2017).

Attrition rate and the high number of injuries should concern anyone involved in sports, including parents and caregivers, coaches, sport administrators, and sport organizations. However, these concerning numbers are contrary to the financial success of sport industries and the sport market. In 2014, the sport industry in general in North America was worth $60.5 billion (Heitner, 2015) while in 2022 it increased to an impressive $80.5 billion (Statista, 2022). In other words, sport has become a lucrative business.

STRESS OF YOUTH SPORTS

Although being active in sports includes many recognized benefits, it also includes some negative consequences on young athletes, including sports-related stress and injuries.

Some injuries can stem from cumulative, repetitive exercises and skills that are performed during a young athlete's time of rapid physical growth with 80 percent of those injuries occurring in the lower extremities (Brenner and the Council of Sports Medicine and Fitness, 2016).

Most injuries are at the connective tissue level. **Connective tissue** refers to ligaments and tendons that connect the muscles to the bones to perform an athletic action. Although ligaments and tendons are trainable just as muscles are, coaches rarely address specific training programs to strengthen these tissues that connect muscle to bone (tendons) and bone to bone (ligaments). Stronger ligaments and tendons can perform mechanical work more efficiently and can more easily withstand the pull of muscle contractions with lower probability of injuries.

In addition to many hours of training during the week, professionalized youth sports can include organized weekend tournaments in many sports, including baseball, softball, basketball, soccer, and tennis. Youth sport organizations tend to imitate the programs of college and professional sports, using the adage *If you want to be good, do what the best do*. Tournaments include travel and two or three games each weekend day. This rigorous schedule leads to lack of free time, proper rest, and hydration, which adds stress to children and their caregivers. Because children are exposed to risks such as heat, heat-related illnesses, nutrition problems, fatigue, and overtraining, they are more susceptible to experiencing acute injuries, such as broken bones and concussions, under high pressure to succeed. Coaches, parents, and caregivers should ask themselves whether most young athletes (under 18) are ready for the physical and mental stresses of training and many months of league games.

SPORT INJURY STATISTICS

The U.S. Consumer Product Safety Commission (2021) has issued the following sport-related statistics specific to children aged 5 to 14 treated in hospital emergency rooms:

- *Basketball:* More than 170,000 were treated for injuries related to basketball.
- *Baseball and softball:* Nearly 110,000 were treated; three or four children die from baseball injuries in each year.
- *Bicycling:* More than 200,000 were treated for injuries related to bicycling.
- *American football:* Almost 215,000 were treated for football-related injuries.
- *Ice hockey:* More than 25,000 were treated for injuries related to ice hockey.
- *Skateboarding:* More than 66,000 were treated for skateboarding-related injuries.
- *Snow skiing and snowboarding:* More than 25,000 were treated for injuries related to these snow sports.
- *Soccer:* About 88,000 were treated for soccer-related injuries (62% were recorded during practice).
- *Trampolines:* About 65,000 children (in this case, they were 14 years old and younger) were treated for trampoline-related injuries.

According to Steinback Chiropractic Clinic (2018), concussions account for 15 percent of all sport-related injuries; the numbers in specific youth sports are as follows:

- Boys' ice hockey: 23 percent
- Girls' lacrosse: 21 percent
- Boys' lacrosse: 7 percent
- American football: 17 percent
- Girls' soccer: 15 percent

MAIN CAUSES OF SPORT INJURIES

Many of the sport-related injuries in youth can be attributed to the following:

- Participating in too many games
- Coaches' limited knowledge of training methodology, particularly regarding strength training
- Too frequent use of high-intensity training

> ## SPORT DROPOUT: A MAJOR CONCERN
>
> Crane and Temple (2014) made a substantial review regarding the reasons children abandon the sports they used to love. After reviewing 557 articles on the topic from 30 sports, they concluded that children abandon sports for the following reasons:
>
> - Too much emphasis on winning
> - Lack of enjoyment
> - Interpersonal and intrapersonal constraints
> - Perception of competence
> - Maturation, friends, and new priorities
> - Injuries

- A frequent attitude of winning at all costs often among sports coaches, who often keep win-loss statistics as a main focus
- Inappropriate use of popular training gadgets that offer minimal physical training effects and can lead to injuries (including **overuse injuries**, injuries caused by exaggerated, repetitive, specific training)

In addition, Johns Hopkins Medicine (2019) claims that most sport-related injuries occur for the following reasons:

- Highly specialized training that does not provide a balanced program and disregards children's needs of fun and enjoyment
- Inappropriate equipment (particularly safety equipment) used in contact sports
- Poor training and conditioning of athletes, particularly physical training before the start of league games
- Inadequate strength training methodology that does not address the needs of young athletes
- Poor hydration before, during, and after training or competitions
- Inappropriate preparatory (preseason) training, leading to most injuries occurring prior to the beginning of league games (36% from running and sprinting; 16.6% overuse injuries) (Jan Ekstrand, M.D. UEFA Medical Committee, Annual Report, 2021)
- Inadequate use of strength training as a tool for injury prevention, particularly for the foot, ankle (leading to injured ligaments), and calf muscles (leading to an injured Achilles' tendon)

Poor playing conditions can also lead to injuries, including field or court conditions.

INJURY PREVENTION

Many coaches, trainers, and parents overlook injury prevention. Some trainers and coaches have superficial or inadequate knowledge in strength training. Consider the following effective methods for preventing injuries:

- Encourage young athletes under 15 (U15) to participate in more than one team sport. Consider a recreational sport as well.
- Do not abuse specificity in training programs for children by only using exercises specific to the selected sport since it has a greater chance of creating overuse injuries (Cain and Maffulli, 2005).
- Select exercises carefully to avoid overstressing the same joints over time, which may result in overuse injuries.

CONCUSSIONS IN SPORT

Among the highest risk of sport injuries is the concussion, a traumatic brain injury (TBI) that occurs mostly in contact sports. If you witness (or even suspect) any injury to the head, you should immediately request the service of a medical professional, ideally one who is on-site. Parents and coaches should also look for symptoms that might not appear immediately after the incident, such as headaches, balance problems, confusion, or loss of memory. The best and safest approach is to have a comprehensive neurological evaluation that includes assessing the athlete's vision, hearing, sensation, coordination, memory, and reflexes.

Prevention techniques and education of coaches, parents, and athletes in this area are two of the best strategies to impede concussions. Appeal to medical specialists as immediately as possible to have an education session with the parents, coaches, and athletes, or at least use online information to be ready to manage concussions. In addition, you may also consider asking your athletes to use protective equipment for head and face (face shield or mask); use head gear in soccer, rugby, and lacrosse; improve the strength of neck and shoulder muscles; and use maximum attention to anticipate collision in sports.

- Ensure that athletes complete a preseason physical examination with their physicians.
- Use proper protective equipment in contact sports.
- Ensure medical coverage by a team physician at sport events as well as that each athlete has insurance coverage.
- Provide proper coaching by focusing on good technique in both technical skills and strength and power training.
- Always ensure a good warm-up before training and competitions.
- Analyze training to make sure each athlete has a training program commensurate with individual abilities.
- Provide well-planned and well-selected exercises according to the prime movers of the sport (dominant muscle groups in the sport), particularly for strength training sessions, during the preseason (preparatory) phase.
- When coaching for strength and conditioning, understand that sprint training must be preceded by good strength training, particularly by maximum strength (MxS). High-velocity sprinting is possible only when an athlete can apply high force against the ground (propulsion phase of the running step). The basis of high-velocity running is a strong push-off against the ground.
- Provide strength training for the ankle. It is the most neglected joint in training programs; in many team sports, most injuries occur at the foot and ankle level.
- Avoid having young athletes participate in weightlifting and powerlifting competitions or lifting maximum loads before they achieve skeletal maturation (ossification), which occurs around age 18 to 20 (Bompa and Carrera, 2015).

Also, injuries can be prevented by concentrating on fitness training in two areas:

1. *Maximum range of motion (ROM).* The maximum degree of flexibility used by athletes during a game (e.g., lifting the leg higher than hip level) must be considered the minimum degrees of flexibility during training. Al ways look for maximum degrees of flexibility.

2. *Maximum strength (MxS).* The maximum load of strength applied against resistance (gravity, opponent) during the contest must be considered the minimum load during strength training. Maximum strength will always serve you well. It will improve maximum speed, power, and agility. By applying this methodology, you will prevent injuries and develop your athletes' essential abilities (Bompa and Buzzichelli, 2021).

You may also consider the following suggestions made by the American Academy of Pediatrics (2017) regarding the prevention and reduction of injuries:

- For recovery purposes, provide time off (at least one day a week and one month per year).
- Have children wear the right gear to protect the face, shoulders, elbows, chest, knees, and shins (e.g., helmet, mouth guard, face guard, pads, protective eyewear).
- Provide adequate training to strengthen the muscles and connective tissue.
- Establish good flexibility for most joints, particularly for ankles, knees, hips, and shoulders.
- Remind children to play safe by following the rules of the game.
- Do not have children play through pain.
- Avoid heat illnesses by providing lots of fluids before, during, and after the game.
- Supervise children during difficult exercises.

The long-term training programs suggested in this book will enhance your athlete's physical abilities for the selected sport and help prevent injuries.

PREVENTING STRESS AND BURNOUT

Stress is usually perceived as an unpleasant emotional reaction to threatening situations or failure to meet performance expectations. Games expose athletes to stress where not every athlete can adequately tolerate physical and psychological strain. Regardless of the level of games, excessive stress has negative consequences, such as insomnia. Winless stretches during competitions are often a source of stress, which can be intensified by pressure from both parents and coaches, and can aggravate the degree of stress children experience. The stress level is higher if the love and approval of parents is contingent on performing well. Pressure from parents, coaches, and peers is often too difficult to cope with, especially for young children. Although training specialists and researchers often refer to the negative effects of competition stress, they less often discuss the strain and pain children experience in training sessions preceding important games. These workouts often produce negative effects that are similar to those experienced during games. However, moderate levels of stress can provide a setting that enhances children's motivation and performance.

Competition-related stress manifests before, during, and after games (Bompa and Carrera, 2015; Gustavsson et al., 2017) in the following ways:

- Precompetitive stress manifests as fears about not playing well, fear that one's contribution to the team's performance will not meet the expectations of teammates, sleep disorders, restlessness, frequent urination, and diarrhea.
- During games, stress manifests as fear of making mistakes, failure to take chances, poor performance due to high anxiety, sensitivity to coaches' or teammates' criticism, lack of **energy** (the capacity to perform work), paleness, and trembling.

- Postgame stress, which can occur after losing a game or after a poor performance, manifests in lethargy, depression, moodiness, irritability, isolating oneself from family and peers, lack of appetite, sleep disorders, and lack of willingness to train or to show up for the next workout.

Burnout, a physical and emotional exhaustion in athletes that can affect the level of performance, is the result of chronic stress induced by training and games. Symptoms of burnout include lack of energy, exhaustion, sleeplessness, irritability, physical ailments, headaches, anger, loss of confidence, depression, and decrease in performance achievement. Often, some athletes may experience burnout during the final competitions of longer tournaments, such as after several races or matches during one weekend, which can affect their overall standings in the tournament.

Athletes can prevent both stress and burnout to a high degree by using the following techniques (Rotella et al., 1991; Raedeke and Smith, 2004; Bompa and Carrera, 2015):

- Have a good time in training and games. Enjoy being with your friends and improving your skills. Set goals for yourself that are not directly related to the outcome of the games.
- Separate overall self-esteem from performance (especially for specific tasks). Failure to win the game does not rest strictly on you. Set goals for yourself that you can achieve. If you have achieved your own goals, be satisfied.
- Develop interests other than the chosen sport. Your life and satisfaction with life must not depend strictly on the performance you achieve in your sport. Have hobbies. Listen to music, paint, socialize, and find other reasons to be happy.
- Play a sport recreationally—just for the fun of it!
- Take time to relax. Enjoy family and friends.
- Remember that the sport is just a game.
- Learn to laugh at yourself, accept and learn from your errors and failures, and enjoy your successes. Sport is just one of many environments in which you are involved. A loss of a game can easily be offset by the next satisfaction you have in other areas of your life.

Coaches can help athletes avoid burnout by doing the following:

- Watch for signs of staleness such as lack of enthusiasm, irritability, and decrease in performance.
- Provide variety and fun in training.
- Encourage athletes to have balance in their other activities outside of practices and competitions, including school activities, work, social events, and time with family. Encourage athletes to have other interests.
- Coaches, athletes, and parents should keep sport in perspective. Satisfaction from participating in sports is a wonderful experience. However, balance your interests for best life enjoyment. There is more to life than sports.
- Emphasize the goal of doing certain skills well rather than worrying about the result of the game.

Parents and coaches can also help prevent or diminish the impact of stress on children by better organizing weekly activities. Table 2.1 and table 2.2 provide suggested weekly schedules designed to strengthen athletes and avoid burning them out.

Table 2.1 Weekly Training Program for U12 to U15

Monday	Tuesday	Wednesday	Thursday	Friday	Saturday	Sunday
Training	Free for socializing with friends	Training	Free play and games	Training	Recreational sports and hobbies	Off

Table 2.2 Weekly Training Program for U17 to U19

Monday	Tuesday	Wednesday	Thursday	Friday	Saturday	Sunday
Training	Training	Free for socializing with friends	Training	Training	Recreational sports and hobbies	Off

WHEN ARE CHILDREN READY FOR GAMES?

In most cases the decision regarding when children should start playing games rests with coaches and parents. However, children generally enjoy playing games and can be very competitive. Therefore, no debate is needed about the age at which children should start playing games. When determining readiness for play, coaches, parents, and caregivers should always consider the following factors:

- Enter children for competitions only when they are ready technically. This readiness includes motivational and physical readiness.
- Ensure that the primary goals are to have fun, they have already learned the fundamental skills, they have acquired basic tactics, and they physically can play for 20 to 30 minutes.
- Children younger than 8 can play in informal, noncompetitive environments.
- Children begin to understand the rules of the game at the U12 level.
- The following number of official games are suggested for different age groups:
    - U10: 5 to 10 informal games
    - U12: 12 to 15 informal games
    - U15: 18 to 20 house league or even formal games
    - U17: 20 to 25 formal games
    - U19: 25 to 30 formal games

LETTING CHILDREN BE CHILDREN

Many challenges related to participation in sports, such as mental health issues and physical injuries, can be improved simply by remembering that children are still developing, and they need to have fun. Taking sports too seriously can lead to overtraining, which in turn leads to mental health problems and physical injuries. Prioritizing fun in youth sports is important for keeping children healthy enough to continue to succeed; therefore, it is not contrary to developing high-level athletes. In fact, it is necessary for sustaining them and should be alternated with intensive training days. Children should be allowed to have fun and to make mistakes and learn how to play a sport in a relaxed and enjoyable environment. A child who makes gross technical errors now might surprise you by becoming an accomplished athlete later. A child athlete is just a young person on the road to becoming a successful professional and eventually also a good athlete. Even when athletes are in their teen years, adults should avoid treating them with rigidity that can stifle their enjoyment of sports.

Winning is fun but not the determinant factor during the early ages of training. Enjoyment, fun, and socializing with their peers is more important than being a champion. Let children be children.

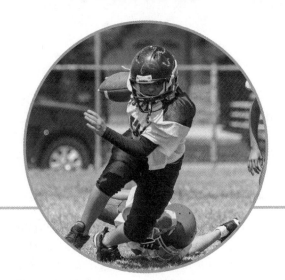

chapter

Guidelines for Long-Term Training

Success in any arena is usually the result of planning, hard work, and commitment, and athletic training is no exception. All successful athletes are trained individuals who excel in a particular physical activity and generally have followed a well-designed long-term training program over several years. In sport, **training** is the process of executing repetitive, progressive exercises or work that improves the potential to achieve optimum performance. For athletes, it means using long-term programs that train and condition the body and mind for the specific challenges of competition and lead to excellence in performance.

Although many coaches are competent at designing seasonal training programs, it is essential to look beyond this short-term approach and plan for the athlete's long-term development. Therefore, proper training should start in childhood. The young athlete can progressively and systematically develop both the body and the mind to achieve long-term excellence rather than immediate success that is followed by burnout.

Often sport programs for children imitate the programs of well-known elite athletes who have captivated the imaginations of young athletes and their coaches. The followers of such programs might think that if a program works for a professional athlete, it should also work for a young athlete. Coaches often employ these programs in detail without evaluating the degree to which they serve the interests of young athletes and with no guiding concepts (e.g., training principles). With the stroke of a key, coaches can download complex programs from a website or article and begin to blindly train their athletes with little consideration for the child's current physical needs.

These coaches and parents do not intend to damage the athlete's development. They want to give their athletes and kids a fighting chance to excel in the extremely competitive environment of sports—sometimes at the detriment of initiating and maintaining a clear focus on development. For instance, it is common for parents to streamline their children into a particular sport or competition. Elijah wants to play in the NHL, or Nevaeh wants to be a professional soccer player and bring home an Olympic gold medal. In both cases, parents can misinterpret a child's early love for a sport as an opportunity to focus programs, coaching, and skill development on one particular sport. Children as young as six years of age have their entire physical development geared around the particular movements of a single sport. Instead, children should be encouraged to play games, perform activities, and participate in multiple sports to optimize athletic development, muscle strength, and neural programming. Children are not simply little adults. They have complex, distinct physiological and psychological characteristics that must be considered.

STRIKING A BALANCE

On one end of the spectrum are child athletes who train excessively; they are specifically training for one sport or doing particular drills while neglecting much-needed **multilateral development** (the development of all abilities of an athlete as required by the selected sport or position played). On the other end of the spectrum are children who are not active or involved in organized sports, and because of their inactivity they might be overweight, undernourished, and detrimentally sedentary.

Childhood obesity gradually increased since 2000 in both the United States (Health Day News, Oct. 20, 2019) and worldwide (World Health Organization, 2019). In 2018, the Centers for Disease Control and Prevention (CDC) reported that one in five children and adolescents are **overweight** (being an abnormal weight for their age or height) or **obese** (having excessive fat accumulation). The World Health Organization (2019) reported that obesity increased globally from 32 million in 1990 to 41 million in 2016. Furthermore, the same source indicates that in 2016 more than 1.9 billion children were overweight while 650 million were obese. Possibly even more damaging to the health of future generations is that in 2019, more than 38 million children aged under five years were overweight or obese.

Trends in obesity and weight gain vary by sex, race, and ethnic group. However, of primary significance is that children are becoming less healthy and less active. For less active children, the program does not focus on what type or intensity of activity is best; rather, it emphasizes that any type of consistent activity—especially in the form of cardiovascular exercise such as walking, running, or cycling—can decrease health risks and improve health outcomes into adulthood.

BUILDING THE FOUNDATION

As athletes reunite in locker rooms and gyms after a short break from competition or training, a saying commonly repeated is *Build the foundation*. Following a hard-fought season or training phase, athlete's' bodies are tired, worn out, and in need of relaxation and—most important—regeneration or replenishing energy stores. Once their bodies heal from the strains of competition, athletes need to take the time to rebuild the foundation of strength, power, endurance, speed, agility, and all the motor abilities that apply to their sport. A strong foundation ultimately leads to optimal performance and less injury.

Some foundational skills are natural extensions of childhood play. From an early age, children can begin building a general foundation of motor skills such as running, jumping, and skipping. They can learn to perform push-ups and chin-ups in their neighborhoods, local parks, and backyards rather than in multimillion-dollar gyms or athlete development centers. However, in today's world of less activity, more screens, and busy schedules, children do not always have the opportunity to learn foundational skills in an informal setting and are coming to sport teams with fewer skills than past generations. Therefore, coaches of entry-level athletes must spend extra time to teach children the fundamental skills of basic motion.

COUNTERACTING THE EFFECTS OF CULTURAL CHANGES AND INACTIVITY TRENDS

A sedentary body can, over time, become obese, sick, and diseased. Researchers at the University of South Australia analyzed the change in running speed and cardiovascular endurance in children aged 9 to 17 years from data collected between 1964 and 2010. Results show that running speed and endurance gradually declined as the years progressed (American Heart Association Scientific Sessions, Tomkinson, 2013). Other sources (Bacil et al., 2015; Dishman et al., 2015; University of Strathclyde, 2019; University of Jyvaskyla, 2019) concur with Tomkinson (2013). This decline can be attributed to many reasons, including the prevalence of gaming and other sedentary habits and the overconsumption of sugar-filled drinks. Although the jury is out on the precise effect of obsessive gaming on health, any activity that limits one's ability to engage in regular physical activity will negatively affect cardiovascular health.

The overall health trend for kids does not look good. Kids are getting fatter and becoming less active. A host of technological advances and behavioral changes such as no longer walking or cycling to school have contributed to our current health crisis. Kids need to get active. We are not talking about long-term athletic development or upper-level sporting camps; we are simply discussing the need for greater movement opportunities. Numerous governing bodies in the United States, including the Centers for Disease Control and Prevention (CDC) (2015) recommend that children get 60 to 90 minutes of physical activity every day in the form of running, jumping, skipping, cycling, and muscle strengthening. The American Heart Association (2020), on the other hand, recommends 30 to 60 minutes of exercise, three or four times per week.

Despite these cultural changes and inactivity trends, "house-league" organized sports can provide a solution. Numerous organizations provide an opportunity for kids to play basketball, soccer, football, hockey, and many other sports for the pure love of exercise and team spirit and without the burden of advancing to a higher league, getting a scholarship, or becoming a professional athlete. If you are a parent who is struggling to encourage your children to become more active and want a suitable form of exercise that will improve their strength and endurance and help build relationships, look to house-league organizations in your area. There is no finer way to get kids active, engaged, and moving and instill the value of being active for a lifetime.

Some benefits of organized sport include the following:

- Promotes healthy living with an emphasis on building skills, strength, and endurance
- Improves mental health and focus
- Teaches important life skills, including self-respect and respect for others, in a safe environment
- Teaches important life lessons about winning, losing, and striving to give one's best effort
- Provides positive role models in coaches, parents, organizers, and other athletes
- Emphasizes fitness and fun because each athlete gets equal playing time
- Represents a great introduction to sport and exercise in a nonthreatening environment, which may motivate participation, growth, and involvement in further levels of sport and activity

The focus of this book is to provide the tools necessary for training and conditioning young athletes—tools that coaches, parents, and athletes can use to better understand the physical necessities of their sport and how to properly train for optimal performance in the short term and the long term. More than 35 million young athletes in the United States play organized sport every year (Nettle and Sprogis, 2011). If athletes are to progress their training from multilateral development and general training and conditioning to sport-specific training and specialization, a proper training philosophy is important to promote improvement and avoid burnout. This chapter discusses four overarching programming guidelines for young athletes: developing a long-term training program, adding training variety, understanding individual characteristics, and increasing training loads appropriately.

DEVELOPING A LONG-TERM TRAINING PROGRAM

For a long time, from about 1900 to 1980, some coaches suggested that performing sport-specific exercises from an early age was the optimal way to train for a sport. They suggested that to yield the fastest results, a training program must do the following:

- Stress the energy system that is dominant in each sport. For instance, a sprinter must do sprints only, and a long-distance athlete must train only the aerobic energy system.
- Follow motor skill specificity. In other words, athletes must select exercises that mimic the skill patterns used in the sport and that involve only the muscle groups used to perform a technical skill.

However, contrary to this methodology, athletic training experts from Eastern Europe dismissed this concept in favor of the following:

- Long-term, progressive training programs
- Multilateral development for young athletes

Even if scientific research demonstrates that specificity training results in faster adaptation and leads to faster increments in performance, it does not mean that coaches and athletes must incorporate specificity training from an early age. In this narrow approach to children's sport, the only scope of training is achieving quick results that do not consider the future of the young athlete. To achieve fast results, coaches expose children to highly specific and intensive training without taking the time to build a good base. It is like trying to erect a high-rise building on a poor foundation. Such a construction error clearly will result in the collapse of the building. Likewise, encouraging athletes to narrowly focus on their development in one sport before they are physically and psychologically ready for that commitment, often results in the following problems:

- It can lead to unilateral, narrow development of muscle and organ functions.
- It can disturb harmonious physical development and biological equilibrium, which are prerequisites of physical efficiency, athletic performance, and the development of a healthy person.
- Over the long term, it can result in overtraining and even overuse injuries. In fact, young athletes should not be encouraged to push through injuries with the misunderstanding that their young bodies can take any kind of stress and eventually bounce back.
- It can have a negative effect on the mental health of the children involved. This type of training and participation in many competitions can create high levels of stress.
- It can interfere with children developing social relationships because of the many hours associated with intensive training. For example, children may fail to make friends outside of their selected sport.

- It can affect the motivation of children because the program can be too stressful, too boring, and lacking in fun. Often young athletes quit the sport before they experience physiological and psychological maturation. Consequently, a talented young person may never find out how skilled she could have become.

Multilateral Development

It is important for young children to develop a variety of fundamental skills, develop motor abilities, and become good overall athletes before they start training in a specific sport. This process is called **multilateral development**, and it is one of the most important training principles for children and youth.

Multilateral, or multi-skill and multi-abilities, development is common in Eastern European countries; in these countries, some sport schools offer a basic training program. Children who attend these schools develop fundamental skills such as running, jumping, throwing, catching, and balancing. The children gain good coordination, and they acquire skills that are fundamental to success in a variety of individual and team sports, such as track and field, basketball, and soccer. Most programs also have a swimming component because swimming helps children develop aerobic capacities while minimizing the physical stresses placed on their joints. Proper understanding of the need to fully diversify programs for child athletes and offer multilateral skill development has spurred the opening of many sport schools—schools dedicated to academic achievement with a heightened emphasis on sport development—throughout North America (Harre, 1982; Faigenbaum et al., 2005; Capranica and Millard-Stafford, 2011; Council of Sports Medicine and Fitness, 2016).

If you encourage children to develop a variety of skills, they will probably experience success in several sport activities. Some will have the inclination and desire to specialize and develop their talents further. When children demonstrate interest in further developing their talents, adults must provide the necessary guidance and opportunities. It takes years of training to become an excellent athlete; young athletes striving for excellence need a systematic, long-term plan based on sound scientific principles.

Figure 3.1 illustrates the sequential approach (from the foundation up) to developing athletic talent over several years. Although the ages vary from sport to sport and from athlete to athlete, the model demonstrates the importance of progressive development.

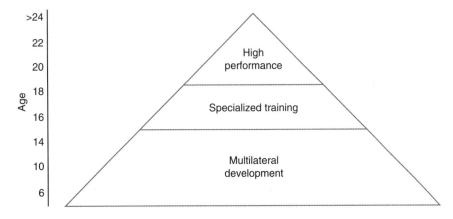

Figure 3.1 Suggested long-term approach to training young athletes.

Reprinted by permission from T.O. Bompa, *Periodization Training for Sports* (Champaign, IL: Human Kinetics, 1999), 39.

The base of the pyramid, which you may consider the foundation of any training program, consists of multilateral development. When the development reaches an acceptable level, athletes specialize in one sport and enter the second phase of development. The result will be a high level of performance.

The purpose of multilateral development is to establish a multi-skilled base and multi-abilities adaptation that covers all physical abilities from strength and speed to endurance. Children and youth who develop a variety of skills and motor abilities are more likely to adapt to demanding training loads without experiencing stresses associated with early specialization. For example, young athletes who specialize in middle-distance running may be able to further develop their aerobic capacities by running, but they are also more susceptible to overuse injuries. Athletes who are capable of swimming, cycling, and running can exercise their cardiorespiratory system in a variety of ways and significantly reduce their chance of injury. If a young athlete wants to become a professional football player, running is not the only cardiovascular activity that athlete should perform. Other skills, such as jumping, skipping, climbing, and cycling, help strengthen the development of muscles at various angles and encourage neuromuscular focus. Most importantly, developing this variety of skills is necessary before the body can begin specializing in specific movement patterns. Furthermore, emphasizing cable or dumbbell movements intended to help the baseball swing (which are often touted as sport-specific movements) at such a young age is not necessary, especially if athletes are struggling to perform fundamental exercises such as push-ups or chin-ups.

Focus on the fundamentals first, and the specifics will take care of themselves. Adults often tell children to slow down and not rush to grow up; the same idea applies to sport. As an athlete matures in age and physiological function, specificity in training will inevitably become the focal point. Sport-specific training programs and the stress of repeating movements that are essential to the desired sport will become necessary. The athletic conditioning required to safely make the transition to and recover from the intensity of sport-specific training will depend on the athlete's overall development of strength and coordination and the preparedness of the athlete's nervous system—the key components of multilateral training.

Young athletes should be encouraged to develop the skills and motor abilities they need for success in their chosen sport and other sports. For example, a well-rounded training program for children and youth would include low-intensity exercises for developing aerobic capacity, anaerobic capacity, muscular endurance, strength, speed, power, agility, coordination, and flexibility. A multilateral training program that focuses on overall athletic development, along with sport-specific skills and strategies, will lead to more successful performances at a later stage of development. As table 3.1 demonstrates, a multilateral program provides many benefits. If you are interested in developing successful, high-performance competitors, you must be prepared to delay specialization and sacrifice short-term results. The following long-term experiment demonstrates this concept.

In a landmark longitudinal (14-year) study performed in the former East Germany (Harre, 1982), children aged 9 to 12 years were divided into two groups. The first group participated in a training program that entailed early specialization in each sport and incorporated exercises and training methods that were specific to the needs of the sport. The second group followed a generalized program; it incorporated overall skills and specific drills, as well as a variety of other sports and skills. As table 3.1 illustrates, the results prove that a strong foundation leads to athletic success.

Table 3.1 Comparison Between Early Specialization and Multilateral Development Programs

Early specialization	Multilateral development
Quick improvement in performance	Slower improvement in performance
Best performance achieved at age 15-16 years because of quick adaptation	Best performance achieved at age 18+ years (age of physiological and psychological maturation)
Inconsistent performance in competitions	Consistent performance in competitions
Common burnout and quitting the sport by age 18 years	Longer athletic life
Prone to injuries because of forced adaptation	Few injuries

Interest in research regarding sports specialization versus multilateral development has grown since the 1990s, yielding results similar to Harre's (1982) claims. With emphasis on universal sport competitions, athletes are subtly encouraged to specialize at an earlier age (Capranica and Millard-Stafford, 2011). Young athletes are now taking on rigorous training schedules that are similar to adult training models. Such schedules, which can include more than 10 hours of training per week and weekend tournaments, can lead to many negative consequences, including physical, mental, and emotional problems.

In a study regarding youth specialization, Baker (2003) found that specialization limited overall motor skill development and promoted imbalance in the joint—particularly in the knee development—such as tightness and inflexibility because muscles and tendons did not increase in length at the same rate as the bones. Baker (2003) also expressed concerns that early specialization resulted in dropouts from participation in sports.

In an article published in *British Journal of Sports Medicine*, Mostafavifar and colleagues (2013) argue that early specialization in one sport can lead to numerous practical and physiological implications, including the following:

- A decrease in motor skill development because focus shifts from general development to sport-specific programming
- Increased risk of injury to the cardiovascular and musculoskeletal systems because of the intensity and volume of training
- Improper recovery because of a lack of knowledge about nutrition and proper macro- and micronutrient ratios
- Early burnout caused by high number of hours of dedication
- Early injury from overuse

In addition, Branta (2013) claims that early specialization limits a child's acquisition of fundamental motor skills, while Feeley et al. (2016) concluded that specialization does not lead to competitive advantages but rather to increased risk of injuries. Several scholarly studies refer to the grave concerns regarding the high numbers of injuries in youth sports (Fabricant et al., 2016; Brenner and the Council of Sports Medicine and Fitness, 2016; Pasulka et al., 2017; Post et al., 2017; Bell et al., 2019). Jayanthi and colleagues (2019) cite that sports medicine organizations recommend against sports specialization for youth because of the risks of injuries and the negative health-related quality of life consequences.

The intent of this chapter is not to discourage a discussion on the viability of early specialization. Rather, the scope is to highlight the adverse effects of prematurely nudging an athlete to train beyond the body's ability to heal and recover. The debate between early and late specialization continues, but the priorities—the long-term mental and physical health of the young athlete and the formula for achieving one's greatest potential with minimal risk of injury—should remain the same.

Although multilateral training is most important during the early stages of development, it results in higher performance benefits (Krasilshchikov, 2015; Granacher and Borde, 2017; Bompa and Buzzichelli, 2021), and it should be part of the training regimen for advanced athletes. Figure 3.2 illustrates that although the ratio between multilateral development and specialized training changes significantly throughout the long-term training process, athletes need to maintain throughout their careers the multilateral foundation they established during their early development.

For instance, consider the case of Maya, a 12-year-old tennis player. Every week Maya engages in 10 hours of tennis training and 4 to 5 hours of other physical and multilateral training such as flexibility, basic strength (using medicine balls and dumbbells), and agility exercises. A parent or a coach might think that more tennis drills would make Maya a more-skilled athlete. However, increasing her tennis training is possible only at the expense of reducing her multilateral training. Maya's tennis skills may improve in the short term, but lack of training in basic physical abilities such as strength, agility, and flexibility would thwart her playing abilities in the long term. A lack of good physical qualities at the age of 18 would result in weaker strokes, slower movement on the court, and decreased agility and quickness, thus lowering Maya's overall tennis-playing potential.

The latter slightly decreases as Maya matures. If Maya is doing 4 to 5 hours of multilateral training per week at age 12, she might do 3.5 to 4 hours per week at age 16. At the same time, her tennis-specific training may increase from 10 hours per week at age 12, to 14 to 16 hours per week at age 16.

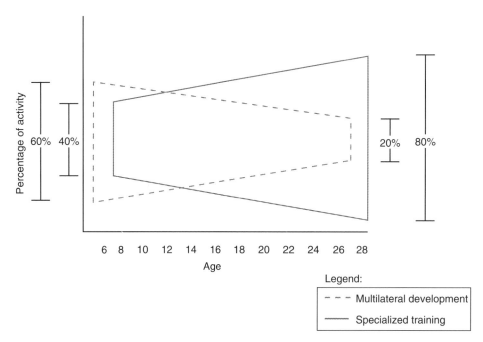

Figure 3.2 Ratio between multilateral development and specialized training for different ages.

Specialized Development

Specialization should usually take place after athletes have developed a solid multilateral foundation and when they have the desire to specialize in a particular sport or a position in a team sport. Specialization is necessary for achieving high performance in any sport because it leads to physical, technical, tactical, and psychological adaptation. It is a complex process. From the onset of specialization, athletes have to prepare for ongoing increments in training volume and intensity.

Once specialization takes place, training should include both exercises that enhance development for the specific sport and exercises that develop general motor abilities. However, the ratio between the two forms of training varies considerably from sport to sport. For example, consider the difference between long-distance runners and high jumpers. The training volume for long-distance runners will consist mostly of running drills or activities that enhance aerobic endurance, such as cycling and swimming. At the same time, a program for high jumpers will consist of approximately 40 percent high jump–specific drills and exercises and 60 percent exercises that develop particular motor abilities (e.g., plyometrics and weight training for developing leg strength and jumping power).

As table 3.2 illustrates, there are general ages at which athletes should start developing skills and specializing in each sport with the hope of eventually reaching a high-performance standard. However, even during the specialization stage of development, athletes should dedicate only 60 to 80 percent of their total training time to performing sport-specific exercises; the balance of their time should be spent on improving most motor abilities related to their selected sport.

Once athletes have decided to specialize, they must prepare to use specific training methods for adapting to the physical and psychological demands of a more competitive sport. The training demands increase significantly, formalized testing begins, and 'coaches plan and schedule organized competitions on a yearly basis.

Specialization takes place at different ages depending on the sport. In sports that require artistry of movement, complex motor skill development, and a high degree of flexibility (e.g., gymnastics, diving, figure skating), athletes should specialize at a young

Table 3.2 Guidelines for the Road to Specialization

Sport	Age to begin the sport (years)	Age to start specialization (years)	Age to reach high performance (years)
American football	12-14	16-18	22-28
Baseball	10-12	14-16	20-30
Basketball	10-12	14-16	20-28
Figure skating	6-10	12-14	18-26
Gymnastics	6-8	12-14	16-24
Ice hockey	8-10	13-14	22-28
Soccer	10-12	14-16	20-28
Swimming	6-8	11-13	16-24
Tennis	8-10	13-14	18-28
Volleyball	12-14	15-18	22-26

Note: The age to reach high performance does not mean an athlete cannot maintain a high level of performance beyond the suggested age range.

age. For sports in which speed and power dominate (e.g., football, baseball, volleyball), athletes can start practicing the fundamental sport techniques at a young age. However, specialization should take place only once athletes are capable of effectively coping with the demands of high-intensity training. In most sports with a focus on speed and power, specialization should take place toward the end of the adolescent growth spurt. For sports in which success depends on the ability to cope with maximal endurance efforts, such as long-distance running, cross-country skiing, and cycling, athletes can specialize at the time that they develop speed and power or later. Some endurance athletes can achieve outstanding performance results at age 30 years or older.

ADDING TRAINING VARIETY

Throughout the long process of their development, young athletes experience thousands of hours of training; they complete exercises and drills many thousands of times to develop their abilities. If training programs are not closely monitored and varied, many athletes will have difficulty coping with the physical and psychological stresses associated with this repetitive action. Therefore, incorporating diverse exercises and developing a range of skills in the training program at every stage of the developmental process not only helps athletes develop new abilities but also prevents injury, boredom, and burnout.

Most team sports, such as hockey, baseball, and basketball, expose athletes to a variety of training methods. To strive for excellence in these sports, athletes must become competent in many skills and exercises. They develop this competence most effectively through training diversity. Other sports, especially individual sports, have less diversity. For example, swimmers rarely participate in other sports and often perform the same exercises, technical elements, and drills for 2 or 3 hours a day, 4 to 7 days a week, 45 to 50 weeks a year, for 20 years. This type of repetitive training may lead to overuse injuries and psychological challenges, particularly the emotional difficulties associated with monotony and boredom.

To overcome these challenges, coaches should incorporate a variety of exercises into each practice session. Using various technical movements from other activities can enrich a coach's list of drills. Coaches can also include exercises that develop the motor abilities needed in the selected sport, such as speed, power, and specific endurance. Coaches who are creative and knowledgeable have a distinct advantage because they can design some workouts with the scope of using variety of exercises and drills. If possible, periodically conducting a session away from the usual training environment can keep young athletes stimulated, interested, and, in some cases, more motivated.

Similarly, performing a variety of exercises also develops muscles other than those the athlete uses specifically in the chosen sport. Too much specificity training may result in overuse injuries. Moreover, it may cause imbalances between the **agonist muscles** (muscles contracting to perform a physical activity) and the **antagonist muscles** (muscles relaxing during a motion). When a strong imbalance exists between these two sets of muscles, the pull of agonist muscles is so strong that it may cause an injury to the tendons and muscle tissue of the antagonist muscles. Therefore, incorporating a variety of exercises that use many muscles of the body can decrease the incidence of injury. Similarly, variations of movement, including practicing other sports, will improve coordination and agility. A well-coordinated and agile athlete will quickly learn difficult skills later.

Coaches who creatively incorporate variety into their training programs will see the benefits. Athletes will remain highly motivated and will be less likely to experience overuse injuries.

UNDERSTANDING INDIVIDUAL CHARACTERISTICS

Every athlete has unique personality traits, physical characteristics, social behaviors, and intellectual capacity. Designing an individual training program is an important step in determining an athlete's strengths and limitations by using both subjective and objective measures. The working capacity of athletes varies significantly. To effectively design training programs for athletes, coaches must consider individual strengths and limitations, individual differences (e.g., stage of development, training background, and experience), health status, recovery rate between training sessions and following competitions, and sex differences between male and female athletes.

Also, it is no longer suitable or acceptable to categorize young athletes strictly based on chronological age because children of the same age can differ in anatomical maturation by several years. Considering anatomical age, biological age, and athletic age is crucial.

Anatomical Age

Anatomical age refers to the several stages of anatomical growth and development children go through during different stages from childhood to maturation that one can recognize by identifying particular physical characteristics. Stated another way, anatomical age is the numerical assessment of a child's growth in relation to chronological age. Table 3.3 summarizes the developmental stages of children and youth. However, keep in mind that many individual differences exist regarding characteristics.

Table 3.3 Stages of Anatomical Age

Phase of development	Chronological age (yr)	Stage	Anatomical age	Developmental characteristics
Early childhood	0-2	Newborn Infant Crawling Walking	0-30 days 1-8 mo 9-12 mo 1-2 yr	Fast organ development
Preschool	3-5	Small Medium Big	3-4 yr 4-5 yr 5-6 yr	Unequal rhythm of development when important and complex changes occur (functional, behavioral, personality)
School years	6-18	Prepuberty	6-11 yr (girls), 7-12 yr (boys)	Slow and balanced development when the functions of some organs become more efficient
		Puberty	11-13 yr (girls), 12-14 yr (boys)	Fast growth and development in height, weight, and the efficiency of some organs; sexual maturation with change in interests and behaviors
		Postpuberty, adolescence	13-18 yr (girls), 14-18 yr (boys)	Slow, balanced, and proportional development; functional maturation
Young adult	19-25	Maturity	19-25 yr	Maturation period doubled by perfecting all functions and psychological traits; athletic and psychological potentials are maximized

Anatomical age clearly demonstrates the complexities of growth and development and helps explain why some children develop skills and motor abilities faster or slower than others do. A child who is more developed anatomically will learn many skills faster than a child who is less developed. Although many children follow similar growth patterns, variations exist. For example, climate, latitude, terrain (mountainous versus flat), and living environment (urban versus rural) can significantly affect the rate at which young people develop. Young people in countries with hot climates mature much faster sexually, emotionally, and physically. As a result, their athletic performance can increase faster between the ages of 14 and 18 than in young athletes who live in countries with colder climates.

Biological Age

Biological age refers to the physiological development of the organs and systems in the body that help determine the physiological potential for reaching a high-performance level in both training and competition. When categorizing and selecting athletes, coaches must consider biological age. Using a rigid classification system based on chronological age will frequently result in misjudgments, faulty evaluations, and poor decisions.

Two athletic children of the same anatomical age who are the same in height, weight, and muscular development could be of different biological ages and possess different abilities to perform a training task. A tall child who looks strong is not necessarily a faster athlete. Similarly, a slightly smaller youngster may be more agile in certain positions in team sports. Whereas anatomical age is visible, biological age is not. One cannot see how efficient an athlete's heart is or how effectively an athlete utilizes oxygen. A less impressive physique may hide a powerful and efficient heart, which is important in endurance sports. To find a child's training potential, you must assess biological age objectively through simple tests.

Without considering biological age, it is difficult to determine whether certain children are too young to perform particular skills or to tolerate specific training loads. It is also difficult to assess the potential of older athletes, who may be considered too old to achieve high performance. Yet, in many sport programs, national and international sporting organizations and coaches still use chronological age as the major criterion for classification.

The following list illustrates some differences in the biological ages of international sport champions.

- Constatina Tomescu-Dita (Romania) was a gold medalist in the marathon at the 2008 Beijing Olympic Games at the age of 38. She is also the oldest Olympic marathon champion in history.
- At the 1964 Olympic Games in Tokyo, Masao Takemoto (Japan) received a silver medal in gymnastics at the age of 44.
- At the 1998 Winter Olympic Games in Nagano, Tara Lipinski (United States) won the gold medal in figure skating at the age of 15.
- Ellina Zvereva (Belarus) received a gold medal in discus throw at the 2001 World Championships at the age of 40.
- In 1988, 15-year-old Allison Higson (Canada) broke the world record in the 200-meter breaststroke.
- In 1991, 12-year-old Fu Mingxia (China) became a world champion in diving.
- Gordie Howe (Canada) was still playing hockey in the National Hockey League at the age of 52. (He played from 1946 to 1971 and again from 1979 to 1980.)
- Tom Brady, the quarterback of the U.S. football team Tampa Bay Buccaneers, was still incredibly successful in 2022, at the age of 44!

This list, which represents only a small percentage of the athletes who have achieved remarkable performances in sport, demonstrates that chronological age does not always represent an athlete's level of biological potential.

INCREASING TRAINING LOADS APPROPRIATELY

Understanding the methods used to increase training loads is essential for creating a good training program. The amount and quality of work that children and youth achieve in training directly affects the amount that their physical abilities will improve. From the early stages of development through the high-performance level, athletes must increase the workload in training gradually according to their individual needs. During adaptation to a particular training load, athletes increase their capacities to cope with the stresses and demands of training and competition. Athletes who develop gradually will likely be more capable of performing work over a long period.

The rate at which young athletes improve their performance depends on the rate and method they use to increase the training load. If they maintain the load at approximately the same level for a long time (standard load), improvements in performance are barely visible. If they increase the load too much, some immediate benefits may be visible, but the likelihood of injuries substantially increases. Therefore, it is important for young athletes to progressively increase the training load. Although immediate, short-term results are difficult to attain; the long-term potential for improved performance is much greater.

Duration of Training Sessions

The duration of each training session can increase from the beginning of the season to the end (e.g., from 60 to 90 min), as table 3.4 suggests.

As the duration increases to 90 minutes, it is important to maintain the children's interest by choosing a variety of drills and activities. Coaches should also include longer rest intervals between drills and exercises so that athletes may more easily cope with fatigue. Note that a training session performed in hot and humid conditions should always be much shorter than a regular session because children become fatigued more quickly.

Number of Exercises

To progressively increase the training load, athletes can also expand the number of exercises and drills they perform per training session over the weeks and years. Increasing the number of **repetitions** (an action that is repeated several times during training) of technical drills or exercises for physical development will certainly improve an athlete's performance. However, as the number of exercises and drills increases, the coach must

Table 3.4 Progression of Training Session Length for a U15 Soccer Team

Month	Duration of sessions (min)
April	60
May	75
June	90
July	90
August	Off

carefully monitor the rest intervals between them. Longer rest intervals allow the athletes to better recover between repetitions and give them more energy to perform all the work planned for that training session.

Frequency of Training Sessions

To constantly challenge the bodies of young athletes to achieve performance improvement, you must regularly increase the frequency of training sessions (the number of training sessions per week). This increase is essential because skills develop during training sessions, not during games and competitions. For young athletes to constantly master the skills of the sport and to develop the motor abilities needed for future competitions, they must have more training sessions than games. Therefore, parents should require that coaches, especially in team sports, have a ratio of two to four training sessions to one game. Such an approach will pay off later in an athletic career because athletes will properly acquire skill fundamentals at the ideal age.

Coaches who extend their season so they have more weeks to prepare before competition begins will likely see positive results. In team sports such as soccer, baseball, and football, children often experience a few weeks of training before games start.

The ideal situation is to practice for most months of the year; it will lead to better development of skills and motor abilities. Coaches and parents can take advantage of a long preseason training period to work with the athletes on skill acquisition without the pressure of playing games on weekends. One problem with current training schedules is that generally athletes are not given an opportunity for downtime; they need a chance to recover from the season and simply engage in fun activities. Parents and coaches are quickly shifting their kids from season play to off-season, sport-specific training camps or to indoor or outdoor leagues with weekend games, depending on the sport. They fear that skill development will stop if the athlete allows the body to move to a lower workload or adds variety in training. On the contrary, the body uses such downtime to strengthen the integrity of the cardiac, neuromuscular, and other vital systems and to refresh the athlete for when training frequency increases. Instead of adding more games or increasing an athlete's workload, coaches should organize general training sessions for the athletes at the end of the regular season.

If coaches cannot organize such a training program, parents should do so. A basement, a garage, an open field, or the backyard are all great places for training simple skills, especially motor abilities. To develop basic strength or endurance, one does not need the most sophisticated facilities.

Young children may commit only a few months to practicing a specific sport, and often these are the months of the competitive season. As young athletes become older and more experienced, they should commit more months to training in a specific sport if they desire high performance results. When young athletes make the commitment to specialize in a particular sport, they will likely be training 10 months or more a year.

Another suggested progression is in the frequency of training. At first the duration of training can increase from two times a week at 60 minutes to two times a week at 75 minutes, then to two times a week at 90 minutes. If you consider it the upper level of the child's tolerance, the frequency of training sessions can then increase from two times a week at 90 minutes to three times a week at 90 minutes. In a later stage of developing the athlete's potential, the frequency can increase to four or five training sessions a week (or even higher for some sports).

As the frequency reaches an upper limit (e.g., three times at 90 min) for that developmental stage, the number of exercises and drills per training session can increase. Consider these two methods:

1. Increase the number of exercises before taking rest (e.g., from 1 set of 8 ball passes, drills, or exercises to 1 set of 10, 12, or even 14). A **set** is the total number of repetitions an athlete performs before taking a rest interval (pause).

2. Decrease the rest interval between sets (e.g., from 2 min to 1.5 min, and then to 1 min).

Step Loading

Standard loading—the same type of training all the time—rarely results in performance improvement. Therefore, improvement in children's abilities is visible only if you increase the load in different parts of an annual training program. The most effective way to increase the training load is to understand and use the **step loading method**. With this method, the load increases in steps; it usually increases for two or three weeks and then decreases for one week to allow for regeneration or recovery. Figures 3.3 and 3.4 illustrate two options. The option shown in figure 3.3 is recommended for young children, and the option shown in figure 3.4 is recommended for athletes in their late teens and young athletes who are advanced in a particular sport. Both models refer to the training weeks when athletes are not in competition.

As figure 3.3 suggests, the training load should increase progressively. During the first two steps, each representing a week, the increased load challenges young athletes to adapt to a greater amount of work. As the athletes become fatigued, the load slightly decreases in the third week to allow for recovery before it again increases further.

As figure 3.4 illustrates, athletes in their late teens (U17 and older) are expected to cope with a more challenging program. During the first three weeks of training, the load increases from week to week, which leads to higher adaptation levels and, ultimately, superior performances. The fatigue level will be high by the end of the third step, so the load slightly decreases in step 4 to allow for recovery. To continue increasing the training load after the third week will result in greater fatigue, which may lead to a critical level of fatigue or, over time, overtraining. If you fail to incorporate a regeneration week into your training plan, athletes may experience fatigue or even injuries, they could lose interest, and they might eventually drop out.

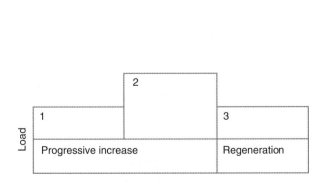

Figure 3.3 Suggested step loading for young athletes (U12-U15).

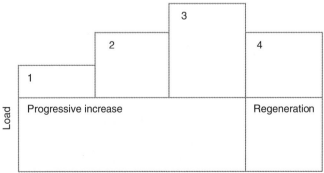

Figure 3.4 Suggested step loading for more advanced athletes (U17 and higher).

Table 3.5 Suggested Progression to Increase Training Elements in the Step Loading Method

Training element	Step 1	Step 2	Step 3	Step 4
Training sessions/wk	2-3	3	4	3
Duration of training sessions (min)	75	90	90-120	75-90
Rest interval between sets of drills or exercises	Standard	Standard	Shorter	Standard

Table 3.5 suggests training elements that you can use to increase the load from step to step or decrease the load for the regeneration week of the four-week cycle without exhausting all the training elements. Note that in table 3.5 the number of training sessions peaks in step 3 to four per week. If you use the three-week step method for children (figure 3.3), then the progression may be two training sessions for the first step and three training sessions for the second step. The number of training hours increases in the same way. Regarding the rest interval, *standard* means the normal periods the coach uses. After step 3 (figure 3.3) or step 2 (figure 3.4), the coach can use a slightly shorter rest period to further challenge the bodies of the young athletes.

The regeneration week is crucial to the step loading method. The athletes are tired at the end of the highest step, and to continue training at the same level of demand is a mistake. For the well-being of the young athletes, the **training demand** (a summation of all the factors used in training or game situations) should decrease during this week (week 4). This will allow the athletes to remove fatigue from the body, relax the mind, and replenish overall energy. Toward the end of this week, the athletes will feel rested and ready for one or two more weeks of increased load increments.

After the regeneration weekends, the step loading method can be applied again but at a slightly higher training demand. At the beginning of the preseason phase, you can increase the workload by 5 to 10 percent. As the athletes adjust to this workload, especially in the second part of the preseason phase, the load increment can be increased from step to step by 10 to 20 percent.

The step loading method is most valid during the preseason, a time when athletes train for upcoming competitions. It is not valid during the competitive season, when athletes are engaged in official or league games at the end of the week. Therefore, during the season, the load of training each week is steady, and a regeneration period is scheduled to remove fatigue after a game. Athletes perform most training during the middle of the week and plan light training for the one day (or maximum of two days) before a game so that they will not experience fatigue that could impair their performance on game day.

Certainly, other options for organizing the weekly program are possible. A coach may organize only two training sessions a week (e.g., Tuesday and Thursday), each one of steady intensity. Each session may be of lighter intensity if the athletes show signs of fatigue. Remember that rested children always play better games.

Training young athletes must be viewed as a long-term proposition in which the load and the overall physical, technical, tactical, and mental demands are increased gradually during the stages of growth and development. Laying the foundation of sound training during childhood through multilateral development rather than narrow, sport-specific training will give young athletes a better foundation for high performance. Providing variety in training, accounting for individual differences among athletes, and appropriately planning the load progression from stage to stage will also result in a more effective training program.

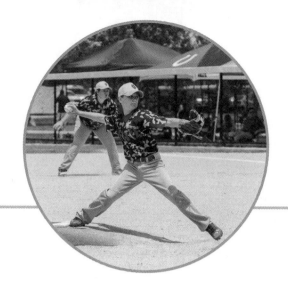

chapter 4

Stages of Long-Term Athletic Development

Sport scientists and highly regarded coaches generally agree that athletes who were exposed to well-organized, systematic training during the early stages of their athletic development have consistently been able to accomplish high levels of athletic performance. Impatient coaches, who push for miraculous results too soon, fail in their athletic dreams for their athletes specifically because young athletes need time to acquire good skills and develop sport-specific physical attributes, such as high levels of speed, agility, and strength or power.

Therefore, coaches should keep in mind that children evolve at different rates. The growth rates of children's bones, muscles, organs, and nervous systems differ from stage to stage, and these developments largely dictate a child's physiological and performance capabilities. Therefore, a training program must consider individual differences and training potential. For example, at the age of 14, the difference between athletes may be so great that some have the athletic potential of 16-year-olds (early developers), whereas others have only the physical capabilities of 12-year-olds (late developers). To neglect such a large range of differences in training potential could mean that an early developer is undertrained while a late developer is overtrained. Training programs need to be individualized as often as possible.

LONG-TERM PERIODIZATION OF TRAINING

The training and conditioning programs proposed in this book account for internationally recognized stages of development; they range from under 12 (U12) to U23 (under 23, but over U21), where exercises and types of training follow a long-term progression. Long-term periodization of training is a gradual, progressive physical training program that, ideally, should lead to a greater possibility of an injury-free athlete.

The term **periodization** derives from the word *period*, which means "time interval" or "phase." For youth sports, it refers to five specific phases (stages) of development of physical abilities such as flexibility, strength, speed, and agility. These five stages (see table 4.1 and the sections that follow) are interconnected in a holistic concept that considers athletes' potential for each age group and assures continuity, progression, and effectiveness.

Table 4.1 Five Stages of Development of Physical Training of Young Athletes

Main objectives	Stages of development	Scope of training	Type of training
Make a child a player.	U12	Initiation stage	Multilateral
	U15	Athletic formation stage: building the foundation for sport-specific specialized training stage	Combined training: multilateral and specialized
	U17	Sport-specific specialized training stage	Sport-specific physical training
Make a player an athlete.	U19	Pre–high performance stage	Sport- and position-specific training, high level of athleticism
	U21-23 and over	High performance stage	Position-specific training, high level of athleticism

Table 4.1 summarizes the concept of long-term periodization and training goals in the five stages of development, which are further divided as follows:

1. *Make a child a player (U12-U17)*. Training objectives are progressive technical and tactical improvement of the main skills of the sport.

2. *Make a player an athlete (from U19 throughout the athletic career)*. Now that the technical and tactical fundamentals are established, the objective of physical training is to reach the highest athleticism possible. While technical and tactical training have the scope of achieving perfection, physical training will be a determinant for a player to become the best athlete possible.

U12: INITIATION STAGE

During the initiation stage, children and youth should be exposed to a low-intensity training program that is commensurate with their potential and also ensures fun, enjoyment, and socializing with teammates. Many skills and exercises at this stage should address all segments of the body to ensure multilateral, overall physical development. Exercises should follow a simple progression. Begin with basic movements of low-intensity strength training; the intention is to adapt ligaments, tendons, and muscles to form the foundation of strength and early stages of developing cardiorespiratory systems needed for stages to come.

Coaches should also consider that during the early stage of initiation, bones are still fragile; ends of bones are still cartilaginous and in the process of calcifying, so they are susceptible to injuries. Children and youth at this stage have a short attention span, but they are also action oriented. Therefore, you should keep theoretical explanations to a minimum. Use variety and creativity to stimulate their attention and concentration.

The initiation stage (U12) is the most important time for developing coordination and flexibility. Therefore, U12 is also called the *rapid gains phase*. At this stage of development, children who are involved in a variety of activities and multilateral training with many skills, drills, or types of activities will make greater gains in coordination compared with those who specialize in only one sport.

Multilateral training enriches skill experience; as a result, it improves coordination dramatically. To experience multiskill activities, encourage children to participate in all kinds of games and play so that they can develop the ability to distinguish between simple and complex skills and exercises. For instance, children invariably dribble a basketball with their dominant hand. As they grow and become more comfortable with the skill, they should also learn to dribble with the nondominant hand. Next, children should learn to dribble between the legs, alternating between the right hand and left hand with both the right and left hands. As their skills improve, athletes must learn how to receive or catch a ball from someone whose skills might be of modest quality, followed by learning how to defend against highly coordinated opponents. The same approach is suggested for most other sports, such as soccer, rugby, ice hockey, and racket sports.

The following guidelines will help you design training programs that are suitable for young athletes at the initiation stage:

- Provide every child with enough time to adequately develop fundamental skills of the selected sport, equal playing time, and activities from other sports.

- Positively reinforce children who are committed and self-disciplined. Reinforce improvements in skill development.

- Encourage children to develop flexibility, coordination, and variety in skill development.

- Encourage children to develop various motor abilities in low-intensity environments. For example, swimming is an adequate environment for developing the cardiorespiratory system while minimizing the stress on joints, ligaments, and connective tissues.

- Select a suitable number of repetitions for each skill—particularly complex skills—and encourage children to perform each technique correctly.

- Modify the equipment and playing environment to a suitable level. For example, some children do not have the strength to shoot an adult-size basketball into a basket that is 10 feet (about 3 m) high using correct technique. The ball should be smaller and lighter, and the basket should be lower. The same can be said about the size of the field in soccer and rugby.

- Design drills, games, and activities to maximize children's opportunities for active participation.

- Promote experimental learning by giving children opportunities to design their drills, games, and other activities. Encourage them to use their imaginations and be creative.

- Simplify or modify rules to help children understand the game or sport.

- Introduce modified games that emphasize basic tactics and strategies. For example, if children have developed basic skills such as running, dribbling a ball with the feet, and kicking a ball, they will likely be ready to successfully play a modified game of soccer.

- During the game, consider introducing the young athletes to situations that demonstrate the importance of teamwork. Teach the athletes all the techniques and tactics of the specific position they play in the team. House leagues are an ideal environment for younger age groups to learn these skills because they can practice in a low-stress environment.

- Provide opportunities for boys and girls to participate together on the same team.

- Make sure that sport is fun. Try to deemphasize the competitive nature of sports and rather create an environment of enjoying play, being with friends, and relishing when a skill is performed well.

- Encourage participation in as many sports as realistically possible.

U15: ATHLETIC FORMATION STAGE

U15 is the first phase of training where the intensity can be moderately increased, setting the stage for higher training demand during the phases that follow. It is called *athletic formation* because it helps acquire sport-specific and position-specific technical and tactical skills, and form the most complex, physical abilities necessary to train during U17 and onward. However, most athletes are still vulnerable to injuries, particularly if coaches believe in the adage of *no pain, no gain*. At this stage of physical development, the cardiorespiratory system has to be continuously developed and athletes must be capable of tolerating the buildup of lactic acid accumulation, specifically for higher-intensity athletic actions.

Keep in mind that variations in individual performance may be the result of differences in growth. Some may experience a rapid growth spurt of up to 5 inches (12 cm), which can cause disturbances in coordination during drills. These disturbances occur mostly because limb growth, especially in the legs, changes the proportions between body parts and their leverage, consequently affecting the ability to coordinate their actions proficiently. In such instances, calmness and patience can be important attributes for both athletes and coaches. In addition, concerns about the *quality, precision, and accuracy of skills are more important to stress than desire to win.*

Also suggested is careful attention to the development of pacing and the rhythm of play, games, or racing; timing of different offensive or defensive actions during the game; and reaction to the tactical moves of the opponents. Every coach should keep a constant visual orientation to the surrounding environment, teaching athletes to sense the actions and technical and tactical maneuvers of teammates and the opposition.

During U15, accuracy of passing and shooting and the timing of most technical skills continue to improve in most athletes. Differences in coordination abilities are visible between early- and late-maturing children. Early maturers go through a slight lapse in motor coordination, which may temporarily affect the coordination of physical actions (Sharma and Hirtz, 1991; Skinner and Piek, 2001; Caprinica and Millard-Stafford, 2011; Bompa and Carrera, 2015). Consequently, because of their fast rhythm of physical growth, early maturers need more exercises to improve coordination than do late maturers. Therefore, you should introduce a variety of exercises that require changes of rhythm and spatial orientation.

Good coaches and parents should always help children who experience these temporary lapses by explaining the nature of motor, physical, and psychological differences and motivating them. They remind young athletes that work will always result in improvement, that over time they will be in control of their actions and skills, and that improvement will indeed come.

The following guidelines will help you design training programs that are appropriate for the athletic formation stage:

- Encourage participation in a variety of exercises from the selected sport and other sports, which will improve athletes' multilateral base and prepare them for games. Progressively increase the volume and intensity of training.

- Design drills that introduce athletes to the fundamentals of a game's or sport's tactics and reinforce skill development.

- Help athletes refine and automate fundamental skills of the selected sport during the initiation stage (U12).

- Emphasize improvement of coordination and range of motion, particularly the flexibility of ankle, knee, and hip joints.

- Encourage children to participate in drills that develop attention control to prepare them for the greater demands of training and competition that occur at this stage.

- Emphasize ethics and fair play during training and games.

- Provide children with opportunities to participate in various challenging environments of the game or sport.

- Introduce them to exercises that develop general strength (anatomical adaptation) as the foundation of the future development of speed, power, and agility needed in the stages that follow (refer to part III for an explanation of these stages).

- Continue to develop cardiorespiratory capacity. A good aerobic base will help them cope more effectively with the buildup of physical and psychological demand and the fatigue of playing the game.

- Introduce athletes to training programs that will improve maximum speed, power, and agility.

- Use complex drills to improve concentration during training and games. Without exaggerating it, you can use these drills to improve athletes' ability to cope with and tolerate fatigue (use complex drills performed under fatiguing conditions).

- Remember to emphasize fun! Children enjoy having fun and enjoyment during training. Use your imagination to create variety, particularly when athletes experience fatigue.

- Provide time for socializing with teammates.

U17: SPECIALIZATION STAGE

During the specialization stage, athletes should be exposed to more specific, higher training demands that increase their capability to better tolerate elevated physical and psychological stress. After several years (U12 and U15) of multilateral and sport-specific training, the programs suggested for U17 need to be more specialized; they should be more specific to the sport and the position. Therefore, coaches have to carefully monitor both the intensity and the volume of training to ensure the risk of injuries is eliminated.

The sport-specific training content needs to ensure that athletes have acquired the technical fundamentals, do not have any technical problems, and are able to contribute highly to tactical abilities. The specialization stage should also allow the coach to move from a mostly teaching role to a primarily training and coaching role. As children approach developmental stages post puberty and adolescence, certain abilities have a different rate of development. Coordination that had slower improvement during puberty will from now on continue to improve at a constant rate. Despite the concentration on sport-specific training at this stage, athletes should still be exposed to a variety of skills that increase maximum speed, agility, power, and strength.

The following guidelines will help you design training programs that are suitable for your athletes at the specialization stage:

- Closely monitor how athletes are coping with increased physical and psychological demand. They can be vulnerable to overtraining.

- Continue to focus on the technical and tactical refinement of the event, game, or position. Now is the time to stress specificity.

- As training and game demands increase, so will the athletes' self-awareness. Top athletes may develop a superiority complex, while those who struggle to keep up with demands of the sport or game may isolate themselves and lose confidence in their abilities. Therefore, you should create an environment that enables team cohesiveness and ensure that all athletes understand the unique qualities each brings to the team. One should not be surprised that those athletes who struggle at this age may become the stars of the team in the future.

- If you think an athlete needs more practice in a particular skill or physical ability, suggest additional training time. Parents, coaches, and caregivers should cooperate together to best support the efforts to help children reach maximum potential in the selected sport or event.

- Check for progressive improvements in the dominant abilities for the sport, such as skills, speed, power, agility, and dynamic flexibility.

- Increase training volume for specific exercises and drills to facilitate performance improvement. The body must adapt to specific training loads to effectively prepare for games.

- At this stage in athletes' evolution, it is important to increase intensity. Ready the athletes to perform skills. Repeat drills with the appropriate rhythm and speed to simulate the rhythm and intensity of the game or event.

- Although fatigue is a typical outcome of higher-intensity training, it is important that athletes do not reach a state of exhaustion. Constantly monitor athletes' reaction to high training and game demand, and use recovery and regeneration techniques to remove fatigue before the next intensive training sessions or competitions.

- Involve athletes in the decision-making process whenever possible.

- Continue to use nonspecific (multilateral) training, particularly during the preseason and preparatory phases. However, most training activities (physical and technical or tactical) should be specific to the sport, game, and position. High playing efficiency will be the typical outcome of specificity in all the aspects of the game.

- Provide opportunities for athletes to learn theoretical aspects of training by sharing the information offered in this and other books.

- Strength training should address the most important muscle groups prevailing in the selected sport or game. Avoid strength training methods that expose athletes to fewer than four repetitions. At this stage, athletes are not ready to use heavy loads. *Heavy* means loads over 80 percent of **one-repetition maximum (1RM)**, also called **maximum strength (MxS)**. Consider using loads of 40 to 60 percent of 1RM.

- Introduce simple, stressless, easy to perform plyometric exercises with a duration of 4 to 12 seconds (skipping rope, jumps over low benches or hurdles) and a longer rest interval (2 min).

- Employ tactical drills and activities where aerobic and anaerobic energy systems are dominant. From this stage on, athletes are capable of tolerating the buildup of lactic acid.

- Select technical and tactical drills that are biomechanically correct and physiologically efficient.

- Improve individual and team tactics using drills that are interesting and challenging; stimulate technical variety; require quick decision-making processes, anticipation, initiative, and self-control; and prolong concentration, competitive vigor, and fair play.

- Although winning becomes increasingly important at this stage, do not overemphasize it.

U19: PRE–HIGH PERFORMANCE STAGE

U19 represents a step toward the stage of high performance; it is a transition to reach efficiency in physical and psychological maturation as well as technical and tactical effectiveness. By 17 or 18 years of age, most athletes have finished their growth in height, and many aspects of physical training are more accessible from this stage on.

Coaches should aim to increase athletes' technical refinement to effectively use technical improvements during the tactical complexity of drills and games. Employ tactical drills to also improve specific speed and endurance—both anaerobic (phosphagen and glycolytic) and aerobic (oxidative).

Continue technical and tactical training to help athletes adapt according to the physiological specificity of the sport or game and the specific requirements of the chosen position.

Before attempting to create a good training program for U19 athletes, consider the following suggestions:

- Increase athletes' ability to tolerate higher training demand by designing a training program that taxes all energy systems present in their sport.

- Organize specific drills for each energy system. The emphasis of each energy system should reflect the specifics of the energy system of the chosen sport.

- Progressively increase intensity of training to higher levels than during the previous stages of athletic development.

- Progressively also increase the volume, duration, and distance covered in training.

- Consistently stress the acquisition of sport- or game-specific abilities to meet the demands of the high rhythm of the game. Emphasize good timing of athletes' actions in the field, anticipation, and quick reaction during all aspects of the game. Practice fast transitions from defense to offense and offense to defense.

- Create tactical drills where you also have psychological objectives, such as concentration, willingness, and determination to achieve your tactical and psychological objectives (e.g., tenacity to be one's best and be effective).

- Find the time to increase the position-specific effectiveness of each athlete and the specific tactics for both the defense and offense.

- Always monitor athletes' reaction to your training. Make the necessary changes in the program according to athletes' physiological reaction to the previous training session.

- Constantly ready the athletes for the training session. Good explanation of your training objectives will always have an equally good and effective reaction from your athletes.

- Plan (once a month, especially during the preparatory phase) formal tests to monitor physical improvement to your training. These tests should be for maximum speed, agility, strength, and power and specific endurance.

- Offer your athletes information about nutrition and meal plans. If necessary, discuss this issue with a nutritionist.

- Train maximum speed with and without the ball or implement.

- Emphasize the development of strength training with loads of 60 to 70 percent of 1RM. Always remember speed, power, and agility are directly dependent on your athletes' improvement in maximum strength.

- Introduce simple tumbling exercises (import them from gymnastics) and bounding (triple jump–like drills from track and field) of four to eight seconds with a rest interval of one to two minutes.

U21 TO U23: HIGH PERFORMANCE STAGE

These two classifications of athletic development represent the entrance of many athletes into the world of high performance, high professionalism, and the apex of athletic satisfaction.

The U21 and U23 levels are grouped together for two reasons:

1. In some sports, the U23 level does not exist; they have only one classification (U21).

2. Minimal differences exist between U21 and U23 in the training objectives and methodology of developing the dominant physical abilities of the sport. The main differences between the two classifications exist in intensity or load of power and strength training, and the individual ability to tolerate work.

As you begin to create specific training programs for athletes at the high performance stage, consider the following guidelines:

- Continue to increase game-specific and position-specific technical finesse in all aspects of the sport or game.

- Improve tactical proficiency based on the strategy you will design for your team or athletes.

- Design game-specific, position-specific tactical drills based on the proportions of energy systems dominant in your sport. These drills should result not only in tactical efficiency; equally important, they should result in the development of the three energy systems:

  1. Phosphagen: High intensity, maximum speed, and agility with and without the ball for a duration of 8 to 12 seconds

  2. Glycolytic: A duration of 30 to 45 seconds but using high intensity (speed, agility)

  3. Oxidative: Medium-intensity aerobic-dominant tactical drill using several athletes and mimicking transition from defense to offense and from offense to defense.

- Use tactical drills for the specific purpose of developing tolerance to lactic acid buildup to overcome fatigue. These drills should be tactically complex and use several athletes to also improve athletes' psychological capacity and willpower.

- Create technical and tactical drills in which athletes are exposed to improving the quality of the game, such as rhythm of the play, pacing and timing, and reaction to opponents' tactics in both offense and defense.

- Create strength training programs (using MxS) that will result in the improvement of maximum speed, agility, and power and specific metabolic elements of the game.

- Regularly monitor athletes' improvement and reaction to your training programs.

- Always train what is important and not what is trendy. Beware of some producers of training equipment and catalog companies who aggressively try to sell products and services that are not applicable to the needs of the sports they claim to help.

The complexity and differences in the growth and development of children from childhood to maturation have to be properly understood by both parents and sports technicians and carefully applied. Patience is a great quality. You'll need it. Apply it with your children and athletes. The most challenging situations are visible in the emotional and psychological behavior, specifically during puberty. Observe, understand, and apply your expertise and find joy in helping a child grow into a decent athlete, but also into a good and productive member of society.

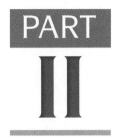

PART
II

NUTRITION AND ENERGY SYSTEM TRAINING

Learn how to produce energy and how to spend it wisely.

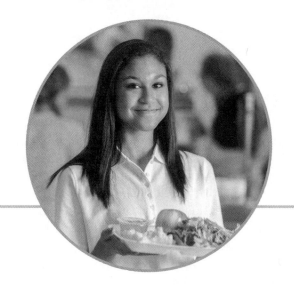

chapter

Nutrition Considerations

Michael Carrera, MS

Proper and progressive training starting at an early age is vital to performance and to the development of sport-specific strength, power, speed, endurance, and other motor abilities. Along with training, sound nutrition (a combination of foods you decide to feed children and inevitably the foods they choose to eat) affects children's overall health on and off the field and helps shape their relationship with food as they mature into young adults. The young athlete's diet differs from that of adults. A young athlete's growing body needs an adequate amount of wholesome carbohydrate, a generous amount of lean protein, and a good source of fat. A young athlete's daily consumption of food should include 50 to 55 percent carbohydrate, 10 to 15 percent protein, and approximately 20 to 25 percent fat. A diet high in nutritious carbohydrate, such as brown rice, pasta, whole-grain breads, vegetables, and legumes (e.g., chickpeas and lentils), is required for optimal energy and sport performance.

Furthermore, athletes must eat an adequate amount of lean protein from animal and plant sources to help the muscles recover from training and competition and to build stronger muscles and bones. Children should also consume good sources of fat such as fish, plants (e.g., avocados and coconuts and the oils derived from them), and nuts and seeds to help develop the skin and hair and strengthen the immune system. Good sources of fat provide fuel for the athlete, insulate the organs, and move the important vitamins A, D, E, and K throughout the body. The bottom line is that young athletes need to eat a variety of whole foods in adequate amounts. A balanced diet that is void of many processed foods will allow the athlete's body to train, perform, and recover well.

Performance relies on good nutrition. Athletes who eat poorly can feel fatigued, have insufficient fuel for training or competing, experience nutritional deficiencies, and jeopardize bone and muscle growth, all of which inevitably affects performance. Parents and coaches can help shape the way kids eat and ultimately influence the foods that make up most of their diet. Kids who balance their diet with nutrient-dense foods report feeling better, stronger, and more energetic. It is up to the adults in their lives to provide the proper path to healthy eating. This chapter discusses five nutritional habits that can help shape young athletes who fully enjoy and appreciate the value of nutritious food, training, and sport.

FUELING HABIT 1: AVOID PROCESSED FOODS

Is it possible to eat plenty of food and still not get the nutrients the body needs? The answer is a resounding yes. In 2003, the American Heart Association reported that children in the United States were consuming seven times the recommended amount of extra sugar (i.e., sugar other than that naturally present in carbohydrate-rich foods such as fruits, oatmeal, bread, and so on) per day. This extra sugar provides no nutritional value, but it fills the belly and prevents the child from wanting to eat foods that provide the nutritional support the body needs (Kavey et al., 2003; Gidding et al., 2005).

Many processed foods, such as snack bars, lunch meats, white bread, and other convenience foods, are filled with calories and are nutritionally poor. Most of these foods taste great and fill an athlete's belly, but they provide few vitamins and minerals (which help the body function optimally) and little protein, carbohydrate, and healthy fat (which aid in muscle growth, bone development, and recovery). Even some supposedly healthy food choices such as fruit juice, milk, yogurt, and cereals can be filled with added sugar, which outweighs the nutritional benefits of regularly eating these foods.

Many processed foods are also filled with sodium, sugar, and other chemicals that satisfy the palate and leave people wanting more. Unfortunately, convenience and lack of time have made these foods a staple of the U.S. household. Avoiding processed foods is a challenge for both adults and children. It is much easier to toss a fruit-on-the-bottom yogurt in your lunch bag than to buy plain yogurt, wash and cut some fruit, and place the fruit in a container to add to the yogurt later. Nutritionists often suggest adding foods containing healthy fats, such as walnuts, almonds, or various seeds, to your yogurt to add more nutrients. In this case, you would need to pack a second container. The fruit-on-the-bottom yogurt with granola included in the container may seem to be a good choice and it is more convenient; unfortunately, it comes with approximately three times the amount of sugar.

The processing of yogurt has further continued in the favor of even more convenience. Because kids are always on the run, why not give them the opportunity to run and eat at the same time? Hence, dairy shelves are filled with sweet liquid yogurts that kids can swallow directly from the tube without making a mess. This convenience comes at a price of extra empty calories from added sugar, fat, corn syrup, and other chemicals.

The effects of processed food on children's physical and mental health are important to consider and merit a longer discussion that is beyond the scope of this book. The purpose of considering them here is to help you train your athletes from early adolescence to the late teens. A plan or training regimen should include adhering to a diet that promotes muscle and bone growth and provides a stable delivery of energy. Thus, it helps athletes participate in numerous activities, recover well, and maintain a healthy body weight and body image as they mature to adulthood. Athletes need to eat, and they need to eat well. An average teenager can consume 2,500 calories a day and maintain a healthy body weight, whereas an active teenager who plays two games and practices four times per week may require at least 5,000 calories a day. Although the caloric requirements of these two teenagers may differ, their nutritional blueprint remains the same. They must eat foods that adequately provide the vital vitamins and minerals along with protein, carbohydrate, and fat that the body needs to function optimally. If they achieve their caloric needs by eating processed foods that are devoid of any nutritional value, they will feel low on energy, they will find it difficult to concentrate, and those who are athletes will find both practice and competition fatiguing. Their diets must consist of whole, unprocessed foods—natural fruits, vegetables, oats, whole grains, and lean proteins—and meal plans that begin at home and can be consistently adapted to their life at school and extracurricular activities.

Kids cannot always eat at home, but they can bring the food values they were taught at home on the road with them.

Everything in Moderation?

You have probably heard the saying *Eat everything in moderation*. Doing so can help you sustain a healthy body weight and prevent cravings or binging episodes that are created when you attempt to abstain from a particular food item. In other words, if you like ice cream, decide to have it occasionally. Moderation may work for some adults, but it does not necessarily work for kids. Kids do not understand the concept of moderation because they are not hardwired to remember every morsel of food that they eat. Kids do not keep track of how many sodas, fruit juices, or cookies they have consumed. In addition, some kids do not handle sugar well and can develop allergies, get sick, or continue to crave unnatural sugary treats.

Parents need to decide what foods they will allow in their homes and what foods to avoid or eliminate. Meals should always include unprocessed food choices consisting of carbohydrate, protein, and vegetables. Processed food items such as ice cream, cookies, or other desserts are best consumed occasionally rather than in moderation. To some, the term *moderation* can mean chocolate chip cookies for breakfast, a double-chocolate granola bar for an afternoon snack, a bag of chips after school, and a soda with dinner. This is not moderation, but it is unfortunately part of the daily North American diet. It is best to choose a specific day of the week for kids to enjoy a dessert or treat, be it ice cream, cake, or another pleasure. Make it an event for the entire family to enjoy. Better to have a specific day that everyone can look forward to than to leave it up to chance. During the rest of the week, choose low-sugar alternatives for snacks. Make your own healthy cookies or cakes (with baked-in goodies such as beets or avocados) or trail mix that includes dried fruit. Turn moderation into an occasion to help the young athlete build a strong and healthy body.

A Word on Sodas

Soda refers to carbonated soft drinks. Soda is a processed food that provides no nutritional value and floods the body with a surge of sugar. Approximately one in five children in the United States consume excess calories from soda and other sugar-sweetened drinks (Rader et al., 2014). U.S. males aged 12 to 19 years consume approximately 12 percent of their total calories per day from sugar-sweetened beverages such as soda and juices (Miller et al., 2013). Soda should not be part of an athlete's diet, either in moderation or on occasion. Studies have shown that soda consumption is linked to childhood obesity (Lim et al., 2009) and diabetes (Miller et al., 2013; Morgan, 2013) and that it can suppress the appetite of a growing child, thus preventing the child from eating vitamin- and protein-rich foods that the body needs. A can of soda can contain more than 50 milligrams of caffeine, a stimulant that can negatively affect a maturing brain (Miller et al., 2013). Furthermore, the acidic nature of soda and its lack of any nutritional quality can affect the alkaline balance of the body, causing inflammation and abdominal upset (Morgan, 2013). All these consequences of drinking soda will prevent the young athlete from functioning at optimal levels and in fact can harm the athlete's long-term health. Although palatable and ingrained in the North American diet, soda is a health concern that should be eliminated from the young athlete's diet. Substitute soda with low-sugar sport drinks and flavored water to promote drinking and hydration.

FUELING HABIT 2: PARENTS AND CAREGIVERS CONTROL THE FOOD SUPPLY

Good nutrition begins at home. Most people know and believe this statement, but the busyness of life has made food preparation and family meals very difficult to adhere to. It is not uncommon for most families to eat separately most days of the week. In today's fast-paced life, meal preparation is often reduced to takeout or simply defrosting some form of prepackaged meal.

Here is a typical scenario: Mom leaves work early to pick up the kid. The kid is starving—not because he has not eaten in hours or because he has been running around all afternoon but simply because he has not consumed the proper foods that satisfy his body's needs. Breakfast was fast and apparently healthy (a pack of instant honey-maple oatmeal and a glass of orange juice). By 10 a.m. the kid was hungry, so he opened his lunch bag and was happy to see a fruit granola bar, a small apple, and a bag filled with gummy candies. He wolfed down the bar, grabbed a handful of candies, and tossed the apple back in the bag for afternoon recess. At lunchtime, the kid made his way to the cafeteria. It was pizza day, so he got a break from chicken fingers and fries. After two small slices of pepperoni pizza, a juice box, and a small chocolate chip cookie, the kid was satisfied. At recess, the kid grabbed the apple and headed outside. He took a few barbecue-flavored potato chips from his friend's bag, kicked the ball around, and took a bite from his apple. When the bell rang and it was time to line up, the kid noticed that the apple was still in his hand, starting to turn brown, and barely eaten. He tossed it in the garbage can as he walked inside the school. At 3:30 p.m., the kid is standing in front of Mom's car feeling hungry. By this point in the day, the kid has consumed approximately 1,200 calories and 80 grams of added sugar. He did take one bite of the apple, but the amount of fiber, protein, whole-grain carbohydrate, and energy-fueling nutrients was minimal.

This scenario highlights an important trend occurring in North America. Approximately one-third of U.S. children and adolescents eat fast food every day. These fast foods, which include hamburgers, pizza, and fried chicken, are packed with fillers and sometimes harmful foodstuffs that rob children of the nutrients that are vital for growth and performance (Bowman et al., 2004). Between 1970 and 1990, the amount of high-fructose corn syrup (HFCS) ingested rose 1,000 percent (Bray et al., 2004). The consumption of sugar and HFCS continued to increase from 1990 to 2000, and use decreased slightly from 2000 to 2004 (Duffey and Popkin, 2008). By 2004, HFCS provided approximately 8 percent of total daily energy intake, and total added sugar provided 17 percent of total daily energy intake (Duffey and Popkin, 2008). HFCS is the primary ingredient in many processed foods, and it is used as an additive in many soft drinks. In fact, fast food and processed foods make up 17 percent of the total calorie intake for many teenage boys and girls (Sebastian et al., 2009). This number is alarming, especially as society battles childhood obesity and an increased risk of chronic disease. To make matters worse, dark green and orange vegetables and legumes make up a very small portion of adolescents' vegetable intake (Kimmons et al., 2009).

Parents and caregivers face a challenge. Not only do they have to sift through the marketing information bombarding television and the Internet; they also must take the time to prepare and properly assess what they are feeding their families. They cannot take the word of food producers and advertisers about what they should be feeding children. For example, a product that is gluten free may be loaded with additional sugar and other foodstuffs. Simply put, parents and caregivers need to take charge and control the food supply. The best approach is to introduce whole foods for the entire household.

According to the United States Department of Agriculture (2015), kids between the ages of 6 and 18 years who eat meals away from home tend to eat at more fast-food outlets, restaurants, and schools compared with kids who eat at home. Furthermore, when dining out, kids drink greater amounts of soda, which increases the consumption of unnecessary and unhealthy sugar.

Consider again the scenario from earlier: After Mom and the kid get home from school, the entire family is out at various commitments within a few hours. Mom may drive the kid to soccer practice while Dad takes the kid's sister to her soccer game. Once again, the busyness of life makes proper meal preparation and planning extremely difficult, and parents succumb to the temptation of ordering out or simply defrosting a prepackaged frozen entree filled with sodium, sugar, and other unhealthy additives. Professionals in the field of athletic development see this scenario often. Parents and caregivers do not know how to overcome such a challenge, and they look to supplements and other products to help improve their children's nutrition. Although many products on the market—including multivitamins, low-sugar protein bars, and whey protein powder—can be useful for kids, these products should not be introduced until the kids are given an opportunity to eat more whole foods and truly taste and feel the difference of eating them.

Building Your Food Supply

Whole foods are foods that are unprocessed and unrefined or have been processed very little; they are foods in their natural state. Such foods are filled with protein, carbohydrate, and fat that body tissues need for growth and regeneration. Many of these foods, especially an array of fruits, vegetables, and legumes, are filled with hundreds of vitamins and minerals that work together to sustain life and keep every cell healthy and nourished. If you look at a typical floor plan of a grocery store, the peripheral walls of the grocery are filled with whole foods such as fruits, vegetables, lean protein, whole grains (e.g., rice, pasta, whole-grain breads), legumes (e.g., lentils, chickpeas), and nuts and seeds. As you look at the middle aisles of the store, you see an unending supply of refined and processed foods.

When building the food supply for your home, try to follow the 90-10 rule: Fill your cart with 90 percent whole foods and 10 percent processed foods. Of course, you can go much lower than 10 percent, but for most parents and caregivers 100 percent whole food is impossible. Kids want to have some lunch meats, some ice cream, and the occasional chocolate croissant, waffle, apple pie, or fast-food treat. In addition, items such as wraps, various styles of whole-grain breads, and energy bars are not considered whole foods but can be part of a kid's diet—especially an active child whose energy intake needs to match energy expenditure. The food supply doesn't have to be perfect, but it should be created with the goal of helping the entire household experience the energy that comes from eating well.

Because whole foods are unprocessed and unrefined, you need to take time to prepare them. Grilled chicken with Greek salad is a wonderful meal. However, someone needs to cut, clean, and cook the chicken; wash and dice the salad; and prepare the salad dressing. Similarly, a dish of pasta with lean meatballs and fresh tomato sauce is a wonderful Sunday lunch, but preparation is required. It is much easier to buy bottled tomato sauce and meatballs and simply boil the pasta, but with the convenience comes a significant price tag of more sodium, sugar, and chemical additives that increase shelf life. Besides that, you lose the opportunities to add your own vegetable blend and spices and to teach kids the value of healthy home cooking. Kids are also able to enjoy a greater quantity of food when consuming whole foods because most whole foods are packed with fiber and protein, which satiate the appetite and prevent cravings for unhealthy snacks and beverages.

Table 5.1 Whole Foods From Different Food Groups

Vegetables	Fruits	Nuts and seeds*	Grains	Dairy	Lean meats	Herbs and spices
• Asparagus • Celery • Pepper (all colors) • Beets • Cucumber • Broccoli • Cauliflower • Eggplant • Spinach • Squash • Sweet potato • Onion (all types) • Kale	• Blueberries (fresh or frozen) • Apple • Orange • Raspberries (fresh or frozen) • Strawberries (fresh or frozen) • Cantaloupe • Watermelon • Grapefruit • Peach • Plum • Banana • Mango • Coconut	• Almonds (unsalted) • Cashews • (unsalted) • Walnuts • Pumpkin seeds • Sunflower seeds	• Brown rice • Wild rice • Millet • Oats • Quinoa (really a seed) • Whole-grain pasta	• Eggs (free range) • Cheese (low fat) • Milk • Yogurt (Greek and plain)	• Grass-fed chicken, beef, lamb, and turkey	• Cinnamon • Turmeric • Cumin • Cilantro • Coriander • Peppermint • Rosemary • Thyme

*You can also get both seeds and nuts in a spread, which is great on breads, wraps, and fruit.

Table 5.1 lists whole foods from the different food groups. This list is not exhaustive; the important point is that all these foods are provided by nature. Organic is arguably better when choosing many of these foods, but simply beginning to include most of these items in both meals and snacks is a great way to optimize your young athlete's health, energy, and recovery.

Planning Your Meals

Although the statement *An ounce of prevention is worth a pound of cure* is intended to emphasize the importance of maintaining a healthy lifestyle and preventing disease, it is also applicable to planning your meals. Eating is important—people need fuel daily—so meal preparation rightfully deserves the time and effort it requires. Without proper planning, people must resort to less healthy alternatives that are sometimes harmful to the waistline, energy, digestion, and overall health. Because people cannot make more time, they must adequately plan to take more time—sometimes from other things—to make meal planning a priority. The following are tips that can help parents to properly plan and deliver high-quality meals for young athletes.

■ **Make a list of items you need for the week, including all fruits, vegetables, legumes, whole grains, snack items, and lean proteins.** If possible, include kids in the shopping experience so that they can understand the difference between a whole food item and its prepackaged alternative.

■ **To help make your food list, think about what meals you would like to prepare during the week.** Start with Monday, keeping in mind the household's work and school commitments. Remember that dinner preparation is the best time to also prepare lunch for the next day. Leftover dinner makes a healthy and satiating lunch.

■ **Include one whole food in each meal (breakfast, lunch, dinner, and snacks).** It will help reduce the number of processed foods your household consumes and ensure that a nutritious portion of whole food is included in every meal. For instance, breakfast on the run may include a granola bar with a banana or apple, and an afternoon snack can be a cup of yogurt and a handful of homemade trail mix (cashews, almonds, sunflower seeds, and raisins). Adding whole foods to the three main meals of the day is easy once you get the hang of it. In fact, if you simply make the commitment to remove processed and prepackaged food and fast-food items, all you are left with are whole foods!

- **Take time to prepare whole foods.** Once you make your meal list, try to arrange some time over the weekend for meal preparation. Wash all the fruit and place it in the refrigerator so the kids can easily access it. Buy fruits in season so that you always have variety. Wash and prepare fruits and vegetables and put them in containers in the refrigerator. This way, you can easily place them in a lunch bag or toss them into yogurt or a stir-fry. Prepare, cut, and marinate lean meats in the refrigerator for a day or two so that you can simply place them in the oven or on the grill during the week. Finally, if you take the time to make sauces or chili, make extra and freeze the leftovers. This strategy will help during busy periods when you just don't have time to prepare a good meal and are tempted to pick up the phone and order a pepperoni pizza. Try to position yourself so that you go out for dinner or get takeout because you want to eat that specific food and not because of a lack of foresight in preparation.

- **You are in charge, so make the list and stick to it.** Try different recipes and various food combinations. If kids just do not like vegetables, dress them up. If you must use dips or a store-bought salad dressing they like, so be it. They are eating their vegetables and getting the necessary fiber and nutrients they need. More important, they are eating whole foods, which will slowly but surely change their palates to desire those types of foods. You do not have to follow a law of all or nothing—whole foods in and everything else out—when it comes to changing how you eat. The important thing is that every meal has a whole-food component; most meals are prepared at home; and kids understand that eating vital fruits, vegetables, and lean protein will help them get stronger, feel better, and improve their focus and concentration. If kids see your excitement about creating a new path for the entire household, they will also get excited about the results. It starts with you; you control the food supply.

- **If you don't cook much or if your kids have specific food allergies or intolerances, find an easy-to-follow cookbook that addresses their needs.** Many books address food allergies and specific food preferences, including vegetarian meals. Buying gluten-free snacks, prepackaged sources of lean protein, and sauces is an easy alternative, but unfortunately, most of these foods are filled with additives and chemicals.

When possible, it is best for families to eat together so that kids understand both the value of eating from a diverse menu and the importance of eating prepared food versus prepackaged or fast food. Also, the dinner table offers a good opportunity to discuss athletic goals and how proper eating can help build a stronger and healthier body. Taking control of the food supply is not about setting restrictive rules, which will most likely backfire; rather, it is about demonstrating to your young athletes the inherent quality of real food and nature's intention in creating it.

FUELING HABIT 3: ALWAYS START WITH A WHOLESOME BREAKFAST

The word *breakfast* is a combination of two words: *break* and *fast*. Because you are sleeping and in essence fasting for 8 to 10 hours during the night (unless, of course, you get up to have a snack), the first food you place in your mouth is considered breaking the fast.

In adults, the importance of eating breakfast first thing in the morning has been challenged in the literature (Halberg et al., 2005; Karli et al., 2007) and in trade publications. A new wave of thought argues for extending the fast and possibly skipping breakfast altogether. The intention is to further stimulate hormonal changes that elicit greater gains in lean muscle mass and improvements in body composition and health. Coaches and parents may be aware of the current literature or theories on fasting and wonder whether they may be applicable to young athletes. The answer is no; they are not.

Young athletes require fuel upon rising, and they need to have a healthy, wholesome breakfast. Many studies have shown that nutritional deficiencies and poor eating habits established during adolescence can have detrimental consequences on health in adulthood (Daniels et al., 2002; Ogden et al., 2002). After 8 to 12 hours of sleep and fasting, a child's glycogen stores are very low. Without eating a proper breakfast, the child can feel lethargic, lack concentration, and not be able to keep up with the activity level required in school.

Of the many reasons children give for skipping breakfast, the main reasons are that they have no time or are not hungry when they wake up (Vanelli et al., 2005). Both reasons are legitimate because, once again, the busyness of life and the demands of work and school chisel away the time available to eat a proper breakfast in the morning. Also, kids may eat a late-night snack, which explains why they are not hungry when waking up. Parents can omit the late-night snack and encourage their children to eat a well-balanced breakfast in the morning. This approach is important for two reasons: First, eating late at night can interrupt sleep patterns and prevent a restful sleep. Second, the snack may not be nutritionally dense or calorically balanced. In essence, the late-night snack may prevent the child from eating breakfast because he is still satiated upon waking. When he gets hungry later in the morning, he may grab a sugar- and fat-filled snack that is calorically dense, nutritionally empty (Nicklas et al., 2000), and void of the many vitamins and minerals that are required for growth and maturation.

Young athletes of all ages need to start the day with a healthy breakfast, and parents and caregivers need to set the example. On weekends (or even during the week if time allows), parents are encouraged to sit down to eat with their children or simply create an environment in which breakfast is an important part of the day. The start of the day needs to be nutritious!

When most people think of breakfast, the first thing that comes to mind is cereal. Breakfast can involve much more than sugary cereals; it can be healthy smoothies, plain yogurt and fruit, eggs and toast, oatmeal, healthy granola bars, and some energy or protein bars. In addition, fresh fruit is great first thing in the morning. Besides being packed with much-needed vitamins and minerals, bananas, blueberries, apples, cantaloupe, and watermelon are filled with fiber and provide immediate energy.

One study looked at the marketing and advertising messages of various cereal brands, which are energy dense and nutrient poor. Children viewed 1.7 cereal advertisements per day. Of these ads, 87 percent promoted high-sugar products, many of which are available at the local grocery store. Furthermore, 91 percent of these ads ascribed extraordinary attributes to these cereal products, and 67 percent showed both healthy and unhealthy eating patterns (LoDolce et al., 2013).

It is no wonder that children—even young athletes in the athletic formation stage—often ask for a particular high-sugar cereal for breakfast. Children who eat a breakfast that is low in sugar and high in fiber show better memory and attention span and fewer signs of frustration two to three hours after eating (Benton et al., 2007). If an athlete wants cereal, look for one that has fewer than 10 grams of sugar and at least 4 grams of fiber per one-cup serving. Because these cereals lack the sugar content that gives them their palatable appeal (some contain 19 to 24 grams of sugar per one-cup serving!), athletes can use vanilla whey protein powder or vanilla almond milk (sweetened or unsweetened) to add flavor. If a child is lactose intolerant, you can choose a plant-based protein powder and dress the cereal with some coconut or nuts for taste.

Although it is always best to consume protein from whole foods, protein powders (especially whey protein, a by-product of milk production) are great for increasing protein intake; they help the body recover from exercise and strengthen the immune system (Krissansen, 2007). Because children tend to get enough protein from whole-food sources, protein powders can be used as supplements and added to shakes or cereals in small quantities. Parents and coaches should do research and choose a high-quality brand of protein powder to guarantee that the manufacturing standards meet or exceed the necessary guidelines of production and that the protein powders do not contain any chemicals or by-products that can elicit an allergic response.

You may also choose to make your own nutritionally dense, high-fiber, vitamin-packed cereal for the entire household to enjoy. Table 5.2 provides a healthy cereal recipe. Because the recipe is low in sugar, you may choose to add flavor by adding any of your favorite toppings, including fresh fruit, seeds, nuts, raisins, and coconut.

Make Breakfast a Priority

Make breakfast a habit for the young athlete. As with every meal or snack, the athlete does not need to gorge on breakfast. It isn't about eating as much food as possible regardless of its nutritional status; it's about eating a balanced meal that includes foods from at least three of the five food groups (grains, fruits, vegetables, protein, and dairy)—real foods that are filled only with the sugar that nature intended. Try to decrease the amount of added sugar by choosing breakfast items that are more nutritionally sound and packed with vitamins, minerals, and fiber. Taste is important, of course, so make better food choices and strive for balance.

Start every morning with one or more of the following options:

■ **A smoothie.** Use one cup (236 ml) of water, skim milk, almond milk (sweetened or unsweetened), or fresh orange juice. Depending on the protein intake of the child and any dietary restriction such as dairy, nut, or legume allergies, you can also add a tablespoon of whey protein powder or a plant alternative. For example, a 12-year-old boy weighing

Table 5.2 Cereal Recipe

Combine 1 cup* of each of the following:
- Organic quinoa puffs or flakes
- Rolled oats
- Kasha
- Sliced almonds

Mix ingredients with 5 tbsp (75 ml) of olive oil in a large baking pan. Roast in the oven at 350 °F (177 °C) for 20 minutes or until browned.
Before eating, add some of your favorite toppings: flaxseed meal, chia seeds, cinnamon, shaved coconut, dried cranberries, raisins, or fresh fruit (e.g., blueberries, bananas).
Add the cereal mixture to yogurt, milk, almond milk, or rice milk.
Once cereal cools, place in mason jars or containers. Eat for breakfast or snack.

*Begin with 1 cup. Once you find the correct mixture for you, add as many cups as you would like.

100 pounds (45 kg) would require approximately 0.45 grams of protein per pound of body weight per day, which equals approximately 45 grams of protein per day. If you assume that the boy eats three meals a day, he will require around 15 grams of protein per meal to fulfill his daily requirements. Therefore, a breakfast smoothie or shake would be an ideal way to incorporate a high-quality protein powder. Given that a scoop of commercial protein powder (around 23-26 g of powder per scoop) contains approximately 18 grams of protein, using half a scoop of protein powder would yield around 7 to 9 grams of protein, which would complement a milk-, water-, or juice-based smoothie. Add fruit of your choice plus nuts, seeds, or a teaspoon of almond butter. The smoothie combinations are endless. It is not necessary that protein powders be added to smoothies. In fact, protein powders are useful to supplement a diet lacking in protein but need not become a general staple in a young athlete's daily diet. What is important is that all smoothies include a protein base (i.e., milk, yogurt, or whey protein powder), some fresh fruit, and a nut or seed butter for some essential fats. In many cases, parents or athletes with good intentions made a smoothie that was too high in sugar and lacked the necessary fat and protein to create a well-balanced, slowly digestible meal. Avoid making a smoothie that includes only fruit and fruit juices and is void of any other nutritional component.

■ **Eggs of your choice (e.g., scrambled, poached, boiled).** Eggs are packed with protein and nutrients, and they are fairly inexpensive when compared with other proteins. Brown and white eggs look different, but they have the same nutritional content. You may choose free-range eggs, but you should know that the term *free range* means that the hens had access to a running area outdoors; it doesn't mean that the hens did run freely. If you live near a farm or farmers' market, buy local eggs; your eggs will be healthier and more nutrient dense. Compared with eggs from the grocery store, the yolks of eggs from local farmers tend to be larger, darker, and more orange. You may also choose to buy eggs that have a higher content of omega-3 fatty acids. Prepare the eggs any way you like, and enjoy nature's goodness. Athletes can eat their eggs with a side of grains (e.g., oats, whole-wheat bread, or whatever bread they like). However, athletes should avoid white bread if possible or simply have it on rare occasions. As a rule of thumb, if you can roll a slice of bread into a ball and it retains its shape, it's probably not very healthful. Add some fruit or slices of tomato or avocado, and you have a wonderful breakfast that is fast, easy to make, and filled with protein, vitamins, and minerals.

■ **Oatmeal and fruit.** Oatmeal is packed with fiber, antioxidants, and minerals such as magnesium, phosphorous, selenium, and copper. Try to stay away from instant oatmeal, which comes in flavors such as brown sugar, maple honey, and apple cinnamon. Although instant oatmeal tastes great, it is often packed with sugar, thus negating the true nutritional benefits of eating a wholesome bowl of oatmeal. Oatmeal can be cooked in water or milk and doesn't have to be dry and tasteless. You can add cinnamon or a bit of natural maple sugar to sweeten it, or you can add some unsweetened applesauce or fresh berries. Pure oatmeal is gluten free, but sometimes oatmeal is made in facilities that also process wheat, so some cross-contamination may occur. Look for brands that are labeled as gluten free, and make oatmeal a staple breakfast option. Use oats to make healthy muffins or to add texture to smoothies (just throw them in raw).

It is very common these days to add protein powder to smoothies for a bit of a protein blast. Ever-popular smoothie and juice outlets offer to add a scoop of protein to any of their products. Protein powder is a fast and easily digestible way to give your body a high-protein boost. When preparing a protein smoothie for breakfast or as a snack for the young athlete, be aware of the athlete's total protein requirements based on age and body weight. Too little protein can weaken the muscles and harm cell growth, whereas too much protein can place stress on the kidneys and be converted to fat. Although the effect of too much protein on the kidneys in adults is a contentious research issue, the effect of excess protein on young athletes is unclear. For this reason, a thoughtful balance is required. Once you have calculated the approximate amount of protein required per day for the young athlete, try to spread the protein intake among three meals and a couple of snacks. Table 5.3 presents a recipe for a whey protein smoothie. This recipe is appropriate for some athletes in the late athletic formation stage and beyond. For younger athletes, modify the amount of protein to a half scoop, and add or remove as needed. It will allow younger athletes to benefit from the wonderful nutritional value of this quick breakfast alternative.

A Word on Protein

Protein is found in many foods, including meats, dairy, legumes, grains, and some vegetables. The body needs protein to build muscles, strengthen the immune system, and help recovery. Because resistance training increases the body's demand for protein for recovery, regeneration, and muscle growth, protein supplements are hyped as a method for increasing the protein demand by making a good source of protein easily available. It can be a challenge to eat enough food to meet the body's demand for calories and protein or to find better food sources. Protein shakes have become very popular among athletes, bodybuilders, and recreational fitness enthusiasts because they are easy to digest and fulfill the athletes' protein requirements. Protein shakes are easy to make and come in many varieties. Whey protein powder is a high-quality protein that is easily absorbed except in those who are lactose intolerant or have a milk allergy. Whole food should always be the primary choice to guarantee intake of a range of amino acids (protein building blocks) and other nutritional components. However, for variety, taste, or simplicity, the young athlete can use whey protein powder or a plant-based protein as part of her nutrition plan. We recommended that young athletes eat whole foods to meet the bulk of their nutritional needs and use protein powders sparingly to add more protein to the overall diet or to supplement (not replace) a particular meal.

Before deciding on the protein needs of an athlete and how to meet those needs, it is important to look at the protein requirements for different age groups (see table 5.4). According to the Centers for Disease Control and Prevention (2015), protein requirements vary with age.

Table 5.3   Whey Protein Smoothie

This whey protein smoothie is packed with dairy, fruit, and grains to provide the energy, protein, vitamins, and minerals the body needs to adequately grow and thrive in schoolwork, fun, and sport.

- 1 cup (236 ml) of skim milk, water, or almond milk (unsweetened or sweetened)
- 1 scoop of high-quality whey protein powder or 1 scoop of plant-based protein
- A few ice cubes (optional; it gives the smoothie a thick texture)
- 1 small banana
- 1/2 cup (75 g) of blueberries or fruit of choice (frozen or fresh)
- 1 scoop (use of the protein scoop) of uncooked rolled oats (optional; it gives the smoothie a nice texture)
- 1 tsp (~5 g) of flaxseeds (optional)

Place all ingredients in a blender, and mix for 20 to 40 seconds or until desired texture is achieved. Enjoy!

Table 5.4 Protein Needs by Stage of Athletic Development

Age (years)	Protein (g/lb of body weight)	Stage of athletic development
4-8	0.5	Initiation
9-14	0.45	Initiation/athletic formation
15-18	0.4	Specialization
18+	0.36	High performance

- Boys and girls aged 4 to 8 years (initiation stage) require approximately 19 grams a day.
- Girls in the athletic formation stage and specialization stage require approximately 46 grams a day.
- Boys in the athletic formation stage and specialization stage require approximately 56 grams a day.

The RDA is a general guideline for protein consumption per pound of body weight. You should follow the recommendations for athletes in the initiation and athletic formation stages of development but allow for a higher total protein content for athletes in the specialization and high performance stages of development. Studies have demonstrated that the protein requirements for young athletes who are involved in intensive training may be higher than those suggested in table 5.4 (Boisseau et al., 2007). Athletes in the specialization stage of development can increase the protein requirements to 0.55 grams per pound of body weight for strength sports and 0.45 grams per pound of body weight for endurance sports. Depending on the level of maturation, strength athletes in the late specialization stage and high performance stage can increase protein requirements to 0.75 grams per pound of body weight, whereas endurance athletes aim for 0.55 grams per pound of body weight.

For example, a strength athlete who weighs 180 pounds (81.6 kg) would require 135 grams of protein per day (180 × 0.75 = 135 g). This number may appear large. However, by spreading out the protein intake throughout the day, starting with a protein-rich breakfast and aiming for 20 to 30 grams of protein per meal, the athlete can meet the requirements needed for muscle growth, recovery, and performance improvements.

FUELING HABIT 4: PROPERLY FUEL THE BODY BEFORE AND AFTER GAMES

Fueling the body both before and after a competition is no different from the usual balanced approach to eating. The foods are still high in wholesome carbohydrate, lean protein, and heart-healthy fat occurring naturally in nuts, seeds, fish such as salmon and tuna, and oils such as olive oil and coconut oil. What changes is when, where, and how to eat these foods.

Pregame Meal

What a young athlete should eat before a game or competition is a common question. Regardless of the sport, all young athletes need to fuel their bodies with the right combination of carbohydrate, protein, and fat before a game. The athletes do not need to engage in carbohydrate loading (a nutritional strategy for increasing glycogen stores). Simply eating a balanced meal at least three hours before the game will top up the energy stores, allow time for digestion, and prepare the body for competition. Because an athletic competition places a lot of stress on the heart to pump blood to the working muscles, you don't want to slow down the body by diverting blood to the stomach for digestion.

Young athletes should follow these guidelines:

- **Between 50 percent and 60 percent of the meal should include high-carbohydrate foods such as whole-wheat or white pasta, whole-grain breads, brown or white rice, or quinoa.** Pasta should not make up the entire meal; you need to include some vegetables and lean protein. A good pregame meal would include whole-wheat pasta with marinara sauce, 4 to 6 ounces (113-170 g) of grilled chicken breast, and broccoli or cauliflower on the side.

- **Eat as much food as is usual—no more and no less.** Simply eat until satisfied. Game day is not a good time to eat more food than the body is accustomed to. Doing so can irritate the digestive system and cause stomach upset. After the pregame meal, have a piece of fruit and sip from a sport drink as game time approaches. Hunger is relatively at bay, and the athlete can focus on the game.

- **Certain foods may need to be eliminated from the pregame meal, even if the foods are part of the daily nutrition plan.** Foods that are high in fiber or fat should be avoided because they are slower to digest and can irritate the bowels, causing stomach upset. For instance, legumes such as chickpeas, lentils, or kidney beans are great sources of carbohydrate and protein but can cause gas and stomach distress. Similarly, high-fat foods such as a hamburger and fries, fried eggs with toast, and high-fat cuts of beef or pork should be avoided in the pregame meal. Table 5.5 lists foods that are good to eat and foods to avoid eating at least three hours before a game. The list is not exhaustive. Each body reacts differently to various foods and food combinations regardless of nutritional value.

Table 5.5 Foods to Eat and Foods to Avoid Before a Game

Eat	Avoid
Whole-wheat or white pasta with marinara	Fruit juices (no need for added sugar)
Brown or white rice	Processed lunch meats (high in sodium)
Whole-grain bread or pitas	Fried foods of any kind
Grilled or baked chicken	High-fiber legumes: lentils, chickpeas, and kidney beans
Potatoes, sweet potatoes, or yams	
Poached, scrambled, or boiled eggs	Spices of any kind
Oatmeal	Soft drinks or carbonated drinks
Fresh fruit: bananas, apples, blueberries, strawberries, grapes	High-fat red meat or pork
Fresh vegetables: broccoli, cauliflower, cucumber, fennel, zucchini	Protein bars or protein shakes (whole food is best for the pregame meal)
Whole-wheat bagels	Candy or chocolate bars
Jams, almond butter, and peanut butter	Hamburger, fries, or pizza (homemade pizza or vegetable pizza with little cheese is fine)
Dairy: milk and plain yogurt	
Salmon and tuna	Cake, pie, and cookies

As a rule of thumb, remember these 10 basic steps to pregame meal planning:

1. Choose foods rich in carbohydrate, including pasta, whole-grain breads, cereals, and rice.
2. Include vegetables that you are accustomed to eating and generally cause little, if any, gas or bloating.
3. Avoid spices of any kind, especially hot spices such as curry, turmeric, and cayenne pepper.
4. Avoid fried foods of any kind, including fried eggs and meats.
5. Avoid soft drinks and carbonated drinks to help prevent abdominal distress and gas.
6. Avoid desserts of any kind.
7. Eat the same amount you are accustomed to eating at everyday meals.
8. Drink plenty of water.
9. If possible, avoid eating on the run or in the car. Sit down to eat, and take your time.
10. Eat whole foods; save the protein bars or snacks for postgame meals.

Common Competition-Day Questions

The following section addresses common questions about fueling before, during, and after competitions.

What Foods Can I Safely Eat Right Before Competition?

Inevitably, some athletes will feel hungry an hour or two before a game. In this instance, they can have a light snack such as fruit or crackers with a tablespoon of peanut or almond butter. If an athlete ate a proper pregame meal at least three hours before the game, she should feel satiated. It is better to eat a bit more at the pregame meal and avoid the snack so that the body can focus on directing blood to the working muscles and not to digestion.

How Do I Properly Eat for an All-Day Tournament?

The pregame principles discussed earlier still apply. The athlete is encouraged to have a suitable and nutritious pregame meal at least three hours before the game. If the first game is at 9 a.m., it is best that the athlete eat a meal that is lighter than usual around 6:30 or 7 a.m. Because the first game is relatively early in the day, the athlete needs to top up the fuel sources and rely on the energy stored from the previous day. A bagel with peanut butter or scrambled eggs and toast is enough to get him through the first game. Then, when the first game is complete, the athlete can eat a more suitable meal of carbohydrate, protein, and fat (as discussed earlier) to help fuel his body for the next game. Pack a few chicken or tuna wraps, some precut vegetables, and fresh fruit for the day. You can also pack some light snacks such as granola or protein bars, water, and sport drinks to help sustain energy throughout the tournament. It is important that the athlete eat carbohydrate-rich foods and continue to eat throughout the day—even if he is not hungry—to prevent a crash in energy. Keep in mind that a high-protein, low-carbohydrate diet is not for young athletes. Young athletes need carbohydrate to sustain energy. If athletes venture to a restaurant between games, they should avoid fast food and fried meals and instead choose a meal that is high in carbohydrate. Choose pasta with chicken, pancakes, waffles, and other starchy foods that are easily digested and that quickly replenish energy stores.

Is It Important to Drink Sport Drinks During a Competition?

For games lasting 60 minutes or less, young athletes should continue to hydrate with water. It is important that athletes continue to sip water before and during the game to regulate body temperature and help the muscles work optimally. After spending hours training, you don't want fatigue or muscle cramps to negatively affect performance because the body is dehydrated. Drink plenty of water as part of a general training lifestyle, and continue to drink water on game days.

If a game lasts for more than 60 minutes or the athlete is participating in a long-distance sport such as cross country or swimming, sport drinks can help replenish and balance electrolytes, including potassium and sodium, both of which are important for muscle function. Choose a brand that is relatively low in sugar, and sip it throughout the game. If you want to avoid having a full bottle of a sport drink, simply dilute the drink by adding water so that you will be inclined to drink more of the fluid before, during, and after the game. During a daylong tournament consisting of multiple games, sport drinks can help prevent blood sugar levels from dipping and causing premature fatigue. Drink responsibly!

How Soon Do I Eat a Postgame Snack?

The soccer match or hockey game is over. The kids are sweating and tired but fired up with excitement and adrenaline. They are still focused on the game and burning off steam by discussing certain plays, goals, and questionable calls by the referee. As they come off the ice or field, they don't feel immediate hunger. However, they have depleted their energy stores and their muscles are ready for protein to help them recover. It is very common at the community-sport level, especially for athletes in the initiation stage and early years of the athletic formation stage, to be given snacks at the end of a sport event. These snacks usually include some high-fructose drink and dessert-type bar, cookie, or cake.

These items are high in sugar and will quickly absorb into the body. However, the body requires a good dose of protein within 30 minutes of the end of a game. Within this 30-minute window the body's ability to replenish energy stores and aid in muscle recovery is optimal, especially when carbohydrate is consumed along with protein. So, if young athletes are given high-sugar treats, they can be allowed to eat them to get the recovery process going, but instead of fruit juices or sugar-filled sodas, they should have an 8-ounce (240 ml) container of skim or even chocolate milk to make sure that they are getting an adequate amount of protein immediately after the game. An 8-ounce (240 ml) glass of milk contains approximately 8 grams of protein and a good amount of amino acids (building blocks of protein) to aid in muscle building. For a postgame treat, athletes in the initiation and athletic formation stages of development can eat a bagel with cream cheese or peanut butter, some dried fruit, and a glass of plain or chocolate milk. Young athletes in the late athletic formation and specialization stages of development can drink a protein shake like the one described in table 5.3, which provides a good dose of carbohydrate and protein. If you don't want to blend the protein drink before the game, simply pack some milk or orange juice in a cooler and place a scoop of protein powder in a container. After the game, mix the powder with the juice. You can also pack a bagel with peanut butter, some crackers, or fresh fruit to complement the protein shake. Athletes in the initiation stage of development can aim to consume between 8 and 10 grams of protein, such as a glass of milk or 1 cup (250 g) of good-quality yogurt, after a game; athletes in the athletic formation and specialization stages can aim for 10 to 20 grams of protein within 30 minutes after the game. As mentioned, all protein should be complemented with a good dose of carbohydrate.

How Soon Do I Eat a Postgame Meal?

The athlete ate a small snack containing protein and carbohydrate after the game, and now it is time to eat a more robust meal. Hours after a game, the body is still healing, replenishing, and growing. Proper care should be taken to ensure that a wholesome amount of carbohydrate, protein, and fat is eaten one to two hours after the game. If the ride home from the game is long, it is best to pack chicken or egg sandwiches or wraps for the car ride home to avoid having to stop at a fast-food restaurant because the athlete is famished. If you have time to eat a meal at home, the balanced approach to eating remains. A meal should include a grouping of complex carbohydrate such as rice or pasta, some grilled chicken or fish, and a generous helping of vegetables. As always, eat to the point of satiation, and snack with nuts, seeds, and fruit (fresh and dried) between meals.

FUELING HABIT 5: KNOW YOUR ATHLETE

Hundreds of books and articles have been written about sport nutrition and about the need to properly fuel the young athlete with wholesome carbohydrate, lean protein, and good fat. However, like most kids, young athletes can be picky eaters. Unfortunately, they have also developed a palate for processed and fast-food items that provide a hefty number of calories, chemicals, and sugars but very little in total-body nutrition. Parents want to provide a variety of foods for their children to eat and plan meals that include a balance of healthy carbohydrate, protein, and vegetables. However, more often than not, kids are determined to eat their own way and thus leave plates filled with good food, opting for chicken fingers and fries or frozen pizza. Growing bodies need good, sound nutrition. The question is how parents, caregivers, and coaches can overcome these barriers to help athletes understand how eating well corresponds to growing well and, ultimately, performing well.

A study conducted in Australia (Odea, 2003) had students in grades 2 through 11 (aged 7-17 years) identify the perceived benefits of and barriers to healthful eating and physical activity and suggested strategies for overcoming barriers. Table 5.6 shows the results of this study.

Although this study was conducted on Australian children, it provides a framework for understanding and acknowledging the benefits of eating well and physical activity for all children. Children in this study understood the benefits of healthful eating, including feeling good physically and psychologically. However, although armed with an understanding of why certain foods are better for health than others, they cited convenience and taste as two barriers to eating well. Adults are expected to (and can) overlook the taste or texture of certain foods for the greater good of health. You may dislike certain vegetables but eat them anyway. You may even purchase a salad greens mixture or supplement with multivitamins to make sure you are getting daily amounts of important vitamins and minerals. This scenario may not be the case with children. Although kids understand the importance of eating whole-grain pasta and Brussels sprouts, unless the foods are prepared a certain way or smothered in a certain sauce, they often say they would rather go hungry than eat some foods their parents have prepared. However, if the pantry is filled with delicious snacks that claim to be gluten free, fat free, lean, and heart healthy—but in fact include 25 grams of added sugar per serving—they may suddenly say they feel hungry again and reach for those snacks instead.

Table 5.6 lists time management, support from parents and school staff, and education as three of the six suggested strategies for overcoming barriers. All three strategies are

Table 5.6 Perceived Benefits and Barriers to Healthful Eating and Physical Activity

Healthful eating		Physical activity	
Benefits	**Barriers**	**Benefits**	**Barriers**
Improvements in cognitive and physical performance	Convenience	Social benefits	Prefer indoor activities instead of outdoor activities
Improvements in fitness	Taste	Enhancement of psychological status	Lack of energy
Improvements in endurance	Social factors	Physical sensation	Lack of motivation
Psychological benefits		Sport performance	Time constraints
Feeling good physically			Social factors

Strategies for overcoming barriers
- Support from parents and school staff
- Better planning and time management
- Self-motivation
- Education
- Restructuring the physical environment
- Greater variety of physical activities

Adapted from J.A. O'Dea, "Why Do Kids Eat Healthful Food? Perceived Benefits of and Barriers to Healthful Eating and Physical Activity Among Children and Adolescents," *Journal of the American Dietetic Association* 103, no. 4 (2003): 497-501.

pivotal to helping kids become better eaters and lovers of healthful foods. Life is hectic and is showing no signs of slowing down. Busyness has encroached on the household and has affected how families dine. After a busy day at work, caregivers don't always want to spend time preparing and cooking a healthful meal. It is much more convenient and palatable to eat a charbroiled hamburger and fries than to grill some chicken and steam asparagus and sweet potatoes. After a long and stressful day, the burger sounds better.

However, a young athlete's body needs the proper nourishment that comes from lean protein and nature's multivitamins (numerous forms of vegetables that are filled with fiber and life-giving antioxidants).

How do you bridge the gap between knowing and doing? The first step is to take inventory of your young athlete. Ask yourself a few questions:

1. What does the athlete like to eat?
2. What does the athlete need to eat more of?
3. What is the athlete eating too much of?
4. How can we work as a household to better prepare meals and snacks so that healthful eating becomes a priority?

Once you have answers to these questions, you can better set a nutritional plan and help educate your young athlete about the importance of eating well. A few years ago, we were coaching a group of 11-year-old soccer players. One of the fathers took a few moments at the end of practice to speak with us about proper nutrition for his son. His son was a typical 11-year-old boy who loved to play sports, was athletic, and detested vegetables or meat that he couldn't smother with ketchup. His father was having a tough time convincing him of the importance of eating better and decreasing the number of sodas and prepared snacks he consumed daily. The problem was that this athlete was fit, healthy, and strong. How do you convince a boy who looks and feels healthy that he should be eating better when he is already experiencing exactly what healthful food is supposed to give you? The kid was reluctant to change his current diet. We asked the father to think about something extrinsic and tangible that would motivate his son to change. He later sent us an e-mail stating that he had found a video interview online in which one of his son's favorite European soccer players discussed what he eats before and after a game. The player talked about how he eats very clean (eating simple, nonprocessed, whole foods without artificial ingredients). The father shared the video with his son. He was pleased by how receptive his son was to understanding the value of nutrition and performance. His son came to believe that the professionals eat well, and he wanted to be like them. Furthermore, the father kept emphasizing this major point to his son: "If you can be that fit and athletic by eating poorly, imagine how much better you will feel and perform if you begin to fuel your body with powerful foods."

You know your young athlete well. Take a moment to think about the changes she may need to make and consider some possible solutions. Remember, your athletes do not need to reach perfection in eating but rather aim for eating well; this pursuit can occur in small, subtle steps. Consider the following tips, which have worked for some athletes and their families:

- **Discuss with the athlete the benefits of eating well, especially during training.** Discuss how giving the body the proper nutrients to grow stronger and move faster will elevate her game.

- **If lack of time is the main challenge with food preparation and you find yourself scrambling to put together a nutritious meal, then forward thinking is the key.** Take one day a week to organize the meals for the upcoming week. Cook a batch of tomato sauce or chili, and freeze it in mini containers so that you can easily defrost it when needed.

- **Grilling is a great way to incorporate vegetables and protein into meals.** You can grill chicken, beef, or other meat, vacuum seal it, and freeze it for later use. Even barbecued chicken can be prepared and frozen. That way, when you need a healthy meal quickly, you can simply defrost the meat and heat it when you get home from work.

- **Toss a lean meat and some vegetables in a slow cooker in the morning before you leave for work.** Many good cookbooks containing recipes for both vegetarian and lean-meat dishes are available. The key steps are planning ahead and purchasing the ingredients.

- **Prepare great snacks that satiate your young athlete and provide the essential fat, protein, and vitamins that he needs.** In a large mason jar, add equal amounts of unsalted almonds, cashews, walnuts, pecans, sunflower seeds, pumpkin seeds, and any other favorite nuts or seeds. Top it off with your favorite dried fruit, such as cranberries, raisins, apricots, apples, dates, or figs. To add a bit of sweetness, you can throw in some chocolate or carob chips. Purchase the items you need at a bulk-food store, and simply mix them together for a delicious and nutritious trail mix. The athlete can take this snack with him in a small container or can eat it at home. Many young athletes are allergic to nuts, including walnuts, almonds, hazelnuts, cashews, Brazil nuts, and pistachios. In this case, nuts can be substituted with seeds (provided that no seed allergy exists), including pumpkin, sesame, and hemp seeds. Dried coconut and dried chickpeas are also wonderful alternatives and mix well with a variety of dried fruit. If you prefer a heartier snack, hummus or another bean or chickpea spread with a variety of raw vegetables packs a good vitamin punch and a healthy amount of plant-based protein. Watch for cross-contamination before substituting a food for a child with allergies. For instance, oats do not contain gluten. However, if oats are processed in a factory that also processes wheat products, a risk of cross-contamination exists, which means that it could harm a young person with a gluten allergy. Many nutritional options are available for kids with food allergies. Once you determine the allergy, seek safe alternatives that provide similar nutritional benefits.

LOSE THE BATTLE, WIN THE WAR!

Seldom does one see a young athlete do a 180-degree turn when it comes to eating better. An athlete is not going to go from junk-food nut to health-food enthusiast. If your teenager didn't like your marinara sauce or the way you made chicken cutlets yesterday, the same will probably apply tomorrow. However, there are things you can do—or battles you can lose—in the hope that you will win the war on food. Here are a few examples:

■ **If your child doesn't like to eat raw vegetables because she finds them boring or tasteless, find a dipping sauce that she likes.** The dipping sauce may have more sugar, salt, or fat than you would like, but if it gets her to eat her raw vegetables, do it. Eventually she will develop a taste and appreciation for the power of eating pure foods.

■ **If you like to make healthy pizza at home instead of ordering out, compromise.** You put time and energy into making spelt or whole-wheat dough and blending vegetables to make your own tomato sauce. The pizza is packed with nutrients. However, your kids don't like the dough and don't care much about the sauce. Try this: Buy the dough they like, but use your sauce on it. Another alternative (especially if they don't want to eat the sauce) is to buy or make the sauce that they do like to eat and simply mix the two sauces together. This way the taste of the sauce they like is not completely altered and you are able to get your nutrient-dense sauce into the mixture.

■ **If they want chicken fingers and fries, try making your own.** The boxed chicken fingers look like chicken and taste like chicken, but 13 chemicals that you can't pronounce are listed on the back of the box. As an alternative, make your own chicken fingers using a breading recipe that you find in a cookbook or online. You may need to add some mayonnaise or other ingredients to make the chicken more palatable, but at least you remove the majority of the chemicals that are present in the prepackaged form. As for the fries, simply cut up your own potatoes, season them for taste, and roast them in the oven or air fryer.

■ **If they like restaurant salad, make it at home with store-bought dressing.** For example, if they like ordering Caesar salad in a restaurant, compromise by buying Caesar dressing to use on the salad of your choice. Add your own grilled chicken and whatever vegetables you desire.

■ **Kids are always looking for convenience, so make healthful food convenient.** When they are hungry or between commercials, they simply scan the pantry and grab whatever is in their sight. If they open the refrigerator to get a snack and they have to wash the apple, cut the watermelon, or peel the carrots, they might opt for grabbing chips, protein bars, or whatever dessertlike treat they find instead. Take time to prewash the fruits and vegetables so they can simply open the refrigerator and reach for a handful of carrots, celery, or fennel, or a piece of watermelon or cantaloupe.

It might sound as if you are being asked to cater to children's bad habits. It may help you think of it as a realistic way to change those habits gradually. It is a request that you concede the battle and make it easy for them to make a good choice. Give them an opportunity to appreciate good food and a chance to feel the difference it makes both physically and mentally. In time, you will win the war on food choices.

CONCLUSION

All young athletes should eat a balanced diet consisting of wholesome carbohydrate, lean protein, and fat, including plenty of vegetables, nuts, and seeds. What the young athlete eats before and after competition is just as important as what the athlete eats in the days, weeks, and months before competition. A healthy, vibrant, and strong body relies on good nutrition every day.

Young athletes must eat whole foods to optimize energy, recovery, and muscle adaptations. Athletes are only as strong and efficient as their recovery, and recovery relies on adequate rest and a supercharged diet that takes advantage of nature's emporium. Don't be fooled by the promises of processed foods. Take the time to plan meals, choose food sources that fuel the body with the necessary nutrients, and create an environment that positively affects young athletes in sport and in life. A healthy young athlete will inevitably mature into a healthy adult.

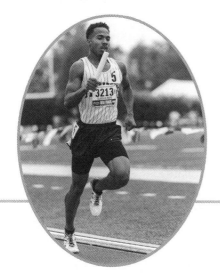

chapter 6

Energy System Training for Sport

In the previous chapter you learned how and when to fuel the needs of young athletes with whole-food energy sources. In this chapter, you will examine the energy systems dominant in team and other sports. A close relationship exists between energy systems and the programming of team-specific and position-specific training programs, so understanding the concepts related to energy systems of the body is essential in training athletes.

ENERGY SYSTEMS OF THE BODY

For an athletic action to occur, the body needs two things:

1. It needs muscles to contract.
2. It needs energy to enable muscular activity.

During training and competitions, the human body utilizes a chemical compound, adenosine triphosphate (ATP), that provides energy.

1. The **phosphagen (alactic, ATP-CP) energy system**, which uses stored ATP and creatine phosphate (CP) to generate energy without the presence of oxygen; it does not produce lactic acid during activity, hence the alternative term *alactic*.
2. The **glycolytic (lactic** or **lactic acid) energy system**, which primarily uses carbohydrate to produce energy without the presence of oxygen.
3. The **oxidative (aerobic) energy system**, which uses oxygen to produce energy, hence the alternative term *aerobic*.

Each system is present if the duration of a physical activity is performed for a relatively long period, for example, an athlete is active continuously for one hour. During the first 10 to 12 seconds of activity, the energy is produced by the phosphagen system. When the phosphagen system is exhausted after the first 12 seconds and up to 90 seconds of activity, the glycolytic system is called into action. From the 90 seconds on, and for up to two

Table 6.1 Characteristics of the Three Energy Systems for Physical Activity

Energy system	Rate of energy production	Duration	Fuel used	Ratio of recovery time per unit of activity
Phosphagen (alactic, ATP-CP)	Very high	10-12 sec	Creatine phosphate	1:12-1:20
Glycolytic (lactic, lactic acid)	High	20-90 sec	Blood glucose; glucose stored in the liver	1:3-1:5
Oxidative (aerobic)	Low	2 min-2 hr	Glucose stored in muscles and the liver; fat; protein	1:1-1:3

The duration of the rest interval for the phosphagen energy system, 1:12, means that for one unit of time (e.g., 10 sec) the rest interval is 12 times longer (120 sec/2 min). The duration of the rest interval for the glycolytic energy system is 1:3, meaning that for a duration of 1 minute of activity the rest interval is 3 minutes. The duration of the rest interval for the oxidative energy system is 1:1, meaning that for 5 minutes of lower-intensity work, the restoration time is also 5 minutes. For higher-intensity aerobic activity, the rest interval is 3 times longer than the activity itself (1:3).

hours or longer, the oxidative system is dominant and supplies energy for the duration.

The phosphagen system primarily supplies energy for quick bursts of fast, explosive actions. Both the phosphagen and glycolytic systems use carbohydrate that is stored in the muscles and in the liver in the form of **glycogen**. The glycolytic system does not produce energy as quickly as the phosphagen system, but it has a higher capacity to produce energy and for a longer duration. As this system is taxed and demand for energy rises, the athlete begins to feel a decrease in movement speed, an increase in fatigue, and a burning sensation in the muscles being used. This sensation occurs because of an increase in the acidity of the muscles, which explains why this system is also called the *lactic acid system*.

Finally, the oxidative, or *aerobic*, energy system produces energy at a slower rate, but it does so for a longer duration than the first two systems. Because this system's energy production relies on the breakdown of carbohydrate and fat, energy production is slower but lasts for hours. Table 6.1 illustrates specific elements of energy systems, rates of energy production, the fuel used for each system, and the ratio of recovery time per unit of time of the preceding activity.

INTERACTION OF ENERGY SYSTEMS

The three energy systems do not act independently. They interact in a specific sequence to generate the necessary energy to sustain physical work, from creating the shortest burst of energy to enduring an exhausting game or race. Coaches' comprehension and imaginative use of these systems has led to the improvement of training science and methodology over the years.

As illustrated in table 6.2, the three energy systems interact to produce the energy required to support physical work. The interaction of the energy systems is directly related to the duration of the activity. Keep these guidelines in mind when planning and designing different types of training to target the individual energy systems, from specific technical and tactical drills to aerobic conditioning methods.

Table 6.2 Percentage Contribution of Energy Systems for Technical, Tactical, and Physical Training

Duration of activity	Phosphagen (alactic, ATP-CP) system	Glycolytic (lactic, lactic acid) system	Oxidative (aerobic) system
5 sec	85%	15%	—
10 sec	50%	40%	10%
30 sec	15%	65%	20%
1 min	10%	40%	50%
2 min	5%	25%	70%
4 min	2%	18%	80%
10 min	1%	9%	90%
30 min	—	5%	95%
1 hr	—	2%	98%
2 hr	—	1%	99%

CLASSIFICATION OF SKILLS AND ACTIVITIES ACCORDING TO ENERGY SYSTEM DEMAND

Team, racket, and combat sports are complex in terms of technical and tactical skills involved and in terms of the dynamic interplay that exists among the energy systems. Various demands are placed on the athletes' bodies and minds when refining specific skills and targeting the various energy systems.

When you plan your training based on energy systems, consider the following two steps.

Step 1: Classify According to Energy Systems

List all the skills and activities for training in your sport, and classify them according to the energy system(s) involved. The classification suggested in table 6.3 represents a general guideline that you can adapt to your specific situation for more effective planning.

The skills and physical training options classified under a given energy system can be trained on the same day because they tap the same energy sources. For practical reasons (fatigue, skill retention, difficulty concentrating on too many training tasks), select only two or three of these training options for a given day, leaving the balance for another time.

Step 2: Alternate Energy Systems

Alternating energy systems ensures that they are not all taxed simultaneously, allowing them each to regenerate fully between sessions. This alternation facilitates a continuous restoration of all three energy systems and allows athletes to recover both physically and mentally. Ultimately, only refreshed athletes will see the athletic improvements they strive to achieve.

The concept of alternation should be considered not only within **microcycles** (a week of training) but also between them. In other words, demanding or strenuous training cycles should be alternated with recovery cycles throughout a training period. Although it is

Table 6.3 Suggested Classification of Skills, Drills, and Physical Training Methods According to Energy Systems

Phosphagen (alactic, ATP-CP) system	Glycolytic (lactic, lactic acid) system	Oxidative (aerobic) system
• Technical skills: 5-12 sec • Tactical drills: 10-12 sec • Maximum speed, power, and agility: 8-12 sec • Power/agility training: a few sets of short duration • Maximum strength: no more than 2 sets, few reps	• Technical skills: 13-90 sec • Tactical drills: 13 to 60-90 sec • Speed training: reps of 15-20 sec • Power endurance*: sets of 20-25 reps nonstop with maximum power and quickness	• Technical skills: >3 min • Tactical drills: 2-10 min • Aerobic endurance: long-duration drills or reps of 2-5 min • Muscle endurance: 1 to 3 sets of reps of 2-3 min performed nonstop

*Power endurance: The ability to perform powerful athletic actions using both the phosphagen and glycolytic energy systems (0-90 sec).

necessary to plan highly demanding microcycles to challenge athletes to greater levels of **adaptation**, especially during the **preparatory phase** (the first phase of a training plan), improvements come only when training is mixed with adequate periods of rest and recovery.

RESTORATION OF ENERGY FROM EXERCISE

A solid understanding of the restoration times required to replenish each energy system lays the foundation for planning rest intervals between bouts of physical effort. Instead of blindly following the traditions of your sport (which may or may not be based on scientific principles), challenge old traditions and view your own training systems with a critical eye. Past notions of *no pain, no gain* are outdated and have little to do with science or methodology. Table 6.4 summarizes the recovery processes and illustrates the time needed for restoring the three energy systems.

Phosphagen

The restoration of phosphagen is quite rapid; 50 to 70 percent is restored during the first 20 to 30 seconds, and the remainder is restored within 3 minutes. Generally, it takes 2 minutes for 85 percent restoration, 4 minutes for 90 percent restoration, and 8 minutes for 95 percent or more restoration.

Removal of Lactic Acid

Removal of lactic acid (LA) requires two phases:

1. Removal of LA from the muscle
2. Removal of LA from the blood

These phases are influenced by the type of activity performed during the rest interval. For example, if an athlete maintains light activity during drills (e.g., 10-15 min of light aerobic activity such as jogging or passing), LA is removed twice as fast as in athletes who rest passively. Considering the demanding and often strenuous game schedules typical of team sports, athletes should be encouraged to use any method available to speed up and facilitate recovery. The faster an athlete recovers, the more energy will be available for the next game. To ensure optimal recovery time, consider the following guidelines.

Table 6.4 Time Needed for the Restoration of the Three Energy Systems

Recovery process	Minimum	Maximum
Restoration of muscle phosphagen	2 min	5 min
Repayment of alactic oxygen debt	3 min	5 min
Repayment of glycogen oxygen debt	30 min	60 min
Restoration of muscle glycogen		
After intermittent activity	2 hr to restore 40% 5 hr to restore 55% 24 hr to restore 100%	
After prolonged nonstop activity	10 hr to restore 60% 48 hr to restore 100%	
Removal of LA from the muscles and blood	10 min to remove 25% 25-30 min to remove 50% 60-75 min to remove 95%	

Adapted from Fox (1984), Powers and Howley (2008), and Bompa and Carrera (2015).

Guidelines for Athletes

- Alternate periods of work with periods of regeneration.
- Try to eliminate all social stressors.
- Follow a sensible diet based on the specific phase of training.
- Participate in active rest, and engage in pleasant, relaxing social activities.

Guidelines for Coaches

- Maintain a positive team atmosphere of calmness, confidence, and optimism.
- Monitor each athlete's health status regularly.

HOW TO TRAIN THE ENERGY SYSTEMS: EXAMPLE 1

Table 6.5 provides an example of the alternation of energy systems during a microcycle with three training sessions a week.

Note that Monday is devoted mainly to training the phosphagen energy system. Of the options suggested for Monday (maximum speed, power, agility, and maximum strength [MxS]), select two or a maximum of three only. At the end of the training session, incorporate elements of power training using medicine balls, plyometrics, or agility drills (e.g., change of direction, stop and go). Concluding the session with 10 to 15 minutes of light oxidative (aerobic) training (specific or nonspecific) stimulates perspiration, which facilitates the removal of metabolites and improves subsequent recovery times.

On Wednesday, plan tactical (TA) training, tapping both the glycolytic and oxidative energy systems, using the values in table 6.3 as a guideline. On the same day, you can plan power-endurance drills (incorporating power training and agility; see chapter 9) using repetitions of longer duration (30-90 sec or longer).

Table 6.5 Periodization of Energy Systems for a Three-Day Microcycle (Weekly Program)

Monday	Tuesday	Wednesday	Thursday	Friday	Saturday	Sunday
• T: phosphagen • Max speed • P/A/MxS	—	• TA: glycolytic and oxidative • PE	—	• T/TA: phosphagen and glycolytic • P/MxS	—	—

T = technical; TA = tactical; P = power; A = agility; MxS = maximum strength; PE = power endurance.

Friday can stress phosphagen and glycolytic forms of training, implementing both specific and nonspecific methods. It is important to train power and maximum strength (MxS) to support continuous improvements in these abilities during the competitive phase.

HOW TO TRAIN THE ENERGY SYSTEMS: EXAMPLE 2

Table 6.6 suggests another training option based on a microcycle of five training days. Monday and Wednesday are devoted to training predominantly the phosphagen energy system whereas Friday is devoted to training both the phosphagen and glycolytic energy systems using both specific and nonspecific training options. To facilitate the removal of lactic acid from the system and aid in a faster recovery for the next training session, schedule 10 to 15 minutes of light oxidative (aerobic) training at the end of these sessions.

On Tuesday and Thursday, the emphasis is on tactical drills, working mainly the oxidative system; it includes a few drills to work the glycolytic system. Again, athletes will benefit from some form of specific or nonspecific oxidative (aerobic) training at the end of the sessions. The phosphagen system is not emphasized at all on these training days during this microcycle.

From analyzing tables 6.5 and 6.6, it is clear that all the energy systems contributing to the sport are trained systematically, and careful attention is given to alternating the energy systems to avoid the potentially debilitating effects of fatigue.

Table 6.6 Periodization of Energy Systems for a Five-Day Microcycle During the Preparatory Phase

Monday	Tuesday	Wednesday	Thursday	Friday	Saturday	Sunday
• T/TA: phosphagen system • S • P/A	• TA: glycolytic and oxidative systems • oxidative system • PE	• T/A: phosphagen system • P/MxS	• TA: oxidative system • Nonspecific, glycolytic and oxidative systems	• T/T/A: phosphagen and glycolytic systems • S • P/A/MxS	—	—

T = technical; TA = tactical; S = speed; P = power; A = agility; MxS = maximum strength; PE = power endurance.

ERGOGENESIS OF SELECTED SPORTS

To create a viable training program for your sport, you must first know the proportions of the energy systems used in the sport, a concept called ergogenesis. **Ergogenesis** is used to describe the proportions (in percentages) of the energy systems used in a particular sport. You must also identify the **biomotor (motor) abilities** (speed, power, flexibility, agility,

strength) required in the sport and try to isolate the most important ones—the so-called dominant motor abilities.

In many cases, the dominant ability identified for a particular sport is actually a combination of two or more abilities, as is the case for power, agility, and **muscular endurance** (the ability of a

muscle to repeatedly exert force against resistance). For example, **power** is the product of **strength** and **speed** or quickness of muscle contraction. Similarly, agility is a complex ability combining elements of speed or quickness, coordination, flexibility, and power, while muscular endurance benefits from the development of both **aerobic endurance** (the ability to exercise at moderate intensity for an extended period) and strength.

The ergogenesis presented in table 6.7 illustrates the proportion of the three energy systems used for team sports (Powers and Howley, 2008; Bompa, 2006). All three energy systems contribute to the energy requirements of athletes during a game, with three excep-

Table 6.7 Ergogenesis of Selected Sports

Sport		Proportion of Energy Systems		
		Phosphagen system	Glycolytic system	Oxidative system
Track: 100 m		53%	44%	3%
Baseball, softball, or cricket		95%	5%	—
Basketball		20%	40%	40%
Field hockey		10%	30%	60%
American football	Linebacker	50%	40%	10%
	Others	30%	40%	30%
Ice hockey		10%	40%	50%
Judo		90%	10%	—
Lacrosse		10%	30%	60%
Rowing		20%	30%	50%
Rugby		10%	30%	60%
Soccer	Men	15%	15%	70%
	Women	0.5%	19.2%	80.3%
Swimming: 100 m		80%	15%	5%
Team handball		20%	30%	50%
Volleyball		40%	10%	50%
Water polo		10%	30%	60%

Adapted from Powers and Howley (2008), Van Someren (2006), Bompa and Haff (2009), and Perroni et al. (2019).

tions (baseball, softball, and cricket), where the phosphagen energy system is dominant. In most cases, the oxidative system provides the dominant source of energy, especially during the final parts of the game. The pace of the game and the tactics applied (all-out pressing from the first minute on), especially between two teams of similar abilities, can always alter the proportions suggested in table 6.7, often in favor of the oxidative system.

Although all three energy systems must be well trained through nonspecific and sport-specific training methods, the oxidative system provides the majority of energy necessary for a strong finish. In addition, a well-developed oxidative system facilitates a faster recovery after competitions and between training sessions. Even if the phosphagen and glycolytic systems supply the majority of energy required during the early part of a high-intensity competition, athletes' effectiveness during the later stages of a competition is impossible without a strong aerobic base.

Energy System Analysis for Soccer

Modern soccer is an intermittent, high-intensity game. During the course of a game, athletes perform a variety of movements such as sprinting, jogging, striding, walking, kicking, and jumping, and they make agile turns and quick changes of direction. Generally, the higher the level of play, the higher the energy demand and overall stresses experienced during the game. However, playing in a high-intensity game is possible only if athletes dedicate adequate time to training and only if coaches design training around the position-specific requirements of the game. The ergogenesis for men's soccer has been estimated at 15 percent phosphagen system, 15 percent glycolytic system, and 70 percent oxidative system; for women's soccer it has been estimated at 0.5 percent phosphagen system, 19.2 percent glycolytic system, and 80.3 percent oxidative system (Perroni et al., 2017) (table 6.8). Furthermore, table 6.8 (Bompa, 2006) illustrates the breakdown of energy systems by position as well as the position-specific motor characteristics required in soccer. Note the differences in energy systems and biomotor abilities between most athletes, especially for midfielders and sweepers.

Energy Sources Demand

Soccer players utilize all three energy systems during a game. With sprints in soccer lasting an average of 4.5 seconds, a good portion of the energy is supplied by the phosphagen system. When these sprints are frequently repeated during the game, the glycolytic system is in high demand.

Low glycogen levels are very common among soccer players at halftime; these athletes often deplete their entire glycogen stores by the end of the game. However, if the demands of the game are low, postgame glycogen levels may remain between 15 and 20 percent of pregame levels. To support their need for energy, athletes must consume a diet rich in carbohydrate for optimal glycogen replenishment.

This replenishment is even more important for athletes who play two or three games a week. Diminished glycogen stores reduce the capacity to play with high intensity and to endure the energy demand for the entire game.

Glycogen restoration is not immediate. About 60 percent is restored in 10 hours, while full restoration takes about 24 to 48 hours. This restoration rate is one reason soccer teams should not play more than two games a week. Ignoring these physiological realities could harm the athletes, resulting in high levels of fatigue, staleness, and even overtraining.

Table 6.8 Ergogenesis and Position-Specific Biomotor Abilities in Soccer

Position	Ergogenesis	Required motor abilities
Goalkeeper	Phosphagen system: 100%	• Power • Reaction time • Movement time
Sweeper	Phosphagen system: 30% Glycolytic system: 30% Oxidative system: 40%	• Starting and jump power • Reaction and movement time • Maximum acceleration–deceleration • Quick turns
Fullback	Phosphagen system: 20% Glycolytic system: 30% Oxidative system: 50%	• Starting power • Maximum acceleration–deceleration • Quick turns and changes of direction • Reaction and movement time
Midfielder	Phosphagen system: 10% Glycolytic system: 20% Oxidative system: 70%	• Power endurance • Speed endurance* • Reaction and movement time • Acceleration–deceleration
Forward	Phosphagen system: 20% Glycolytic system: 20% Oxidative system: 60%	• Power • Starting and jump power • Maximum acceleration–deceleration • Reaction and movement time

*Speed endurance: The ability to perform sprints and fast athletic actions of 15-30 seconds, where both the phosphagen and glycolytic systems are used.

Travel Distance Demand

The distance covered per game is position specific, and it may depend heavily on the rhythm and pace of the game. Highly competitive games tend to be more physically and mentally demanding. In some of these games, top athletes have been known to cover distances of about 10 kilometers (6 mi). Midfielders, the so-called engines of the team, usually cover more distance than other players—an average of 11 kilometers (6.8 mi) per game. The longest recorded distance run by a soccer player so far was French athlete Henri Duquette. In 1989, he covered 15 kilometers (9 mi) in a single game, and he currently holds the record. Next in line are the forwards, who average 9.5 kilometers (5.9 mi) each game, followed by fullbacks, averaging 8.5 kilometers (5.3 mi) each game. Considering their specific tactical responsibilities on the team, it is no surprise that except for goalkeepers, sweepers cover the least amount of ground, with an average of 6 kilometers (4 mi) each game. These values vary from game to game, depending not only on the pace of the game and levels of fatigue but also on the skill level of the athletes and varying climatic conditions (Horsfield, 2015; Thorpe et al., 2017).

Table 6.9 includes data compiled from several studies on the subject. It illustrates the average distance soccer players cover in a game, their different positions, modes of movement, and the intensity of movement. In addition to the modes of movement shown in the table, athletes also tackle, jump, and kick the ball with varying force from different distances. Players perform an average of 9 tackles, and the most active players are involved in about 18 to 20 tackles each game. The intensity of the game often depends on the skill level of the athletes.

Table 6.9 Average Distance Covered (km), Mode of Movement, and Physiological Demands for Soccer Players (by Position)

Position	Average distance covered (km)	Mode of movement					Physiological demand/ intensity (% per game)	
		Walking	Jogging	Striding	Sprinting	Other	High	Low
Forward	9.5	2.5	4.0	1.25	0.8	0.95	40%	60%
Midfielder	11.1	2.8	5.0	1.5	1.0	0.8	50%	50%
Fullback	8.5	2.5	3.5	1.1	0.6	0.8	30%	70%
Sweeper	6.0	2.1	2.5	0.6	0.5	0.3	30%	70%

Adapted from Ekblom (1986); Bangsbo, Mohr, and Krustrup (2006); Bangsbo, Iaia, and Krustrup (2007); and Thorpe, Atkinson, Drust, and Gregson (2017).

The higher the league or level of play, the higher the game intensity. Of the total distance covered, individual athletes perform about 10 percent at maximum speed, with sprints varying from 20 to 40 meters (about 22-24 yd). If sprints and striding or cruising are considered together, higher-intensity running approaches 2.5 kilometers (1.5 mi). The rhythm of the game, the conditioning level of the athletes, and the air temperature and humidity affect performance intensity. Games in hot or humid conditions tend to be played at lower intensity, but they arouse heightened levels of physiological stress.

The intensity of a game is also reflected in the amount of weight athletes lose (generally through increased perspiration) during a game. Games played at a faster pace or rhythm or in higher temperatures or humidity tend to elicit greater weight loss. In temperate climates, such as those in northern Europe and the United States, weight loss per game can range between 1.5 and 2 kilograms (3.5-4.5 lb) per game. However, in warmer climates, such as those in the southern United States, South America, Africa, southern Asia, and southern Europe, dehydration levels can reach up to 5 kilograms (11 lb) during high-intensity games. This level of dehydration can severely affect speed and especially endurance.

Heart rate can also be an accurate indicator of game intensity. Heart rate values for high-caliber athletes can often exceed 180 beats per minute (bpm) during a game. Depending on the pace of the game, the heart rates of highly involved athletes can rise to between 184 and 186 bpm 12 to 16 times in a single game, demonstrating the high levels of intensity to which a soccer player may be exposed. Horsfield (2015) provided this additional information regarding the heart rate during a match:

- Playing for 28 to 30 minutes taxes 85 to 90 percent of maximum heart rate (HRmax).
- Playing for 18 to 20 minutes taxes 90 to 95 of HRmax.
- Playing for 8 to 12 minutes taxes 95 to 100 percent of HRmax.
- Playing for 60 to 70 minutes, athletes are functioning at over 85 percent of HRmax, which is a visible high demand for most athletes.

Another indicator of game intensity is the LA concentration in the blood, which can range from 8 to 12 millimoles per liter. Games of lower intensity yield lower levels of blood **lactate** (a salt formed from lactic acid) concentration.

Muscular Strength Demand

Muscular strength, the capacity of an athlete to perform work or overcome a resistance, is more important in soccer than most coaches recognize, especially in the lower limbs and torso. Strength is not only required for jumping to head the ball frequently throughout the game, it is also essential for the improvement of speed, quickness, and agility—not to mention the ability to withstand the pushing and shoving that goes on in the penalty area as athletes position themselves for corner kicks.

Aerobic Endurance Demand

Tables 6.7 and 6.8 demonstrate that the oxidative energy system is dominant in the game of soccer. A high level of aerobic endurance is an absolute necessity because athletes are expected to display the same quality of play at the end of the game as they do at the beginning. A high level of aerobic endurance allows athletes to cope successfully with fatigue during the game, but it also enhances an athlete's rate of recovery after the game and between workouts.

The average **maximal aerobic power** (maximum rate at which oxygen can be used during intense exercises) of soccer players increased on average from 55 milliliters per kilogram per minute (ml/kg/min) in the late 1970s to an average of 60 ml/kg/min by the mid-1980s. More recent data indicate an increase to 65 ml/kg/min and higher (Bangsbo et al., 2006; Horsfield, 2015; Thorpe et al., 2017).

A strong foundation of aerobic endurance must be established to prevent the negative effects of fatigue. Low endurance levels decrease athletes' ability to perform at a high rate and intensity and negatively affect concentration, tactical judgment, and the ability to perform technical skills such as passing and shooting. More important, a lack of endurance puts athletes at increased risk of injury.

Although soccer is an intermittent, high-intensity sport, its complexity places a high demand on all athletes; it requires good flexibility, maximal speed and power, agility, and high aerobic power. Sound planning and periodized training programs with strong preparatory phases will produce higher-quality athletes with increased technical proficiency and the ability to cope with fatigue effectively.

Dominant Motor Abilities in Soccer

As in most team sports, soccer players must be able to repeatedly sprint with maximum speed for 20 to 40 meters (22-44 yd). This task requires **speed endurance**. Power represents an important element in soccer; it becomes apparent in such game situations as sprinting, changing directions quickly, jumping, and jostling for position (mostly inside the penalty box). However, because powerful actions are repeated many times during the game, athletes must also train for **power endurance** (ability to repetitively perform powerful actions for a long time). It is important to understand that increased power from year to year is impossible without first increasing maximum strength (MxS).

POSITION-SPECIFIC TRAINING

How often do coaches create position-specific training programs? Except for baseball pitchers or goalkeepers in various sports, coaches often tend to train all athletes in the same way regardless of the physiological or motor ability requirements of a given position. However, the use of the same training program for all athletes is inefficient and scientifically ineffective.

Team sport coaches must understand the game- and position-specific physiological demands of a sport in order to design effective individual training programs. You can best understand these demands by doing your own time–motion analysis of the sport. Simply take a stopwatch and follow an athlete for a specified period. Record the time (in seconds) the athlete spends in different types of activities, such as walking, maximum-velocity running, standing, jogging, and striding (running with long strides but at only 75% of maximum velocity). Although such an analysis may have different nuances and variations, a standard analysis (for basketball) is presented later in this section.

Table 6.8 shows the specifics of the energy systems and the modes of movement in the sport of soccer. This table illustrates the differences between the energy system requirements by position. How many coaches actually keep these specific physiological differences in mind when designing a training program? Consider some examples from other sports to better illustrate these differences and to make a case for the need for position-specific training.

Following are selected comments about some characteristics of other team sports.

■ *American football*: Visible differences in the physiological and motor ability requirements of various positions in American football also exist. A wide receiver is actually a pure sprinter dressed in a football uniform. During the game, he runs like a sprinter, with incredible footwork and changes of direction, to finally catch a ball at the end of a fine display of athleticism. Also keep in mind that this same wide receiver runs at maximum velocity for 25 to 40 segments of 25 to 50 yards (about 23-46 m) over the 3-hour duration of a game. This information has important implications regarding the specifics of training for wide receivers. They should be great sprinters, but considering the number of times they need to repeat the distance, they should also be trained to have great speed endurance. In contrast, an offensive lineman's mission on a football team is to hold off the opposition. He plays the role of a bulldozer—displaying the greatest amount of force over a period of 2 to 5 seconds, trying to demolish everything in front of him. In this case, the need to train endurance in the form of a 3-mile (5 km) run is a waste of time. A football quarterback, on the other hand, has the qualities of a javelin thrower—a strong arm and a great display of throwing power. However, he must throw with the great precision and finesse of a dart player.

■ *Ice hockey*: An elite ice hockey player skates at high velocity for more than 5 kilometers (3 mi) each game. Goaltenders, on the other hand, do not require such high levels of endurance; their game is based on concentration, flexibility, and lightning-quick reflexes.

■ *Volleyball*: Attackers in volleyball have an impressive vertical jump that is envied by many other athletes. However, do you realize that attackers jump an average of 200 times each game? In contrast, the libero, who is very mobile, with excellent reflexes on defense, and a great contributor on offense, may be considered the epitome of agility and quick reaction.

■ *Basketball*: The differences between various positions in team sports is illustrated by motor ability characteristics and test results for different positions in basketball, shown in table 6.10.

Adapted from Van Someren (2006); Pain and Hibbs (2007); Carling, Bloomfield, Nelson, and Reilly (2008); Horsfield (2015); Thorpe, Atkinson, Drust, and Gregson (2017); Douglas et al. (2019); and Colomer et al. (2020).

Table 6.10 Test Results for Different Positions in Basketball

Position	$\dot{V}O_2$max (ml/kg/min)*	600 m run (min)	Maximum-velocity run repeated to exhaustion** time (sec)	20 m sprint (sec)***
Guard	54.3	2.15	31.0	3.46
Power forward	50.7	2.13	32.2	3.67
Small forward	47.4	—	31.4	—
Center	50.9	2.21	32.9	3.81

Adapted from Erčulj (1997), Naumovski (2001), and Urbach (2001).

*$\dot{V}O_2$max: The amount, or volume, of oxygen an athlete uses during high-intensity exercise.

**A maximum-velocity run is performed back and forth between two lines and repeated to exhaustion.

***18-year-old subjects.

TIME–MOTION ANALYSIS OF BASKETBALL

The following data highlight several game-specific activities involved in basketball. Coaches as well as strength and conditioning professionals looking to create unique fitness training programs for basketball can use this information.

A time–motion analysis of basketball (Urbach, 2001) reveals the following:

- Total played time (PT): 26.3 minutes
- Longest period of work: 23 seconds
- Shortest period of work: 1 second
- 56 activities performed at high intensity
- 96 activities performed at moderate intensity
- 25 activities performed at low intensity
- 72 periods of active recovery (walking)
- 7 periods of passive recovery (time-out)
- Duration of high-intensity actions: 3.64 seconds
- Duration of moderate-intensity actions: 9.73 seconds
- Duration of low-intensity actions: 9.6 seconds
- Duration of active recovery: 26.7 seconds
- Duration of passive recovery: 42.4 seconds

- Duration of technical or physical actions:
  - Dribbling: 3 to 10 seconds
  - Passing: 1 to 2 seconds
  - Shooting: 1 to 2 seconds
  - Defensive slides: 3 to 10 seconds
  - Sprints: 3 to 5 seconds
  - Jumps: 1 to 2 seconds
  - Cuts: 3 to 5 seconds
  - Combinations (run/jog/walk): 4 to 20 seconds

For female athletes, research shows the following heart rate values (Urbach, 2001):

- 61 percent of PT spent at 85 percent of HRmax
- 30 percent of PT spent at 90 percent of HRmax
- 9 percent of PT spent at 95 percent of HRmax

For male athletes, the following data were reported (McInnis et al., 1995):

- 75 percent of PT spent at 85 percent of HRmax
- 10 percent at low intensity
- 15 percent at high intensity
- Blood lactate: 6.8 millimoles per liter for elite athletes, demonstrating a high reliance on the glycolytic system

Adapted from Urbach (2001) and McInnes, Carlson, Jones, and McKenna (1995).

ERGOGENESIS MODELS FOR TEAM SPORTS

This section analyzes examples of ergogenesis for the most popular team sports. The analysis refers to these elements:

1. Dominant energy system(s): The dominant system or systems used in the selected sport
2. Ergogenesis: The contribution of each energy system for the sport (expressed as a percentage)
3. Limiting factors of performance: The dominant physical qualities of the sport that, if improperly developed, will limit the progress of your team and athletes. (If you want to improve the game and the way your athletes play, you have to first stress the development of the limiting factors of performance to decrease the abilities that keep the athletes from achieving maximum potential.)
4. Training objectives for each sport: A list of your training objectives for the future based on analyzing your athletes, prioritizing the dominant abilities, and evaluating how well they are developed

Baseball, Softball, or Cricket

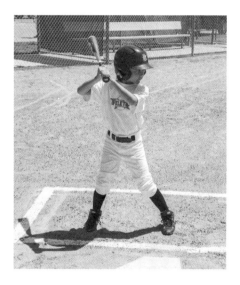

- Dominant energy system: phosphagen
- Ergogenesis: phosphagen = 95%; glycolytic = 5%; oxidative = 0%
  - High bursts of energy
  - Longer periods of recovery
- Limiting factors of performance: Throwing or batting power, acceleration, agility, and reaction time

Training Objectives

- Develop the phosphagen and glycolytic energy systems.
- Develop the aerobic base to enable faster recovery between workouts and after the game.

Basketball

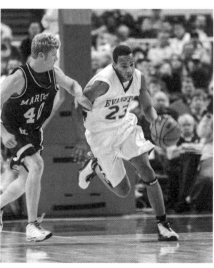

- Dominant energy systems: phosphagen and oxidative
- Ergogenesis: phosphagen = 30%; glycolytic = 40%; oxidative = 30%
  - High bursts of energy between different jumps and dunks, with short periods of recovery
  - High accelerations and decelerations and other variations of running (3-4 mi/5-7 km) per game, followed by approximately 280 quick changes of direction
- Heart rate average: 167 bpm; 25% of the time over 180 bpm
- Limiting factors of performance: Acceleration and deceleration power, take-off power, agility, coordination and ball handling, reaction time, and movement time

Training Objectives

- Develop all three energy systems with game-specific means of training.
- Develop a good aerobic base to help the team play effectively for the duration of the game (especially in the later stages) and to enable faster recovery between workouts and after the game.
- Develop maximum strength as the foundation for the refinement of power, acceleration–deceleration, agile actions during the game, and faster and highly coordinated footwork.
- Develop power endurance.
- Develop maximum speed with effective running, high-frequency footwork, reaction time, and movement time.

Field Hockey

- Dominant energy system: oxidative
- Ergogenesis: phosphagen = 10%; glycolytic = 30%; oxidative = 60%
  - Short bursts of intense athletic actions, repeated many times during the game, with medium-duration periods of recovery
  - Strong aerobic capacity that allows athletes to repeat powerful actions for the duration of the game
  - Limiting factors of performance: Acceleration and deceleration powers, agility, reaction time, and movement time

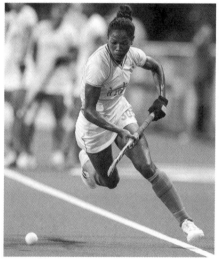

Training Objectives

- Develop all three energy systems, with emphasis on aerobic endurance for the needs of the game and improved recovery rate.
- Develop maximum strength as an element for increased power, agility, acceleration and deceleration, and changes of direction.
- Develop maximum speed with a good and relaxed form.

Berengui/DeFodi Images via Getty Images

Football (American)

Linebacker

- Dominant energy systems: phosphagen and glycolytic
- Ergogenesis: phosphagen = 50%; glycolytic = 40%; oxidative = 10%
  - High bursts of explosive energy (2-5 sec) and attempts to withstand the opponents' strength
  - Brief periods of recovery: 25 to 40 seconds

Training Objectives

- Develop maximum strength and increased muscle hypertrophy (where needed).
- Develop explosive leg power.
- Develop reactive power.

Wide Receivers, Defensive Backs, and Tailbacks

- Dominant energy systems: phosphagen, glycolytic, oxidative

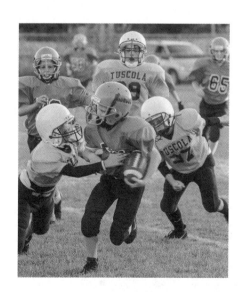

- Ergogenesis: phosphagen = 30%; glycolytic = 40%; oxidative = 30%
  - High display of quickness, agility, and maximum speed and power
  - Brief periods of recovery except for wide receivers, who have a slightly longer time to recover
- Limiting factors of performance: Acceleration power, agility, reactive power, and starting power

Training Objectives

- Develop maximum acceleration with effective running form.
- Develop speed endurance for wide receivers so that they are able to repeatedly run segments of 25 to 50 yards (about 23-46 m) 25 to 40 times per game.
- Develop a high level of agility, quick footwork, reaction power, starting power, and maximum strength.

Ice Hockey

- Dominant energy systems: phosphagen, glycolytic, oxidative
- Ergogenesis: phosphagen = 10%; glycolytic = 50%; oxidative = 40%
  - High bursts of energy from 5 seconds to 3 minutes
  - Shifts of about 40 seconds, repeated 12 to 20 times during the game
  - Rest between shifts: about 3 minutes

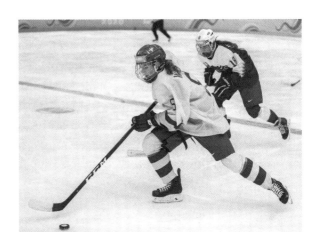

Linnea Rheborg/Getty Images

  - High display of power and speed interspersed with battles for the control of the puck along the boards (Elite athletes skate at high velocity for about 3 miles [5 km] per game.)
- Limiting factors of performance: Acceleration power, power endurance, and shooting power

Training Objectives

- Develop all three energy systems with emphasis on the phosphagen and oxidative systems.
- Develop maximum strength as the key element needed for quick acceleration, quick stoppages, powerful shooting, and winning battles for loose pucks.
- Develop maximum acceleration and the ability to repeat it numerous times during the game.

Lacrosse

- Dominant energy system: oxidative
- Ergogenesis: phosphagen = 10%; glycolytic = 30%; oxidative = 60%
  - Fast and powerful actions with high bursts of energy for longer offensive drives
  - Short rest intervals during the game
- Limiting factors of performance: acceleration and deceleration, quick changes of direction, starting and shooting power with a high degree of accuracy, agility, quick footwork, and fast reaction time and movement time

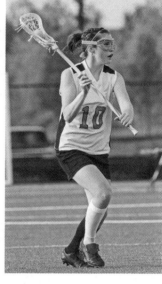

Training Objectives

- Develop all three energy systems with emphasis on the glycolytic and oxidative systems.
- Develop a good aerobic base for a forceful and equal rhythm in the later part of the game and to enable faster recovery between workouts and after the game.
- Develop maximum strength as the determinant for improved speed, agility, shooting power, and power endurance.

Rugby

- Dominant energy system: oxidative
- Ergogenesis: phosphagen = 10%; glycolytic = 30%; oxidative = 60%
- Limiting factors for performance: Acceleration and deceleration with quick changes of direction under the high demand of lactic acid and aerobic endurance (Power and power endurance are in high demands for the duration of the game.)

Training Objectives

- Develop all three energy systems, with emphasis on aerobic endurance.
- Develop maximum strength as the main ingredient for the development of starting power and power endurance.
- Develop agility, with emphasis on quick footwork.
- Develop acceleration and quick changes of direction.

Soccer

- Dominant energy system: oxidative
- Ergogenesis: phosphagen = 15%; glycolytic = 15%; oxidative = 70%
  - High energy demand, with high accelerations and quick changes of direction
  - Rest periods during the game: interruptions of 5 to 15 seconds (or longer for defense, when the game is played in the opposite end of the field)

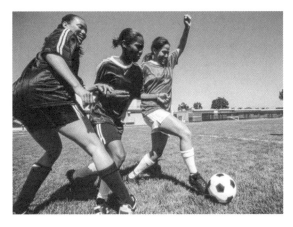

- Limiting factors of performance: Acceleration and deceleration power, agility in the form of quick footwork and quick changes of direction, reaction and movement time.

Training Objectives

- Develop all three energy systems based on a strong, specific aerobic base
- Develop powerful legs (and torso)—as the foundation for high acceleration, deceleration, and changes of direction.
- Develop starting power and jumping power.
- Develop position-specific agility for all three energy systems.

Team Handball

- Dominant energy systems: glycolytic and oxidative
- Ergogenesis: phosphagen = 20%; glycolytic = 30%; oxidative = 50%
  - Fast and explosive actions with high bursts of energy, repeated 20 to 40 times per game
  - Short periods of recovery (3-7 sec) during stoppages
- Limiting factors of performance: Acceleration and deceleration, quick changes of direction, quick footwork, throwing power, and ball handling

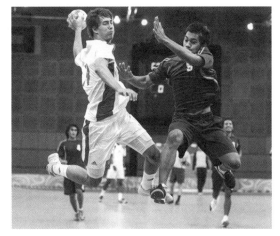

Mark Dadswell/Getty Images

Training Objectives

- Develop all three energy systems, based on a strong but specific glycolytic and oxidative base, to sustain a consistently fast pace throughout the game.
- Develop maximum acceleration and deceleration and quick changes of direction.
- Develop position-specific agility, reaction, and movement time.
- Develop maximum strength as the source of developing speed, agility, quick footwork, and ball handling.

Volleyball

- Dominant energy systems: phosphagen and oxidative
- Ergogenesis: phosphagen = 40%; glycolytic = 10%; oxidative = 50%
  - Fast and powerful actions, with explosive off-the-ground spikes, blocks, and dives
  - Short periods of recovery (9 sec average) after two rallies, or longer during time-outs
- Limiting factors of performance: Take-off power, reactive power, movement time, power endurance, and agility

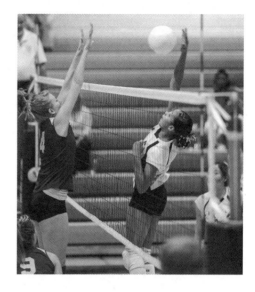

Training Objectives

- Develop maximum strength as the foundation for increased take-off power, spiking power, and agility.
- Develop power endurance to sustain take-off power for the duration of the game.
- Develop position-specific agility, reaction, and movement time.

Water Polo

- Dominant energy system: oxidative
- Ergogenesis: phosphagen = 10%; glycolytic = 30%; oxidative = 60%
  - High energy expenditure, with high-velocity sprints, powerful actions, and shooting
  - Short recovery time during penalty stoppages
- Limiting factors of performance: Starting power, acceleration power, and shooting power, all relying on a solid aerobic base

Training Objectives

- Develop all three energy systems, emphasizing the oxidative and glycolytic systems.
- Develop maximum strength as the foundation for all the powerful actions of the game, from sprinting to shooting.
- Develop maximum speed based on the force applied against water resistance.

The level of athleticism, intensity, and complex use of energy systems during training and competitions is very high in most sports. From team, racket, and contact sports to most individual sports, the level of skills and demand in physical potential is so high that there is no room for innocence.

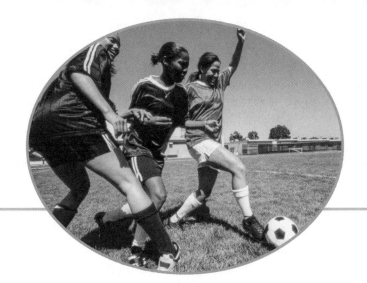

chapter 7

Model Training for Team Sports

Modeling as a sport science concept has a foundation in mathematical methods of modeling. Jiri Vanek, physiology professor at the Charles University in Prague, Czechoslovakia, promoted model training in the 1960s. Since then, an array of scholarly publications followed through the 1990s and into the next millennium. In terms of both theoretical development and practical application, model training is still in its infancy.

As a theoretical concept, a **model** is an abstract form of a concept to be used in the future, while **modeling** is the actual process of creating a model.

When applied to physical training, modeling has the potential to simulate training of technical and tactical strategies that should be reproduced during the game. These strategies prepare athletes for different game situations and social environments. Modeling has been applied in many areas of sport science, including the following:

- Statistics and game analysis (Avalos et al., 2003)
- Modeling the coaching process (Cushion, 2007)
- Computer simulation for tapering (Luc et al., 2009)
- Organizational tool for professional sports (Cyrenne, 2009)
- Modeling sports tournaments (Cattelan et al., 2012)
- Using imagery in sport psychology (Post and McCullagh, 2017)
- Modeling performance excellence in sport psychology (Aoyagi et al., 2018)
- Applying computational models in learning science, sport psychology, biomechanics, and game analysis

Modeling is also used during training to mimic technical and tactical elements and skills (physical and psychological) that will be used in the upcoming tactical plan for the next competition or game.

As you (the coach) make the game plan, consider how the athletes' abilities can be integrated into the team's philosophy and how individual athletes fit into the overall game plan. A game or competition plan can never be complete unless you also consider the strengths and weaknesses of the opposition and the strategies necessary for adapting your own game to that of the opposition.

Finally, you should plan specific training sessions to ensure a game-specific adaptation that ultimately will improve game effectiveness and result in a superior performance.

INTEGRATED GAME OR CONTEST MODEL

Before coaches begin working with an athlete or team, they must have a general guideline that dictates the team's future training. This guideline, the integrated game or contest model (table 7.1), is considered the cornerstone of a team's overall program. It guides all activities throughout a year of training. In addition, it serves as a general guideline for all mini models that coaches create in preparation for league competition.

A coach's first responsibility is to set *performance objectives* for the athletes and team; these objectives must be realistic and attainable while also challenging. In setting these objectives, the coach has to consider the quality of athletes available for each position, the system of play to be used, and the athletes' range of technical and tactical abilities. Before setting these ranges the first step is to create an overall game model. The scope of this model should share with athletes all the details of the overall model (traveling to the venue, meal times, etc.). The game model also refers to the overall tactics and strategies for the team—including offensive and defensive and individual plans for each athlete—all of which should be integrated into the overall game model for the entire team. Similarly, there should be a psychological model for the team for prior to, during, and after the game. A physical preparation model should be included also as part of the overall game model and explains how to ready athletes for competition including athletes' reactions and adaptation to the intensity and physical demand of the game or contest.

The environmental model refers to the following:

1. The circumstances under which the athletes will perform. These circumstances include equipment, time of the game, quality of officiating, and whether the athletes had a chance to have a workout on the field or at the gym before the official game or contest.

2. The sociopsychological climate (how the spectators may affect the athletes' and team's performance). Often, an unfavorable environment leads to high tension that disturbs psychological processes such as concentration, self-control, combativeness, perception, lucidity, reaction time, and decision-making process. A friendly audience could stimulate these traits, resulting in a better performance.

Steps for Developing an Integrated Game Model

Creating a game model follows several steps (see table 7.2). It commences with thorough analysis (*analysis phase*) of the effectiveness of last season's training and game plan (e.g., how successful were the team's and individual athletes' achievements?). Based on this analysis, training elements are retained or replaced with new concepts in all elements of training (technical, tactical, physical, psychological, and social).

In the next step, new qualitative elements (training volume and duration, number of repetitions, etc.) are introduced (*introduction phase*). The new game model is then tested in training and later in exhibition games (*testing phase*). If not totally satisfied with the team's performance during the testing phase (*validation phase*), coaches still have an opportunity to take any necessary changes before the league games start, and, as such, to finalize the model (*finalization phase*) to be used in the upcoming competitive season (*application phase*).

The best time to create a new model is during the off-season (transition) and the new preseason (preparatory) training phases, when the stresses of competitions are absent.

Table 7.1 Integrated Game or Contest Model

Performance objectives • For the entire team • For each individual athlete
Game model • Formations and positions • Between lines or groups • Transitions from offense to defense and from defense to offense

Tactical model
• Offensive model to be employed
  • Counterattacks
  • Positional attacks
  • Flexibility in adapting the model to the opposition's system of play
• Defensive system to be employed
  • Defense against fast breaks
  • Defense against positional attacks
  • Special game situations

Technical model • Skills necessary to apply the tactical model   • Predominant skills used in offense and defense
Physical preparation model (Modeling the physical demand of the game) • Your team's model • The opposition team's model
Environmental model (Modeling the game's environment) • Time of the game, eventual delays • Hostile crowd • Intimidating strategies • Equipment; playing conditions; quality of the field, court, or ice; water temperature; etc.
Psychological model • Psychological skills required prior, during, and after the game • Model the expected organizational details and conditions of the game to be played • Quality of officiating: how to react to bias officiating
Monitoring and analysis • Evaluate the model. • Analyze the athletes' application of technical, tactical, physical, and psychological models. • Conclusions for the future: positive, negative • Proposed changes for the future

This time is ideal for a comprehensive and critical retrospective analysis of the previous year's game model, including reevaluating whether the objectives, tests and standards, and training parameters were set and accomplished adequately. Similarly, analyze how the athletes coped with stresses of training and competition, and find ways to improve responses in the future. Then, objectively select the methods and means of training that will materialize in the new game model, eliminating those that were ineffective.

Table 7.2 Steps (Phases) of Developing a New Game or Contest Model for the Next Season

Phase	1. Analysis phase	2. Introduction phase	3. Testing phase	4. Validation phase	5. Finalization phase	6. Application phase
Action	Analyze past season.	Introduce new training elements.	Test the model.	Validate the model.	Finalize the model.	Apply the model in exhibition contests and games.

It is possible to make changes to the basic model during league play according to the team's new performance. If the team does not match performance expectations, you have to adapt by altering the model.

SIMPLE MODELS FOR SIMULATION TRAINING

The aim of simulation training is to replicate fundamental elements of a competitive game, to establish specific technical and tactical schemes, and to standardize certain parts of the game plan with the ultimate goal of increasing the team's effectiveness. It is equally important that coaches use individual methods to evaluate whether the simulation models translate well to game situations and whether athletes are effectively following the tactical model. A coach may use the following simulation models:

■ *Simulation of the team's tactical offensive and defensive actions.* This simple simulation considers athlete placement on the field, court, or ice; the main principles of ball and athlete movement during the game; and offensive and defensive strategies for special situations, such as in-bound plays, jump balls, face-offs, odd-number situations, and tactics after scoring. In other words, specific tactical elements are repeated frequently during practice to produce typical actions that are likely to be used in upcoming games or tournaments.

■ *Simulation of the interaction between two or more athletes but also the tactical schemes.* Interaction and tactical schemes include the role of the playmaker(s), the tactical support given to teammates in scoring position, and tactical approach after a successful or unsuccessful offensive sequence. To achieve maximum benefits, this model must be repeated many times during training to make sure that athletes forming a specific unit or line become familiar with each other's roles on offense and how to cover each other on defense.

■ *Simulation of the game's technical demand.* This simulation must consider the roles of offensive and defensive athletes (who often differ considerably) in both the technical and tactical abilities. While the defense may be concerned mainly with disrupting the offensive tactics of the opposition (e.g., breaking up an organized attack), offensive athletes must become adept at using a variety of technical skills to create an effective offensive drive, such as executing clever fakes and demonstrating finesse in controlling or passing the ball or puck. Therefore, allot adequate time during workouts to rehearse these specific skills.

■ *Simulation of individual tactical actions.* This simulation can be specific both to an athlete's position and her role within the overall team game plan. However, it must also consider those athletes who are given a greater degree of tactical freedom during the game, both on offense and defense. Particularly on offense, these types of athletes have to be flexible tactically, possess tactical intelligence, and demonstrate originality in response to the dynamics of the game.

■ *Simulation of the game's physical demands.* Quickness, agility, power, and speed are some of the many physical attributes required to perform during a game or competition. These abilities must be trained during the preparatory phase and should follow specific periodization schedules throughout the year. Make sure these physical abilities are incorporated into workouts within the context of simulating specific tactical maneuvers.

■ *Simulation of signs used to communicate specific tactical actions during the game.* Such communication rests with the playmaker in most team sports (e.g., point guard in basketball, quarterback in American football, setter in volleyball). To develop an optimal level of communication among athletes, plan specific parts of the workouts to rehearse the signs and signals to be used during the game.

■ *Simulation of the game environment.* Performing well under adverse circumstances and overcoming biased officiating, particularly during away games, require special training strategies. Consider the following points when preparing your team for unfavorable playing conditions:

- Remind athletes about officiating rules in advance, and alert them to the possibly biased application of these rules.
- Familiarize athletes with the specific conditions of the field, gym, court, or ice.
- Prepare athletes to deal with common problems such as poor playing conditions, equipment (deteriorated playing surface, wet field, unfamiliar goals, or balls), and an unfamiliar time of the day the game may be played.
- Prepare athletes for dealing with the opposing team's crowd, which may be hostile, loud, and biased against your team.

Any training program can be modeled to coincide with a coach's objectives for training. Therefore, creating a model for a given training program provides an advantage for the coach and athletes because a certain physical quality (skill) can be developed according to the specifics of the game. The training models described in the following section refer only to the training sessions, microcycles, and annual plans.

MODELING THE TRAINING SESSION

Each training session can be planned to target specific objectives, whether technical, tactical, or physical in nature. Accomplishing these objectives successfully depends largely on how the session is organized. As a coach, you should resist the temptation to structure training sessions the same way every time. A varied approach to training prevents boredom and keeps athletes motivated to improve. The following training session models and plans were designed with variety in mind.

Modeling Training for Skill Acquisition

To enhance the acquisition and refinement of new skills, or to perfect passing and shooting accuracy, consider the following training structure.

1. Warm-up: 15 to 20 minutes
2. Technical and tactical drills that teach or refine a skill or improve the accuracy of passing and shooting: 60 minutes

3. Physical training (improve or maintain strength): 30 minutes
4. Cool-down: 10 to 15 minutes

The benefits of such a training model are not difficult to justify. Specific skill training should occur before the central nervous system (CNS) becomes fatigued because fatigue affects skill development and retention. Therefore, drills for skill acquisition or accuracy should immediately follow the warm-up when athletes are still fresh. Do not plan skill activities for the end of a training session when the athletes are more likely to be fatigued.

Rest intervals should be long enough to prevent fatigue and to facilitate maximum skill retention. The only training objectives for this part of the session are skill retention and improved accuracy in passing and shooting.

Because such a training session taps the phosphagen (also called alactic, ATP-CP; see chapter 6) energy system, you may plan two or three sets of maximum strength during the preparatory phase. Under these conditions, the same energy system is tapped; the glycolytic (also called lactic or lactic acid; see chapter 6) system provides additional energy.

Modeling Training for Skill Acquisition Under Conditions of Fatigue

If you intend to train skill refinement and accuracy under different physiological conditions, the following training plan is recommended.

1. Warm-up: 20 minutes
2. Technical and tactical drills that tap the glycolytic and oxidative (also called aerobic) system: 50 minutes
3. Speed or power training using specific or nonspecific exercises and drills: 20 minutes
4. Technical and tactical drills to improve accuracy of passing and shooting under conditions of fatigue: 20 minutes
5. Cool-down: 10 minutes

The main goal of such a structure is to train the athletes' technical and tactical proficiency for the later stages of the game, when fatigue starts to set in. Athletes must train under conditions of fatigue to adapt to such conditions and perform well under a similar physiological state during the game.

Modeling Training for Speed and Power Development

If the objective of training is the development of speed, quickness, agility, power, and explosiveness, the structure of a training session can be organized as follows.

1. Warm-up: 20 minutes
2. Specific or nonspecific drills and exercises for the development of power, speed, and agility: 30 to 40 minutes
3. Technical and tactical drills for skill automation (repetitions of technical and tactical drills with the plan to have them become an automatic reflex): 45 to 60 minutes
4. Cool-down: 10 to 15 minutes

Like skill development, training aimed at developing maximum speed, agility, power, or explosiveness should be performed immediately after the warm-up, when the CNS is not yet fatigued. Training these abilities under fresh conditions is essential because the signals from the CNS (in the form of nerve impulses) need to be fast and fluid, which is impossible when an athlete is fatigued.

Modeling Training for Speed and Power Development Under Conditions of Fatigue

Team, racket, and some combat (e.g., fencing, martial arts) sports are typically speed and power dominant; they involve mostly fast and explosive actions. Performing fast and powerful actions in the early stages of competition is not a challenge for most athletes. However, performing these same moves in the later stages of a competition under conditions of fatigue may present a different set of challenges. Just as most mistakes are made late in a competition when athletes are tired, the ability to perform fast and explosive actions is affected by an increased level of fatigue at the end of the competition.

In many cases competitions are won or lost at the end. Athletes are expected to sustain a high tempo throughout a competition while maintaining consistently quick and powerful actions, but fatigue often interferes with their intentions. Unless you organize a training structure that facilitates speed and power training under conditions of fatigue, do not expect miracles from your athletes in crunch time. To overcome these potential barriers to performance and to improve the team's performance in the later stages of competitions, try the following model.

1. Warm-up: 20 minutes
2. Technical and tactical drills of longer duration that tap the oxidative system and fatigue athletes: 60 minutes
3. Speed and power drills performed under conditions of fatigue: 30 minutes
4. Cool-down: 10 minutes

After the warm-up, organize 60 minutes of technical and tactical drills of longer duration that are typical of lactic acid (glycolytic) endurance (30-60 sec or longer). The scope of this part of training is to fatigue athletes. Because this type taps the glycolytic system and cumulatively also the oxidative system, athletes will experience fatigue levels similar to those encountered toward the end of a game. With this base level of fatigue established, you should then organize 20 to 30 minutes of technical, tactical, and physical drills and exercises that demand quickness, agility, and power. If technical and tactical drills are performed, instruct athletes to concentrate fully and to perform every pass and scoring attempt with maximum accuracy.

This training plan is specifically designed to improve performance at the end of the competition, when under conditions of fatigue, athletes are expected to increase the tempo, to move quickly, to concentrate, and to maintain the accuracy of passing, shooting, or spiking. Such a structure stresses both the physiological and psychological aspects of training through maximum nervous system concentration, willpower, determination, and resilience.

Modeling Training for Tactical Pressing

Pressing has been utilized as a tactical weapon for many decades. This tactic has two simple variants: total pressing throughout the game, and partial pressing during different parts of the game, particularly at the end of the game (like the finish in some individual sports). Partial pressing is the most effective because total pressing requires a complete commitment and strong conditioning. Partial pressing, particularly in the last 10 to 20 minutes of a game, is recommended with a relatively simple model to follow: Usual training throughout the session with a visible increase in the tempo of every type of training for the last part of the session.

Tactically, pressing used for the last part of the game is recommended in these two cases:

1. In a tie game, with the intention of pressing the opposition to create chances for scoring and winning the game
2. When your team is losing, with the intention of pressing to overcome the opposition and tie or win the game

Modeling Training for Controlling Program Arousal

To achieve and maintain maximum efficiency during games or matches, athletes must reach an optimal state of arousal (physiological and psychological alertness). A short workout before the game may develop the team's optimal arousal level as well as reduce their anxiety level while helping athletes overcome feelings of excitability and restlessness. During the pregame morning practice, promote calmness and controlled confidence among the athletes. The following model would be beneficial for fostering an optimal level of pregame arousal.

1. Short and light warm-up: 10 minutes
2. Short, explosive, and fast technical and tactical drills with the ball or puck, and with longer rest intervals than usually used: 10-15 minutes
3. Cool-down, including stretching: 10 minutes

Depending on the specifics of the sport and position played, athletes can perform a few repetitions of powerful, explosive, fast actions, such as a few throws with a lightweight medicine ball, or two to four repetitions of half-squat jumps with a low load (30%-50% of 1RM). These short actions that do not produce fatigue can maximize performance by increasing the contractibility of the muscles involved and arousing power production before the competition. To avoid the accumulation of fatigue or potential interference with the process of **supercompensation** (a physiological condition that allows the athlete to use maximum physical potential for the game), activities should be of short duration with longer rest intervals; this approach ensures that full recovery is achieved before the next repetition is performed.

During the pregame arousal activities, ensure a relaxed atmosphere and controlled optimism. These activities provide an effective use of time before the competition.

MODELING THE MICROCYCLE

The concept of modeling can also be applied to planning, particularly to the methodology of planning microcycles (weekly training plans) with a varied number of games per weekend.

Modeling a Microcycle Ending With an Exhibition Game

The standard format of a microcycle is illustrated in table 7.3, where the days of the week (first row) are numbered because some exhibition games do not always follow a standard week's days. The second row refers to training objectives, the third row suggests how to plan the energy systems to correspond with the training objective, and the fourth row suggests training demand for each day.

Table 7.3 Suggested Training Model for a Microcycle Leading to an Exhibition Game

Day	1	2	3	4	5	6	7
Training objectives	Recovery and regeneration	T/TA	T/TA/S/P/A/MxS (30 min)	T/TA longer-duration drills	T/TA/S/A/MxS (30 min)	TA model training	Exhibition game
Energy system(s)		Oxidative	Phosphagen/glycolytic	Oxidative	Phosphagen/glycolytic	Oxidative	All
Training demand		M	H	M	H	M	H

T = technical; TA = tactical; S = speed; P = power; A = agility; MxS = maximum strength; M = medium training demand; H = high training demand.

The time noted for some training (i.e., 30 min) refers only to posttraining conditioning.

An exhibition game should be planned only when the team is ready, usually at the end of the preparatory phase (one or two per week). The main scope of these games is not victory; rather, it is for testing and monitoring all aspects of the game and individual athletes, from collaborations between different lines or compartments of the team to the efficiency of transition from defense to offense and vice versa. Therefore, the demand of training for the week is slightly higher than the demand preceding league games.

Logically, planning of the exhibition games should be progressive, from a team of a lower standard to teams that offer a good opposition. Enter each game with specific objectives in mind, each goal being an intrinsic part of your game plan. Modify and refine your game model based on your observations and conclusions from the exhibition game with the intent of taking the time to change and validate your game plan.

Modeling the Microcycle With One or Two League Games

The structure of the training model for one league game at the end of the week is like the model for exhibition games, except the last day before the game has a low (L) demand. The big difference arises when a team must play two games a week; before and after each game, you have to plan low training demand to rest for the game and facilitate supercompensation.

After the game, the primary goal is to remove fatigue from athletes' systems through recovery, regeneration, and physical therapy techniques. A short aerobic activity to produce perspiration may aid in removing the fatigue from the system because perspiration facilitates the removal of metabolites.

As shown in table 7.4, during the league games the only time you can train maximum speed, agility, power, and strength is at the end of days 2 and 5. This model is a maintenance-type program for retaining the abilities you have trained during the preparatory phase. (For training methods and programs suggested for each dominant ability, see chapters 9-12.)

Table 7.4 Suggested Training Model for a Microcycle With Two Games

Day	1	2	3	4	5	6	7
Training objectives	RR	T/TA/A/P/MxS (20 min)	Game	AM: RR PM: T/TA	T/TA/S/P/MxS (30 min)	TA model training	Game
Energy system(s)		Phosphagen/glycolytic	All	Oxidative	Phosphagen/glycolytic	Oxidative	All
Training demand		M	H	L	H	L	H

T = technical; TA = tactical; A = agility; P = power; S = speed; MxS = maximum strength; AM = morning session; RR = recovery and regeneration; PM = afternoon session; M = medium, H = high; L = low.

Modeling Weekend Tournaments

Model training is the most effective method for training the athletes to cope with the specific physiological, psychological, and social stresses that arise during tournament games. In most team sports, especially basketball, handball, lacrosse, hockey, baseball or softball, volleyball, and water polo, weekend tournaments are a tradition. During these tournaments, teams usually play at least three games.

As illustrated in table 7.5, modeling a training program for weekend tournaments involves organizing two or three microcycles that mimic the future tournament structure, ensuring readiness for the tournament. The model includes three or four high-demand training sessions on three consecutive days. It is the only way to adapt successfully to the specific physiological demands of the tournament and be able to cope with the psychological fatigue associated with three days of challenging games. If you expect to play two games each day, such as Saturday and Sunday, that tournament structure needs to be modeled over two or three weekends.

Table 7.5   Suggested Training Model for a Microcycle With a Weekend Tournament

Day	1	2	3	4	5	6	7
Training objectives	Recovery and regeneration	T/TA longer-duration drills	T/TA/S/P/A/MxS (30 min)	Creating and validating the composing elements of a TA model to be implemented in the next tournament	Model training for the next tournament (T/TS/A [20 min])	Same as day 5	Same as day 5
Energy system(s)		T/TA longer-duration drills	Phosphagen/glycolytic	Oxidative	All	All	All
Training demand	L	M	M/H	L	H	H	H

T = technical; TA = tactical; S = speed; P = power; A = agility; MxS = maximum strength; AM = morning session; RR = recovery and regeneration; PM = afternoon session; M = medium, H = high; L = low.

Suggested Training Model for a Long Tournament

In some team sports, long tournaments (e.g., championship tournaments; national, continental, or world championships; the Olympic Games) can last up to three weeks. In many cases, teams play every second or third day. A major concern for coaches involved in such tournaments is how to prepare for them; however, equally difficult is the type of training and daily activities to organize during the extended game schedule. Table 7.6 illustrates the type of training to consider during a major tournament lasting two weeks or longer.

Physical training is not simple. On the contrary, it is a complex activity in which coaches are exposed to a high variety of conditions from training athletes (in technical and tactical strategies, physical and psychological skills, nutrition) to the needs of monitoring behavior, athletes' improvements or stagnation, and reactions and prediction of future events. Modeling is one of the best organizational activities that can help the coach, staff, and parents to cope with the myriads of challenges that sport offers.

Table 7.6 Suggested Activity During a Long Tournament

Day	1	2	3	4	5	6	7	8	9	10	11	12
Activity	MT	MT	G	RR O2	MT	G	RR O2	MT	G	RR O2	MT	G

MT = model training, 45-60 min: warm up, rehearse elements of the tactical plan you will use for the next game; G = game; RR = recovery and regeneration, plus 30 min low-intensity aerobic activity (O2) and simple, low-intensity T and TA training. (*Note:* a simple, low-intensity aerobic training session enhances recovery and glycogen restoration much better than an off day with no physical activity at all.)

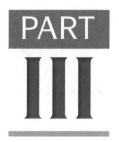

TRAINING METHODS

If your methodology of training is good,
so will be your athletes.

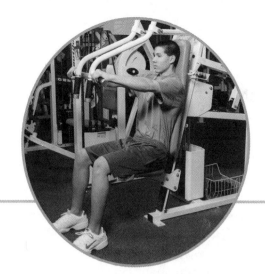

chapter 8

Science-Based Strength Training Methodology

The world of sports training is constantly exposed to changes. Some of those changes are based on science and methodology; others originate from sports equipment or catalog companies. At any time, you can find countless self-proclaimed experts who enthusiastically share their different theories of the moment on the Internet. All these sources share novel training methods for the development of strength, power, speed, agility, and specific endurance, but those methods may have nothing to do with sound research or science-based methodology. This constant change and abundance of conflicting information can leave some strength and conditioning coaches confused about which theories they should follow.

COMMON PITFALLS OF CONTEMPORARY TRAINING

This book shares science-based training concepts to offer better and more efficient training methodology and methods. The following list summarizes an analysis of the present state of training of young athletes.

- The determinant physical abilities in team, racket, or martial arts sports are power, speed, agility, and sport-specific endurance.
- Most programs for developing the physical attributes of athletes in team sports have good intentions, but they miss the mark.
- Training of speed and agility is organized in bouts of 4-8 or 10 seconds. However, games in team sports usually last 60 to 90 minutes. How can you train the physiological needs of these games with energy generated by the phosphagen (alactic) energy system? The glycolytic (lactic acid) and oxidative (aerobic) energy systems are dominant in many team and other sports; when and how do you train them?
- Energy requirement is a scientific reality, but some strength and conditioning coaches emphasize the wrong energy system.
- Strength, power, maximum speed, and agility are also trained with some exercises of short duration, targeting the phosphagen energy system. However, coaches often neglect developing maximum strength (MxS) and power endurance.

STRENGTH AND CONDITIONING COACHES AND THEIR TRAINING

Many strength and conditioning coaches are enthusiastic professionals, and they come from diverse backgrounds. Some have a four-year college degree; others completed a certificate program from an online course or from a one-week seminar. If you are a sport coach seeking a strength and conditioning coach for your athletes, or if you want to become a strength and conditioning coach, keep in mind the following:

- Some strength and conditioning programs focus on teaching as many exercises as possible. However, quantity of exercises does not mean a quality program.
- Exercises are necessary as a *means to target the prime movers* (the essential muscles needed to perform a certain athletic move), but prime movers are not the only important part of training athletes.
- Knowledge in exercise physiology, particularly in neuromuscular physiology, is determinant in becoming a successful strength and conditioning coach.
- Understanding the fundamentals of sport science and science-based training methodology is essential to effective training.

The methodology of training young athletes, which is essential for the formation of future champions, appears to be an area of neglect and in need of revamping. Improving youth sports begins with information from biology, growth, and development during the childhood and teen years; energy systems training; methodology of developing age-group motor abilities; sport psychology; and nutrition.

Furthermore, personal experience and opinions of former top athletes and sport coaches are helpful, but equally important for selecting the best training methods is to validate your own convictions with science and methodology. Ask yourself what works for you and what does not, and seek to understand why.

Strength training is one area of training that is often misunderstood and improperly applied. Gadgets and training methods are promoted as effective, but they might not be validated by science. Consider these physiological realities (see chapter 9):

- Power, maximum speed, and agility increase only after maximum strength (MxS) has increased.
- MxS increases the recruitment of fast-twitch (FT) muscle fibers, which are essential for the improvement of power, speed, and agility.
- Strong muscle contractions that occur as a result of sliding the myosin and actin filaments are a determinant for developing power, speed, and agility.
- Athletes can increase speed and agility only when capable of applying high amounts of force against the ground during the propulsion (push-off) phase of the running step.

AN INVESTIGATION OF CONTEMPORARY TRAINING METHODOLOGY

We (the authors of this book) performed an investigation to compare contemporary training methods to the methods we promote in this book to determine which approach has the greatest impact on the development of physical qualities dominant in team sports. The organization and methodology of our investigation are presented in this section.

- *Research hypothesis*: A science-based strength training methodology will result in the superior development of sport-specific dominant abilities, such as strength, power, maximum speed, and agility.
- *Subjects and duration of experiment*: Two groups of 14 male U17 soccer players were selected from local youth championship teams.
  - ◻ The experimental group was formed by the ASU Polytechnic Timisoara (Romania) soccer players.
  - ◻ The reference group were soccer players from the Sports High School Timisoara team.
- *Duration of the experiment*: 12 weeks (The training programs started in mid-January 2020 and ended in mid-April of the same year; this period coincided with the preparatory phase for the local championships.)
- *Number of training sessions per week*: 3 for both groups
- *Testing*: Standard test-retest format for both groups
- *Experimental group (ASU Polytechnic) training program*: Periodized strength, power, agility, and maximum speed training
  - ◻ Anatomical adaptation (AA) training for 3 weeks
  - ◻ MxS training for 6 weeks using a progressively increased heavier load of 50%-70% 1RM
  - ◻ Power, agility, maximum speed training for 3 weeks
- *Reference group (Sports High School) training program*: A contemporary type of training program for soccer
  - ◻ Maximum speed runs of 10-30 m
  - ◻ Agility runs consisting of slalom and zigzag movements, agility ladder drills, and agility rings on flat terrain and over low hurdlers of 4-10 sec
  - ◻ Resistance training using a speed sled
  - ◻ Circuit training consisting of jumps over boxes, pull-ups, push-ups, and lunges into BOSU balls
  - ◻ Medicine ball throws
  - ◻ Strength training (using resistance bands) consisting of pulls and presses for the arms and legs
- *Testing protocols*
  - ◻ *Testing power using the Myotest*: The Myotest is a portable instrument that is equipped with sensors to record any movements the athletes make. It is used to measure force and power with a strong positive correlation ($r = 0.96$) and a high probability ($p < 0.05$) (Comstock et al., 2011; Orange et al., 2019). The Myotest has an accelerometer that analyzes the following measurements:
    - Duration of contact time (duration of athletes' feet on the ground during maximum speed and take-off to perform a jump)
    - Reactivity (proportion of jump height and duration of contact time)
    - Stiffness (proportion between the force applied against the ground and the degree of vertical deformation during sprinting and jumping; poorly trained athletes with low strength capabilities often cannot overcome the force of gravity to react quickly between landing and take-off during sprinting and repetitive jumps)

MYOTEST

The Myotest has been used for testing counter-movement jumps (CMJ) and reactive jumps. It has also been used to assess force, power, height, and speed. Performance in a CMJ is directly correlated to sprinting capabilities and 1RM. Plyometric jumps (PJ) can provide information regarding the duration of contact on the ground, the contractile properties of the muscles, reactivity, and muscle stiffness—all of which are essential to improve athleticism and performance in the chosen sport.

◻ *Testing MxS*: Finding 1RM is essential for knowing athletes' MxS and to calculate the load for the duration of training for MxS. Three tests were used for the major muscle groups used in soccer:

- *Leg press* assesses the 1RM for hip and knee extensors (gluteals, hamstrings, and quadriceps).
- *Calf press* targets the most important muscles in team sports for running and jumping (gastrocnemius and soleus).
- *Bench press* is used to train the upper body muscles that are used to block out opponents during a game.

◻ *Testing maximum speed and agility*: Speed and agility are essential qualities in team sports. Assessment includes the following:

- *Maximum speed test*: 30 m sprint from a standing position
- *Illinois agility test*: The test is performed on a flat surface (grass or gym) using 8 cones to mark the turning points during the test. Athletes start the test from a resting supine (on their backs) position on the floor. At a signal they get up and run as fast as possible, following the design of the test.

Test Results and Discussions

The results from the testing protocols are presented in tables 8.1 through 8.4 so that you can make direct and relevant comparisons between the experimental (ASU Polytechnic) and reference (Sports High School) groups. We were selective with different tests, focusing mostly on testing the major abilities specific for team sports. Specific and relevant discussions are provided for each test, along with an explanation of the correlations between some of the tests based on the dominant abilities of team sports, such as maximum speed and agility.

CMJ Test Comments

For the first test, no significant difference was observed between the two groups. However, the retest scores revealed a consistent improvement for the experiment group in the tests for height (2.8 cm vs. 0.8 cm), power (4.7 W/kg vs. 3.7 W/kg), force (2.7 N vs. 0.9 N), and speed of CMJ (16.35 cm/sec vs 10.17 cm/sec).

CMJ Test Conclusions

The significant improvement for power and force tests for the experimental group also explains why height and speed of CMJ were better than for the reference group. For practical purposes, the most important improvement appears to be the speed of CMJ; it will assist an athlete in being more reactive and moving faster in various aspects of the game.

Table 8.1 Mean Testing Results for Each Group of Athletes for the Countermovement Jump (CMJ)

	Group	Test	Retest
Height (cm)	Experimental	32.71	35.47
	Reference	32.59	33.35
Power (W/kg)	Experimental	40.59	45.32
	Reference	43.19	46.68
Force (N)	Experimental	23.74	26.43
	Reference	24.75	25.61
Speed of CMJ (cm/s)	Experimental	223.41	239.76
	Reference	221.16	231.33

W = Watts; Force (N) = force in Newtons. (Unlike the measure of force in kilograms or pounds, the advantage of using N is that it also considers the mass—the weight of the subject.)

Table 8.2 Mean Values per Group for Plyometric Jump (PJ) Test

	Group	Test	Retest
Duration of contact time (ms)	Experimental	174.75	170.66
	Reference	160.41	159.75
Stiffness (kN/m)	Experimental	35.95	35.18
	Reference	41.75	39.57
Power (W)	Experimental	34.33	31.54
	Reference	30.4	30.36

ms = milliseconds; N/m = Newton/meter; W = Watts.

PJ Test Comments

Duration of contact time decreased the time by 4.09 milliseconds for the experimental group and 1.34 milliseconds for the reference group. This decrease proves that a significant correlation exists between improvement in leg strength and the decrease in the duration of contact time. In practical terms, it means that these athletes can run faster, turn around more quickly, and change direction more quickly with faster reaction times during the dynamic parts of the games.

PJ Test Conclusions

The results of the PJ test demonstrate that improvement in power directly correlates with the decrease in the duration of contact time. The shorter the duration of contact time, the faster and more reactive and agile the athletes will be.

MxS Test Results and Comments

The results of MxS tests have demonstrated the highest (high significance) difference between the mean scores of the experimental and reference groups (26.5 kg) for the leg press. The same differences were visible for the calf press (10.6 kg). These differences represent a demonstration that the training program followed by the experimental group has resulted in visible gains in all the tests where strength, power, and jumping abilities have been assessed. The MxS tests, the leg press and calf press, have significantly improved for the experimental group (by 33.16 kg for leg press and by 15.58 kg for calf press). At the same time the improvement of MxS for the reference group was marginal (6.7 kg for leg press and 5 kg for calf press). Considering the modest improvements recorded for the reference group, improving speed and agility (the determinant abilities in soccer and most other team sports) is unlikely. The results of the bench press had a similar trend: 10.34 kg for the experimental group and lower improvements (2.92 kg) for the reference group.

Maximum Speed and Illinois Agility Test Results and Comments

While the scores for the reference group were relatively flat for both tests, the experimental group showed improvement (0.25 sec for the maximum speed test and 0.41 sec for the Illinois agility test). The discrepancy between the two groups demonstrates that the experimental group has improved the speed and agility performance simply because the strength–power scores have improved. Gains in strength and power have been translated into improvements in speed and agility.

Table 8.3 Mean Values for the MxS Tests

	Group	Test	Retest
Leg press (kg)	Experimental	96.67	129.83
	Reference	76.64	83.33
Calf press (kg)	Experimental	84.00	99.58
	Reference	54.58	59.58
Bench press (kg)	Experimental	58.41	68.75
	Reference	53.33	56.25

kg = kilograms.

Table 8.4 Mean Values for the Maximum Speed and Illinois Agility Tests

	Group	Test	Retest
Maximum speed test (sec)	Experimental	4.74	4.49
	Reference	4.61	4.60
Illinois agility test (sec)	Experimental	16.55	16.14
	Reference	16.36	16.42

Applications

The scope of this experiment was to compare contemporary fitness training used in soccer with a science-based training methodology, promoted in this book. Two groups of players U17, an experimental group (following a science-based training program) and a reference group (exposed to contemporary training methodology) were used for this investigation.

The initial tests did not reveal a significant difference for the test scores between the two groups. However, the retest data demonstrated a statistically significant difference for the improvement of strength between the two groups ($p = 0.032 < 0.05$, and a validity of 95%). Evidence is clear that our working hypothesis has been proven to be correct. Test results have demonstrated that the increase of athletes' strength (experimental group) has resulted in visibly improved maximum speed and agility, the two determinant abilities in team sports.

What does this information mean for sport coaches and strength and conditioning coaches? A strong correlation exists between improving strength and power and increasing maximum speed and agility. In other words, athletes can be fast only if they first improve their strength and power. Therefore, if you want to improve your athletes' maximum speed and agility, improve their MxS and power.

CONCLUSION

Contemporary training methodology in soccer, where most of the fitness training is an array of short sprints and agility drills lasting 4-8 or 10 seconds, is far from addressing the needs of energy systems in soccer. Fitness trainers use different designs to perform their drills, without realizing that the physiological benefit of the program is minimal. Respectfully, we want to suggest to coaches and fitness instructors from all sports to review their training methodology and programs in an attempt to find more effective methods that could result in superior physical qualities specific to the needs of their sport.

It is our opinion that coaches and fitness specialists might want to review the type of fitness training they use. There is ample possibility of improvement in training for the development of dominant abilities in most sports by resorting to a better organized strength training. *MxS is poorly understood and underutilized.* The use of MxS in your training regimen will result in higher improvements in strength, power, speed, and agility. *Improvements in speed and agility are possible only if strength, particularly MxS, is utilized.*

We invite you to carefully read chapter 9, with particular attention to the section titled Mechanism of Muscular Contraction. You will learn more about why you should use MxS in your sport, and the result, which is a visible increase in your athletes' power, speed, and agility.

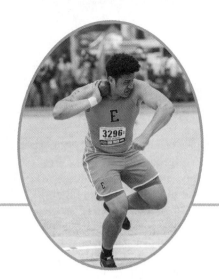

chapter 9

Training Methods to Develop Strength and Power

Power, agility, speed, and quickness are among the most important abilities of successful athletes in most sports. Athletes have progressively become faster and more dynamic, reflecting increased skill levels and strength. As a result, the importance of strength and power for performance has shot to the forefront of training.

Since 1990, numerous studies have highlighted the important role strength training can play in the physical and emotional development of young athletes. Benefits include increased bone density, self-esteem, power, speed, and fat-free mass (Dahab and McCambridge, 2009; Behm et al., 2017; Radnor et al., 2017). Previous concerns regarding related injury and growth plate issues have been set aside; recent publications and scholarly studies clearly summarize the efficacy and benefits of strength training for young athletes (Behm et al., 2008; McCambridge and Stricker, 2008; Faigenbaum et al., 2009). In addition to improving performance, strength training decreases the chance of sport-related injury. It also creates a foundation for maintaining an active lifestyle and protecting against the onset of diseases as children mature (Rivier et al., 2017).

WHY STRENGTH AND POWER MATTER IN SPORTS TRAINING

For many years, several U.S. team sports (football, baseball, rugby, ice hockey, lacrosse) and other sports (track and field, Alpine skiing, wrestling) have adopted strength training as an important tool for overall performance development. Although it still has great room for improvement, strength training has become a fixture in many sports. The time is ripe for other team sports to get on board and take full advantage of the benefits of strength and power training to maximize athletes' physical potential and performance quality.

CHOOSE YOUR STRENGTH TRAINING PROGRAM WISELY

Many strength and conditioning professionals and parents are confused about strength training in general and how it applies to young athletes in particular. When they get advice from people (solicited and unsolicited, in person and online) who profess theories and exercises that are not supported by science and methodology, they become more confused about how to help young athletes. Further, athletes need to be protected from commercialism, where exercises used for trained athletes are promoted to young athletes who do not have the needed training or experience in strength training to perform the exercises appropriately or safely.

When deciding the type of strength training young athletes should be exposed to, some coaches do what they did when they were athletes, which can result in injuries. For example, a former weightlifter may teach children to lift heavy weights, which their bodies are not ready to do. Weightlifting moves are not compatible with young athletes before bone maturation, which occurs around 25 years or older (American Academy of Pediatrics Council on Sports Medicine and Fitness, 2008; Mora and Gilsanz, 2010; McQuilliam et al.,

2020). Make sure that prior to heavy-load strength training you expose young athletes to exercises that strengthen the spine (intervertebral muscles) and the knees, where the muscles, ligaments, and tendons are vulnerable. In fact, the entire structure and its progression of the training program proposed in this book is based on solid science and methodology. Beware of people who advise exercises such as shoulder press or snatch, which are not needed for the majority of sports. Instead, focus on exercises that are specific to your sport.

When introducing strength training to young athletes, using modern strength training machines is the best option. Today's gyms are equipped with machines that allow an appropriate load progression. They also mimic the moves that target the most important muscles in team sports, the leg muscles. For example, some machines can target the triple extensors—ankle (plantar flexion and dorsiflexion), knee (extension), and hip (extension). They also work the hamstrings (knee flexion), which are important in running, a common activity in team sports.

Athletes in team sports have a lot to gain from regular strength and power training. The most important reasons to consider incorporating such training into an overall training regimen are listed next.

- *Injury prevention*: Although it has long been viewed as an important benefit of strength training, strength training for injury prevention is not well understood or used as frequently as it could be. As a coach, you should focus on the following:
  - *Develop both agonist and antagonist muscles.* The muscle or group of muscles producing a desired effect in strength training is known as the **agonist muscles**, or the **prime movers**; the muscle or group of muscles opposing the action is called the **antagonist muscles**. Choose balanced exercises that focus especially on those muscles involved in overuse injuries; for example, focus on the rotator cuff muscles for pitchers in baseball or the knee ligaments for soccer, basketball, team handball, and racket sports.
  - *Strengthen tendons and ligaments.* Most of the injuries caused in sports tend to occur at the tendon and ligament level because those connective tissues are weaker than the force of the contracting muscles themselves. Muscles work in perfect synchrony; when one muscle contracts (shortens) to move a bone, another muscle relaxes, allowing the bone to move.

- *Improved game and sport-specific abilities for young athletes, such as:*
  - *Increased speed*: Speed depends directly on strength, particularly the propulsion (push-off) phase of the running step (gastrocnemius and soleus muscles). The more powerful the push-off phase, the higher the velocity achieved. Speed cannot be increased unless the force application against the ground, ice, or water is also increased.
  - *Improved agility*: Agility is the ability to quickly accelerate (concentric, or shortening the muscle while they contract), and decelerate (eccentric contraction, or lengthening the same muscles during action), and change directions.
  - *Faster reaction time*: **Reaction time** (how long it takes the neuromuscular system to respond to a stimulus) in response to a wide range of game situations can also be improved by increasing limb power. The speed of an athlete's reaction to a specific signal or stimulus (e.g., a passed ball) depends on the time elapsed between reception of the signal and propagation of the nerve impulse through the central nervous system (CNS) to the muscles involved. Once the nerve impulses have reached the muscles, the speed of the limb action depends on the power of contraction, or how many fast-twitch (FT; see Overview of Strength Training Science) muscle fibers have been recruited. The higher the number of FT fibers recruited into the action, the faster the movement.
  - *Improved passing and shooting accuracy*: Passing and shooting accuracy in sports including ice or field hockey, soccer, volleyball, rugby, and lacrosse can be improved with increased levels of power in the relevant limbs. For example, a soccer ball, handball, or water polo ball has a higher probability of reaching its intended target if the pass or shot is executed with superior force. Passing the ball with greater force implies that the ball is passed with greater speed. The higher the speed of the ball, the lower the probability that the ball will be intercepted by someone on the opposing team.
  - *Increased confidence*: When your strength capabilities are high, so is your confidence.

STRENGTH AND POWER TRAINING FOR SPORTS

In many sports, the belief persists that sport-specific training (through technical and tactical drills) is sufficient to develop and maximize the physical potential of athletes. While there is some truth to the fact that enhanced speed and powerful jumps are best trained by repeating running and jumping exercises, particularly for younger athletes, the development of the highest physical abilities (strength, speed, endurance, flexibility) occurs in two phases:

1. *Improvement phase.* In this phase, young athletes see rapid improvements as they adapt quickly to organized training. Such development may continue in athletes for several years, all the way up to the national level.

2. *Plateau phase.* As its name suggests, this phase is one of stagnation. Unless the athletes are stimulated by means other than sport-specific training, such as strength training, they eventually reach a plateau. From this point on, improvements come very slowly or not at all.

Because of the plateau phenomenon, improvements in physical abilities have to use some other methods, not just technical and tactical training. If athletes expect to become faster and more powerful, develop more agility, and get quicker on their feet, the only way to stimulate further these improvements is to expose athletes to strength and power training.

Misconceptions About Strength Training for Power Development

Although many coaches have come to realize and appreciate the need for strength and power training, knowledge is still lacking on many levels. Often people confuse strength and power training for sport performance with bodybuilding, which leads to misconceptions such as the following:

- *Strength training increases muscle size.* Although some increase in muscle size is a normal physiological adaptation, it will not occur to the degree of making an athlete heavier and slower. Many traditional coaches would be surprised to learn how much strength training with heavy loads long jumpers do. The best male long jumpers run the 100-meter (about 109 yd) sprint in 10.4 to 10.8 seconds and test high in the vertical jump (50-75 cm [20-30 in.]). Who would not want a wide receiver, winger, power forward, or striker in soccer with these athletic abilities?

- *Strength training decreases speed.* If you train athletes in bodybuilding, you should not expect them to be fast. The physiological reason is simple. To increase muscle mass—the actual scope of training in bodybuilding—bodybuilders use medium loads (60%-70% of 1RM), and every set has to be performed to exhaustion. Under these conditions, the speed of contraction is performed slowly with medium-duration rest intervals (not full recovery). Bodybuilding has little (if any) positive transfer to most athletes in team, martial arts, or contact sports. However, strength and power training increase the speed of contraction and the recruitment of a high number of muscle fibers simply because they use medium-heavy loads (60%-95% of 1RM), performed as quickly as possible with long rest intervals to allow for high levels of recovery. These types of training result in increasing athletes' power, speed, and agility.

Changing Need for Strength and Power Training in Team Sports

Whether achieved through improved training methods or simply superior genetics, team athletes are undeniably bigger and more powerful today than they have ever been in the past. As a result, games have become visibly faster and many athletes increasingly aggressive. In ice hockey, offensive athletes do not dare venture out in front of the opposition's goal unless they are prepared to absorb a strong dose of bodily punishment. Some teams even include athletes on their rosters whose primary role is to intimidate and wear down the opposition through aggressive physical play.

In basketball, the battles for position and rebounds under the basket can be equally fierce. Drives to the basket often end with bodies hitting the floor, and opponents are increasingly unforgiving in the amount of physical punishment they dole out. Similar physical play is visible in soccer as well, where pushing, shoving, tugging, and jockeying for position in the penalty area on corner or free kicks have become a part of the game. The big struggle in rugby is present throughout the field, where strength and power endurance often determine the winner. Team handball is also full of physical challenges, where the inside of the 9-meter (about 9.8 yd) zone feels like a war zone. A similar situation occurs underwater during a water polo match. In other words, athletes need to be strong not only to increase power, maximum speed, and agility but also for their own physical protection.

The desire for strength and speed has tempted some coaches and athletes to consider many options, including purchasing ineffective equipment and making unethical choices (e.g., using performance-enhancing drugs). A better, healthier option for all athletes is to take the time to learn about and adopt scientifically proven strength training methodology.

The search for better training methods has opened the doors to unethical products promoted by some disingenuous producers and catalog companies. For example, gimmicky balance training equipment and exercises performed on a BOSU ball have not demonstrated visible benefits for improving athleticism. Similarly, elastic cords cannot replace traditional strength training. Finally, misleading over-speed gadgets that contradict science, the mechanics of running, and the Newtonian laws of motion (the laws of acceleration, action, and reaction) cannot improve maximum speed.

Soccer is one of the best examples where some fashionable, but ineffective, exercises have replaced sound physiological training. In the instance of several young Romanian and Central and South American soccer teams, gimmicky exercises and unskilled fitness coaches created a scenario where some players are fragile; as such very few players were able to integrate in the Western European teams.

OVERVIEW OF STRENGTH TRAINING SCIENCE

High athletic performances involving power, maximum speed, and agility are achieved under two specific conditions:

1. Genetic inheritance
2. Specialized training

People are born with different proportions of muscle fiber types, which have different biochemical (metabolic) functions and characteristics (see table 9.1). Some are pale or white and are called **fast-twitch (FT) muscle fibers**; others are red and are known as **slow-twitch (ST) muscle fibers**. When FT fibers are prevalent, the athlete is naturally suited for sports in which speed and power are dominant. Conversely, when an athlete has a higher proportion of ST fibers, aerobic, long-duration activities may come naturally because ST fibers are effective in transporting oxygen to the working muscles. For instance, a marathon runner has 82 percent ST fibers whereas an ice hockey player has only 58 percent ST fibers, the balance being FT (Costill et al., 1976; Van Someren, 2006).

Specialized strength training, such as maximum strength (MxS) and power, exposes athletes to quality neuromuscular training, which results in high levels of neural adaptation. Consequently, neuromuscular training improves the efficiency of neural transmissions to the working muscles while MxS increases the recruitment capabilities of the same, giving such athletes the potential to apply superior force during athletic contests. This is why coaches should be more concerned about muscles' physiological potential (higher application of force) rather than form and size of muscles.

Mechanism of Muscular Contraction

To best understand how strength training enhances athletic performance or improves your game-specific physical qualities, you need to know the science behind it; specifically, you should understand the physiology of muscle contraction, known as the **sliding filament theory** (Huxley, 1954; Enoka, 2015). For more information on the sliding filament theory please refer to figures 9.1 to 9.4 and their accompanying text.

Table 9.1 Comparison of Fast-Twitch (FT) and Slow-Twitch (ST) Muscle Fibers

	ST fibers	FT fibers
Metabolic function	Aerobic	Anaerobic
Fiber type characteristics	• Appear red • Are slow to fatigue • Have smaller nerve cells (innervate 10-180 muscle cells) • Develop long, continuous contractions • Are used for endurance • Are recruited during low- and high-intensity work	• Appear white or light • Are fast to fatigue • Have large nerve cells (innervate 300-500+ muscle fibers) • Develop short, forceful contractions • Are used for speed, power, and agility • Are recruited only during high-intensity work

Adapted from Fleck and Kraemer (2004); Zoladz et al. (2005); Trappe et al. (2006); McArdle, Katch, and Katch (2007); and Bompa and Haff (2009).

Figure 9.1 illustrates the structure of a skeletal muscle, from the tendon—where it originates from—to the muscle fiber, and it ends in the smallest element of a muscle, the muscle filaments. These two muscle filaments are the essential elements of muscle contraction, called **actin** (thin filament) and **myosin** (thick filament).

When a muscle contracts, the myosin heads (**crossbridges**, extensions from myosin toward the actins) are activated, binding them with the actin and pulling against it (see figure 9.2). This action results in the overlapping of myosin with actin, producing the muscle contraction (shortening of the muscle), which generates the force necessary to produce an athletic action.

The overlapping and sliding of actin and myosin produce the necessary force to overcome gravity, the weight of an implement, or the force of an opponent. Force produced by this sliding action is also at the base of moving fast or with agility. None of these athletic

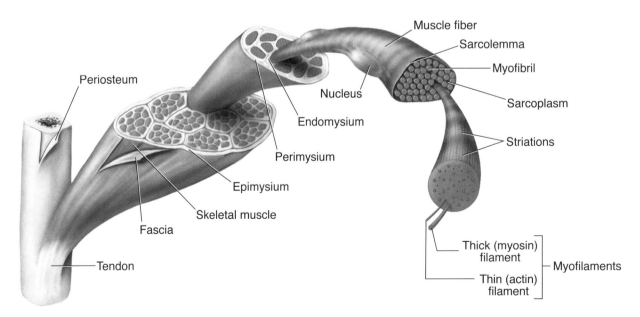

Figure 9.1 Muscle structure, starting from the bone attachment to the tendon and ending with the muscle bundle and muscle filaments.

abilities are possible without first developing maximum strength (MxS). The result of training athletes for MxS is the increase of the thickness of the myosin filament that, in turn, results in a stronger pull (figure 9.3). **The thicker the myosin, and the higher the number of myosin heads (crossbridges), the higher the capability of the athlete to produce force.** What is the athletic consequence? A stronger, faster, and more agile athlete and her skills or actions.

Figure 9.4 illustrates the effect MxS training has on the muscle filaments and crossbridges of athletes: Athletes who are not exposed to MxS training have thinner muscle filaments and a lower number of crossbridges, while athletes who are exposed to MxS training have thicker myosin and a higher number of crossbridges.

To produce faster, more agile athletes, you need to expose them to a progressive and well-organized strength training program that develops thicker myosin and a higher number of myosin heads; in other words, train for MxS. If instead you try to train athletes by using the same number of repetitions of speed work or agility drills with the same intensity, you will improve speed and agility only during the first few weeks of training. Furthermore, if training for MxS is absent from your power- and speed-training program, the result will be a plateau. Toward the end of the playing season, it can even decrease the quality of speed and agility.

The sliding filament theory is of determinant importance in strength training, particularly in MxS training. Please remember that most athletic actions and technical skills require a specific type of strength, power, or agility. Find out the type of strength training that prevails in your sport, and create your own plan that can best improve performance. Please remember, MxS should always be part of your plan. If it is missing, you'll have a high difficulty achieving your athletic goals.

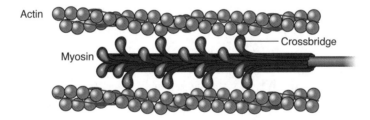

Figure 9.2 The sliding filament theory of muscle contraction.

Reprinted by permission from T.O. Bompa and C.A. Buzzichelli, *Periodization of Strength Training for Sports*, 4th ed. (Champaign, IL: Human Kinetics, 2022), 26.

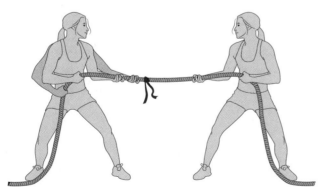

Figure 9.3 Training for maximum strength (MxS) increases the thickness of myosin and the number of myosin heads (illustrated by more arms on the subject on the left). Which athlete can generate higher force and quickness of muscle contractions?

Reprinted by permission from T.O. Bompa and C.A. Buzzichelli, *Periodization of Strength Training for Sports*, 4th ed. (Champaign, IL: Human Kinetics, 2022), 26.

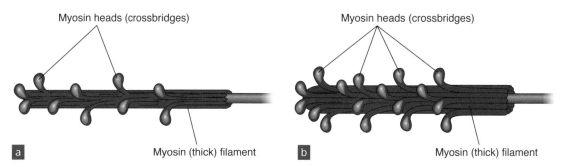

Figure 9.4 Two myosin filaments of two hypothetical athletes: (*a*) An athlete who was not exposed to MxS; thinner muscle filaments and lower number of crossbridges. Such an athlete does not have the physiological capacity to perform strong, fast, and agile athletic actions; (*b*) The intimate elements of the muscle filaments of an athlete exposed to MxS: higher number of myosin heads and much thicker size of myosin. Clearly this athlete can generate higher pull between myosin heads and actin; as a result, the athlete can produce higher force, higher maximum speed, and quicker agility.

Reprinted by permission from T.O. Bompa and C.A. Buzzichelli, *Periodization of Strength Training for Sports*, 4th ed. (Champaign, IL: Human Kinetics, 2022).

Neuromuscular Strategy for Strength Training

Until the 1980s, some sport professionals believed that strength was determined mainly by the cross-sectional area (size) of the muscle. For this reason, strength training was used to increase muscle **hypertrophy** (an increase in muscle size). However, exercise scientists no longer believe in this theory. Muscle is important, but many research studies in this area show that the main factor responsible for increase in strength (not size) is neural adaptation to strength training, such as improvement in intermuscular and intramuscular coordination, both of which are load related and are defined as follows:

- *Intermuscular coordination* refers to the ability to synchronize all muscles of a kinetic chain (movement) and depends strictly on learning (technique) by repeating the same exercises many times. When you use lower loads (30%-70% of 1RM), you improve the capacity of the muscles involved in a chain to work together to achieve your training goal (intermuscular coordination).

- *Intramuscular coordination* represents the capacity to voluntarily recruit as many motor units as possible in an athletic action. Every time you use heavy loads (defined as more than 80% of 1RM), you train the capacity to recruit a high number of FT fibers to cooperate in action to overcome heavy weights or high resistance (intramuscular coordination).

When an athlete executes a fast and powerful action, such as a very fast sprint, jumping and throwing, a powerful swing in baseball or softball, a dunk in basketball, shooting in team handball, or a spike in volleyball, the neuromuscular system responds in the following manner:

- At the beginning of an action, FT muscle fibers are recruited to overcome the force of gravity, the inertia of a piece of equipment, or the weight and force applied by an opponent. The greater the number of FT fibers recruited, the easier it is for athletes to overcome external forces acting against them.

- These initial responses are followed by increased acceleration and fast, powerful actions, which are made possible through an increase in the firing rate (the quickness of contraction) of FT fibers. This quick application of force is the basis of any fast and powerful athletic action, and it is impossible to achieve without first increasing the ability of the neuromuscular system to recruit the greatest number of FT fibers possible.

BENEFITS OF HEAVY LOAD STRENGTH TRAINING

Heavy loads always increase the myosin thickness and the number of crossbridges. The higher the number of crossbridges and the greater the thickness of myosin, the stronger the pull and, consequently, the faster the athlete's action. To be powerful, fast, and agile, an athlete must increase MxS.

Tendons and Their Importance in Sports Requiring Power, Speed, and Agility

The force exerted by muscles depends not only on the activity of crossbridges but also by the elasticity of the tendons. Figure 9.5 illustrates the calf and the foot; the most powerful skeletal muscle of the body, the gastrocnemius, connects to the Achilles tendon, which inserts to the heel bone (calcaneus).

Coaches and fitness instructors should consider the following points regarding the gastrocnemius and the Achilles tendon:

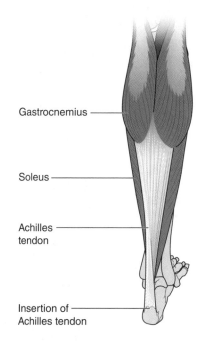

Figure 9.5 The gastrocnemius muscle and where the Achilles tendon is inserted to the calcaneus bone.

- The gastrocnemius is the strongest skeletal muscle of the body. It consists of 1,120,000 muscle fibers and 1,934 innervation numbers that can be recruited during maximum speed or high jumps/agility (Enoka, 2015). For a comparison of gastrocnemius muscle to quadriceps, please also refer to the selection of exercises in part IV.

- From ballet to any leg push-off or propulsion action, gastrocnemius contributes with over 51 percent of the force necessary to produce such actions. As a comparison, the quadriceps muscles participate only with 18 percent (Enoka, 2015). Therefore, **to increase speed, agility, and any jumps, concentrating on calf presses is more effective than squats and step-ups**.

- The vertical ground reaction force for the gastrocnemius is 940.75 Newtons (N) or 95.8 kilograms (211.2 lb), while the horizontal ground reaction force is 132.2 Newtons or 13.5 kilograms (29.7 lb) (Richards et al., 2013).

- When horizontal power (horizontal force produced by an athlete while sprinting) was compared between sprinters and soccer players, the latter scored only half of the force the sprinters were capable of applying: 15.7-17.9 Watts/kg (W/kg) vs. 7.9-11.9 W/kg) (Colyer et al., 2018). This demonstrates that sprinters have a more specific strength training program, are stronger athletes, and, therefore, are faster than soccer players.

- The gastrocnemius, which is a powerful and determinant muscle for sports and actions requiring speed and power, is innervated with the highest number of nerve plates of all muscles (about 2,000) (Enoka, 2015). The higher the number of nerve plates, the higher the force and velocity an athlete can generate. Nerve plates are attached on muscle cells and stimulate them to contract.

- Tendons store and release the highest mechanical energy.

- When the gastrocnemius muscle contracts, it has to transmit mechanical force to the bone to initiate a physical motion through the Achilles tendon.

- The Achilles tendon can transmit the highest force (4,900 N or 510 kg [1,124 lb]) (Enoka, 2015).
- Enoka (2015) specifies that the Achilles tendon also has the most stiffness of all muscles (2,857 N/cm or 291 kg/cm [641.5 lb/in.]). This stiffness is determinant for any reactive activities, changes of direction, or reactive jumps, and it is directly dependent on the force of the gastrocnemius.
- Powerful muscles always have a thicker cross-sectional area of a tendon and, therefore, can transmit muscle force to the bone to initiate an athletic action, such as sprinting and jumping and agility moves.
- Long tendons, such as the Achilles tendon, have a higher capacity to store elastic energy that can be used during athletic actions, such as sprinting and jumping.
- As a result of specific training (e.g., sprinting, plyometrics, bounding exercises, rope jumps, step running, reactive jumps), the insertion of the Achilles tendon on the calcaneus bone is larger. A strong Achilles tendon has an insertion area of 65 square millimeters or more (Enoka, 2015). The stronger and larger the insertion of the tendon, the better insurance the athlete has against injuries.
- If the tendon is weak, the transmission of high mechanical force is nearly impossible; it results in discomfort and even in injuries.
- The elastic properties of the Achilles tendon are stored in this tendon and used during high-velocity sprints, jumps, or quick changes of direction.
- Regularly expanding the range of motion (ROM), or flexibility, of the Achilles tendon is essential. Limited ROM may result in tearing or even breakage of this tendon.

PERIODIZATION OF STRENGTH AND POWER

Maximum effectiveness of a training program is impossible without good organization. In training methodology, this organization is called **periodization**, or the structuring of training in specific training phases, each with clear training goals. Gains in power do not occur overnight but rather cumulatively, over time, in a specific and predictable sequence, and following well-designed training plans.

Power is a function of MxS; the higher the gains in MxS, the greater the benefits to power. During the MxS phase, the FT fibers are trained to be recruited maximally in order to overcome high resistance; during the power phase, the same muscle fibers are exercised to be able to contract quickly, discharging faster and more explosively in order to perform a quick athletic action. As more FT fibers are recruited in action and trained to discharge faster, power, speed, and agility improve.

Table 9.2 illustrates the basic model of the periodization of strength, power, speed, and agility using the three traditional training phases: preparatory (preseason), competitive (in-season), and transition (off-season). The purpose of this model is to arrange specific strength and power training phases so that maximum power, speed, and agility will be achieved before and during the competitive season. Therefore, the periodization of strength is in essence a neuromuscular strategy that ensures the development of the dominant physical abilities of a sport at the highest level possible.

The sequence of strength training phases is essential for achieving improvements in power. The sequence and duration of these training phases are presented next.

Table 9.2 Basic Model of Periodization of Strength, Power, Speed, and Agility

Training phase	Preparatory (preseason)			Competitive (in-season)	Transition (off-season)
Periodization of strength	AA	MxS	Power Speed Agility	Maintenance of strength and power	Balanced development
Neuromuscular strategy and benefits	Adaptation	Increase in recruitment of FT fibers	Increase in discharge rate of FT fibers	Maintenance of the ability to recruit FT fibers	Rest recovery (AA)

AA = anatomical adaptation; MxS = maximum strength.

Note: This model of periodization is presented conceptually, illustrating the neuromuscular strategy to follow to achieve the essential physical qualities dominant in team sports. Similarly, the duration of each phase is arbitrary; it does not refer to the duration of each phase in weeks. Adjust this model to fit your needs and competition dates.

The periodization of strength follows the neuromuscular strategy that should enhance the development of the main physical attributes necessary for all athletes. After the adaptation phase (AA), you have to plan the MxS stage, where the scope of training is to increase the capacity to recruit in action a high number of FT muscle fibers. The MxS phase should always precede the development of power, maximum speed, and agility. Physiologically, it means that after a muscle is trained to recruit a high number of FT fibers using heavy loads (>80% of 1 RM), the next phase has the purpose of improving the discharge rate (the speed of contraction) of the same muscles, the prime movers. From the end of the MxS phase onward and during the power, speed, and agility phase, athletes will be able to contract their muscles fast and powerfully, and they will be able to successfully execute fast, explosive sprinting and agility actions.

Phase 1: Anatomical Adaptation (AA) Training

The neuromuscular strategy illustrated in table 9.2 begins with **adaptation** (positive changes in the functions of the body because of training). The AA phase consists of progressively increased demands in strength training; the goal is to strengthen and prepare ligaments, tendons, and muscle tissue for subsequent phases, when loads have increased and the anatomical stresses are much higher. The type of training planned for this phase is typical AA training; loads are lower, and each set is terminated at the instant the athlete feels discomfort. During the early part of an annual plan, and specifically for U12-U15, discomfort might mean stress. At this age, stress is far from being a desirable feeling. The precise duration of the AA phase should be age specific; it should take four to six weeks for U12 to U15 athletes and three to four weeks for athletes in U19 and up. Younger athletes need a longer AA training phase to allow sufficient time to gain the full benefits of adaptation without the pressures of official games.

The main objectives of the AA training phase include the following:

- Increase working capacity of all athletes with progressively increased cardiorespiratory training.
- Progressive adaptation to enable the young athletes to tolerate work, physical, and psychological difficulties.
- Increase general conditioning, endurance, and anatomical adaptation strength training.
- Adapt the ligaments, tendons, and muscle tissue for the strength training phases to follow.

You can effectively plan two or three training sessions each week in conjunction with technical and tactical training. A training session could last 60 to 75 minutes (not including the warm-up) for U12 to U15 athletes and longer for athletes in U19 and up (90-120 min).

Every athlete beginning the preparatory phase must go through an overall conditioning program that involves endurance training. Working capacity cannot increase without dedicating adequate time to endurance training, which provides the aerobic base athletes need to endure the long competitive phase. Well-developed endurance will also enhance athletes' rates of recovery and regeneration in response to the high volume of nonspecific and specific training programs.

Tables 9.3 and 9.4 offer examples of circuit training that represent what most coaches need to train during the AA phase. Both examples are set in a gym, but you can create different variations of these programs depending on the facilities that are available to you. Table 9.3 is recommended mostly for U15 athletes; table 9.4 is recommended for U15 to U17 athletes.

Phase 2: Maximum Strength (MxS) Training

By now, the needs and benefits of MxS training are clear. Stronger athletes will become more powerful, faster, and more agile—abilities that will always result in improving the quality of most sports. Improvements of MxS will help athletes overcome the force of gravity, apply higher force against the ground (push-off phase of the running step), improve speed, absorb the shock of landing, improve reactivity, and overcome aggressive

Table 9.3 Sample AA Circuit Training Program for a Gym Setting—Body Weight or Light Equipment

Station	Exercise	Duration/repetitions (reps)	Rest interval (RI) between stations
1	Lunges: forward, diagonally, and to the side	30-45 sec	1 min
2	An abdominal exercise	8-10 reps	1 min
3	Between-legs (2-3 kg/~5-7 lb) medicine ball (MB) forward throw	10-20 throws	30 sec
4	Push-up	6-12 reps	1 min
5	Two-leg slalom jump	20-45 sec	1 min
6	MB (2-3 kg/~5-7 lb) chest/overhead throw	10-20 throws	30 sec
7	Trunk twist on an incline bench, with a 20 kg (~44 lb) weight held above the chest	8-12 reps in each direction	1 min
8	Chin-up	8-15 reps	1 min
9	Step-up	1-3 min	1 min

Notes: Number of circuits: 1 or 2, depending on athletes' training potential. Rest interval between circuits: 2 min. After the first 2 or 3 weeks, advanced athletes may perform the program nonstop, the RI being employed only between circuits. Progression: Build training demand progressively by increasing the number of circuits per session, increasing the duration of activity per station, decreasing the RI between stations, increasing the repetitions per exercise, and increasing the rhythm of performing an activity. Exercise 7 (a typical core exercise) is performed on an incline bench; arms are extended. The trunk rotates to the right before returning to the starting position; the action is repeated to the left.

Table 9.4 Sample AA Circuit Training Program for a Gym Setting—Weights and Aerobic Exercises

Station	Exercise	Week 1	Week 2	Week 3	Rest interval (RI) between stations (min)
1	Aerobic (min)**	3-4	5	5-7	2
2	Leg press or half squat	50/15/3*	60/12/3*	60/12/3*	2
3**	Bent-knee sit-up	To discomfort	To discomfort	To discomfort	1
4	MB (3 kg) chest throw	20 × 3 sets	20 × 3 sets	25 × 3 sets	2
5	Shoulder press	50/10/2*	60/10/2*	60/12/2*	1
6	Aerobic (min)**	3	5	5-7	1
7	Seated row	50/10/3*	60/12/3*	70/10/3*	1
8	Bench press	50/10/3*	60/12/3*	70/10/3*	
9	Leg curl	50/10/2*	50/12/2*	60/12/2*	2
10	Aerobic (min)**	10	10	10	1

*First digit of a weight program refers to load in percentage of 1RM; second digit specifies number of reps; third digit refers to number of sets.

**Depending on availability, cardio training includes stationary cycling, running on a treadmill or track, Nordic skiing, and rowing machine. For exercise 3, athletes stop at the first signs of discomfort. During the first week, test for 1RM for exercises 2, 5, 7, 8, and 9. Test the highest weight each athlete can lift in one attempt and calculate the percentage suggested in the program for each week. Adapt the suggested program to the team's and athletes' needs and potential.

THE BENEFIT OF MXS

Of all types of strength training, MxS has the highest contribution to the improvement of performance in power, speed, and agility.

In strength training, a 100-percent performance, expressed in kilograms or pounds, is an athlete's maximal performance in 1RM for a specific exercise targeting the prime movers (the muscles responsible for performing a technical move). For example, if an athlete's 1RM for a leg press exercise is 200 kilograms (440 lb), then 80 percent is 160 kg (352 lb).

opponents. The development of MxS involves the use of heavy loads that usually range from 70 percent to 95 percent of one's maximum capacity, which is determined by using the 1RM. For young athletes (U15-U17/U19), the range of loads used in training is lower (50%-70%). From U21 and up, higher loads can be carefully used.

The goal of MxS training is to increase athletes' ability to recruit the greatest number of FT muscle fibers into action; this recruitment enables athletes to overcome external forces in the playing environment. Stimulating a high percentage of FT muscle fibers is possible only by using heavy loads in training. Sport-specific training involving traditional skills such as sprinting, jumping, throwing, Alpine skiing, rowing, kayak or canoeing, and batting cannot achieve the top results without using MxS. Neither can high performance be achieved by using elastic cords and balance trainers. When using those skills and exercises, plateaus in training adaptation occur relatively quickly once athletes reach an advanced skill level. A more effective way for athletes to prevent potential adaptation plateaus is to apply the proposed neuromuscular strategy and the periodization of strength and power training (see table 9.2).

Highly trained athletes in American football, rugby, baseball, track and field (short duration events), rowing, kayak or canoeing below the 1,000-meter events, and other sports may use much higher loads than those suggested in table 9.5. Once again, the duration of the MxS phase depends on the background of individual athletes and the duration of the preparatory phase, which is usually three to nine weeks. The MxS training phase can be shorter for the uninitiated and longer for advanced athletes who are familiar with training with higher loads. However, for best training benefits, to ensure that neuromuscular adaptation does occur, the MxS phase must exceed three weeks.

Consider two examples of MxS training shown in tables 9.5 and 9.6: The first is suggested for U17 to U19 athletes and the second for U21 to U23 athletes. When training for MxS, no rigid formula exists. As a coach you should use the best training information and learn to adapt suggested programs to suit the needs and potential of individual athletes, specifics of the sport, and specifics of the of position played.

Table 9.5 outlines a possible progression to follow for a six-week MxS program geared toward training the prime movers in racket sports, some martial arts, or team sports such as soccer, rugby, handball, volleyball, or ice and field hockey. The program can be repeated two or three times each week, depending on the training capabilities of your athletes. Because this particular program is not exceptionally challenging, training loads can be boosted for more advanced athletes or exercises can be added or changed to suit the specific needs of the individual or sport.

The leg press develops the knee and hip extensors, while the reverse leg press is intended to strengthen hamstring muscles. Exercises 3, 4, and 6 in table 9.5 target the development of the core muscles, while exercise 7 (calf press) strengthens the plantar flexors and the

Table 9.5 Sample Six-Week MxS Training Program for U17-U19 Athletes

#	Exercise	Week 1	Week 2	Week 3	Week 4	Week 5	Week 6	
Training demand		L	M	H	L	M	H	**RI (min)**
1*	Leg press	60/10/2	60/10/3	70/8/3	70/10/2	75/8/3	80/6/3	3-4
2	Reverse leg press	50/8/2	50/10/2	60/6/2	50/10/2	60/8/2	70/8/2	2
3	Abdominal crunch	To discomfort	To discomfort	To discomfort	To discomfort	To high level of discomfort	To high level of discomfort	1
4	Trunk twist	8 × 2 sets	10 × 2 sets	12 × 2 sets	10 × 2 sets	12 × 2 sets	12 × 2 sets	2
5	Front lat pull-down	60/10/2	70/8/2	70/10/2	60/8/2	70/8/2	75/8/2	2
6	Trunk extension	60/10/2	60/8/2	70/10/2	70/8/2	70/8/2	75/8/2	2
7	Calf press	70/8/2	70/8/3	80/5/3	70/8/2	80/4/3	80/6/3	2

*For exercises 1, 2, 5, 6, and 7: First digit refers to load in percentage of 1RM; second digit specifies number of reps; third digit specifies number of sets. Training demand is based on the principle of step loading: L = low; M = medium; H = high.

gastrocnemius muscles, which are prominent in sprinting, jumping, and agility actions. Finally, exercise 5 (front lat pull-down) targets the latissimus dorsi, which is responsible for the arms' drive backward. Remember that the arm drive determines the frequency of arm actions during sprinting. The stronger the arm drive, the higher the leg frequency. Therefore, to increase leg frequency, you should concentrate on the frequency of the arm drive.

Table 9.6 presents a suggested MxS program for U21-U23 athletes in sports requiring strong, powerful legs and trunk rotator muscles (from football, rugby, to throwing events in track and field). Performing a low number of exercises allows athletes to complete a higher number of sets, which is essential in the development of MxS for these sports. The added bonus is that athletes need to spend less time in the gym.

The heavy medicine ball (MB) side throw in table 9.6 is specific and necessary for sports involving throwing a ball, such as baseball, softball, rugby, football, and water polo, and some contact sports, such as martial arts. The first trunk rotation exercise (exercise 1) is performed from a standing position; athletes drive a power ball (figure 9.6) to one side and back for one full side rotation. The forward rotation should accelerate through the entire range of motion, reaching maximum acceleration at the instant of release (when the ball is considered thrown). The action is then repeated on the opposite side.

A power ball is similar to a medicine ball, but it comes with a handle (and in some cases this handle is made of rope). A power ball is available in weights ranging from 1 kilogram (about 2 lb) to 10 kilograms (about 25 lb). Exercises involving the power ball should be chosen and performed carefully and depend on the experience, strength, and power potential of athletes. Some athletic goods stores also offer heavy bags made out of a plastic shell filled with pellets or sand that also have a handle for easier carrying. The power ball or its equivalent can be used for power training, lateral throws, and overhead throws. The rope handle extends the leverage (arm of force) from the shoulder joint to the ball, allowing the athlete to generate higher centrifugal force, thus throwing the implement at longer distance. The longer the arm of force, the higher the centrifugal force.

Table 9.6 Sample Six-Week MxS Program for U21-U23 Athletes

#	Exercise	Week 1	Week 2	Week 3	Week 4	Week 5	Week 6	
Training demand		L	M	H	L	M	H	RI (min)
1	Heavy MB side throw	10 × 3 sets	12 × 4 sets	15 × 4 sets	12 × 4 sets	12 × 5 sets	8 × 6 sets	1-2
2*	Leg press	70/10/3	80/8/4	85/5/4	75/8/3	80/3/4	85/2/5	4
3	Reverse leg press	60/10/2	60/12/2	60/12/3	60/10/2	70/8/3	70/8/3	3
4	Abdominal crunch	To discomfort	To discomfort	To discomfort	To discomfort	To high level of discomfort	To high level of discomfort	3
5	Calf press	70/12/3	75/8/4	80/3/4	75/6/3	80/3/4	90/2/4	2
6	Front lat pull-downs	20 kg/8/2	20 kg/10/3	30 kg/6/3	30 kg/8/2	30 kg/8/3	30 kg/8/3	2

*For exercises 2, 3, and 5: First digit refers to load in percentage of 1RM; second digit specifies number of reps; third digit specifies number of sets; 10 × 3 means 3 sets of 10 reps. Training demand: L = low; M = medium; H = high.

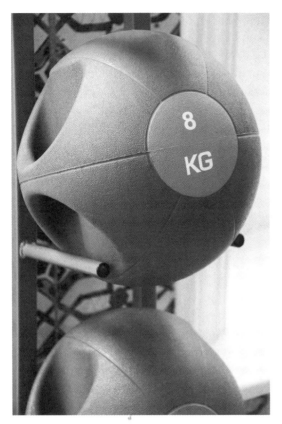

Figure 9.6 A power ball.

BreatheFitness/iStock/Getty Images

The leg press, reverse leg press, and calf press in table 9.6 recruit in action the triple extensors (calf muscles, quadriceps muscles, and gluteal muscles), which are essential for running and movements requiring agility or quick feet. Note that for the reverse leg press exercise, which specifically targets the hamstrings, the load and the number of reps and sets are lower than for other muscle groups. The hamstring muscles are usually not as well trained as the quadriceps (which creates an imbalance), and they have greater innervation (higher nerve end plates per square centimeter) than most muscles (Enoka, 2015). Therefore, be careful because the hamstrings are more prone to injury.

Finally, athletes must perform abdominal crunches to discomfort—even high discomfort—to maximize development of abdominal strength. You can adapt this exercise to incorporate abdominal exercise machines that can be set for specific loads.

Athletes at the U23 and higher levels are constantly exposed to many stressors. They also need a lot of time for recovery and regeneration after games and between demanding training sessions. Thus, they should spend the shortest time possible in the gym. An MxS training program (table 9.7) for these athletes has only three essential exercises, using heavy loads to yield high neuromuscular benefits. A program for the maintenance of MxS can be done in 25 minutes (which should also include the rest interval of maximum 4 minutes).

Table 9.7 Sample MxS Training Program for U23+ Athletes

#	Exercise/microcycle	1	2	3	Rest interval
1	Leg press	75/2-3/6*	80/4/6	85/4/4	4
2	Front lats pull-down	70/2/6	80/4/6	85/4/4	4
3	Calf press	80/3/5-6	85/4/6	85/4/4	3

*For exercises, first digit refers to load in percentage of 1RM; second digit specifies number of reps; third digit specifies number of sets.

Speed of execution: The load is high, so the rate of motion is slow to medium. However, since the application of force should be very active, the recruitment of FT muscles is high, increasing the discharge rate of FT muscles. To avoid eventual anatomical discomfort, always encourage best posture.

GASTROCNEMIUS ANCHOR

In order to target the prime movers of the leg (mostly the gastrocnemius and soleus muscles), squats, half squats, or step-ups (with a barbell on the shoulders) are often suggested. This approach is wrongly influenced by the sport of powerlifting. During the squat exercise, the most involved joints are the knee extensors (rectus femoris muscles), while the ankles are just partially active. In other words, the most important muscle used during running and agility, the **gastrocnemius, is not efficiently targeted in squatting exercises**.

Effectively targeting the gastrocnemius requires a calf press (at the leg press machine). Remember that the gastrocnemius contributes more than 50 percent to the force necessary to achieve maximum speed in running, best jumping performance, or maximum quickness in agility actions, while the rectus femoris contributes only 18 percent (Enoka, 2015). Therefore, to efficiently train the muscles needed for maximum speed, running, and agility, use the calf press.

Phase 3: Power Training

In simple terms, power is defined as the ability to apply force against resistance in the shortest possible time. In team sports, field events in track and field, racket, martial arts. and even combat sports, power manifests itself in many ways. Examples include executing a strong push-off against the ground, ice, or water to move quickly in the desired direction, executing a powerful take-off in basketball or volleyball, and blocking a charging linebacker or forward in rugby, handball, or lacrosse. Similar powerful actions are visible in soccer, water polo, and hockey, and when athletes attempt to choose tactical positions in an offensive zone or during a scrimmage in rugby. While speed, agility, and quickness depend on the level of power development, **power has to be seen as a function of MxS**. The higher the force applied against resistance (the ground), the faster an athlete's action or agility move. **The source of quickness is force, or power. In other words, nobody can be powerful without first being strong**.

Improvements in power are achieved during the power training phase. By using lower loads (<70% of 1RM), athletes are able to perform faster movements as the discharge rate and contraction of the FT muscle fibers increase. Another effective means of developing power and quickness of muscle contraction is MB throws, and **plyometric training**, which involves performing a variety of jumps, heaves, hops, or bounding. Power training results in higher overall velocities, increased muscle elasticity, faster reaction times, superior displays of power during specific athletic actions, and improved agility.

As noted already, when MxS increases, power increases as well, manifesting itself in displays of high speed, quickness, and agility. Unfortunately, the converse is also true: When MxS decreases, so does power. The decrease of power over the course of a competitive season results in reduced velocity, quickness, and agility. When athletes begin to show signs of losing speed and agility, strength and power training are effective in getting them back on track.

For the power training phase, the neuromuscular system is conditioned to increase the discharge rate of FT fibers. In other words, FT fibers are stimulated to contract faster and in larger numbers. An athlete who has adapted well to power training will be fast, powerful, and able to execute explosive actions with improved agility. The success of this phase directly depends on the previous MxS phase, where the FT fibers have been stimulated and conditioned for maximal recruitment into action. The training objectives of this phase can be achieved in three to four or five weeks, with two or three sessions each week.

The objective of the power training phase is to enhance the discharge rate of the FT muscle fibers, which results in faster, increasingly more agile, and powerful athletes in all phases of the game or sport. The power training phase, which lasts three to four weeks, is scheduled just before the competitive phase begins in order to maximize the benefits of the periodization of strength and power (table 9.8).

When reviewing table 9.8, keep in mind the following:

- *Jump squat*: Athletes begin by holding a dumbbell or a heavy MB at the shoulders. They jump vertically and should land carefully, in a slight amortization of the eccentric phase. For the purpose of shock absorption during the landing, the first contact should be on the balls of the feet, followed by flexion of the calf, knees, and hips.

- *MB throws and power ball throws* should be specific to the athlete's sport and position. Athletes perform side, chest, or between-the-legs throws, depending on the primary muscle groups used in the sport. Carefully select the ball weight to reflect the athletes' abilities and needs.

- *Reactive jumps*: Athletes jump down from a box 20 to 30 inches (50-75 cm) high; they touch the ground first with the balls of the feet before immediately jumping upward, without touching the ground with the heels. The same exercise can be executed with an increased load, such as holding a medicine ball or light dumbbell in each hand.

- *MB acceleration–deceleration*: Hold the ball in front of your chest while running and changing direction of motion.

- *Training demands each week*: Calculated training demand together with the demand of speed, endurance, and technical or tactical training. Therefore, you must consider not only the fatigue induced by power training but also the total fatigue induced by all facets of training planned for a given training session.

- *Training sessions per week*: The number of training sessions per week depends on age category, background, facilities, and phase of training.

Table 9.8 Sample Four-Week Training Program for the Development of Explosive Power for U21-U23 Athletes

#	Exercise	Week 1	Week 2	Week 3	Week 4	
Training demand		L	M	M	H	RI (min)
1*	Jump squat	50/8/3	60/8/3	60/8/3	60/10/3	3-4
2	MB throw	10 × 3 sets	12 × 3 sets	12 × 3 sets	15 × 3 sets	2
3	Reactive jump (plyometrics)	6-8 × 3 sets	8 × 4 sets	8 × 4 sets	8 × 4 sets	3
4	Power ball throw	6-8 × 3 sets	8 × 4 sets	8 × 4 sets	8 × 4 sets	3
5	MB acceleration–deceleration	10-15 m × 6	10-15 m × 6	15 m × 6-8	15 m × 6-8	3-4

*For exercise 1, first digit refers to load in percentage of 1RM; second digit specifies number of reps; third digit specifies number of sets.

Training demand: L = low; M = medium; H = high.

- *Individualized programs*: Adapt the load, number of reps, and sets to individual athletes' potentials.

- *Proper form for the jump squat*: It is important that athletes perform the jump squat properly to avoid injury. To avoid knee strain, emphasize a cushioned landing (i.e., decelerating upon impact) and always a vertical upper body.

- *Plyometric exercise level*: Select plyometric exercises according to athletes' previous adaptation to similar types of power training.

When power increases, it manifests itself through displays of high athleticism. However, power can—and should—also be trained to reflect the specific needs of the athlete and sport. Therefore, power can be trained in the form of explosive bursts of energy, in the execution of specific skills (such as spiking in volleyball, pitching or batting in baseball or softball, or shooting in water polo or team handball). Similarly, it can also be trained in the form of power endurance (e.g., the ability to jump to spike, block, or rebound more than 200 times during a volleyball or basketball game, or to repeatedly accelerate and decelerate or change directions quickly).

During many power-type of sport activities, such as stop-and-go, changes of direction, or plyometric exercises, muscle fibers contract concentrically (shorten) or eccentrically (lengthen), a physiological manifestation called the **stretch-shortening cycle (SSC)**. Enhanced performance resulting from SSC most likely occurs because of stored elastic energy during the eccentric phase of a muscle contraction. Enoka (2015) claims that the strong Achilles tendons can store up to 500 N (50.1 kg; 112.4 lb), demonstrating the great capability this tendon has to transmit force from the powerful gastrocnemius muscle to the ground to perform a push-off. The same tendon is also responsible for the quick reactivity of an athlete during landing from a jump and immediately rebounding during a game. **Do you want to increase reactivity? Improve MxS and power**.

The better the quality of strength training (mostly MxS), the better an athlete can activate the SSC (Richards et al., 2013; Enoka, 2015; Pandy et al., 2021).

In addition, the authors in the citations mentioned in the previous paragraph suggest that the duration of the SSC and the duration of ground contact can offer information regarding the athletes' potential.

- *Duration of SSC*: For fast athletes, it was less than 250 milliseconds; for slow athletes, it was more than 250 milliseconds.

- *Duration of foot contact on the ground*: For sprinting, contact lasted 80 to 90 milliseconds; take-off in long jump lasted 140 to 170 milliseconds; multihurdle jumps lasted 150 milliseconds; countermovement jumps lasted 500 milliseconds.

Power Training for Acceleration–Deceleration

Although most coaches stress the importance of acceleration in training, deceleration is at least as important as acceleration. The ability to decelerate allows athletes to change directions quickly when eluding a defender or getting open to receive a pass. The primary muscles involved in deceleration (quadriceps, gastrocnemius, soleus, and tibialis anterior) contract eccentrically.

As you organize your power training sessions, keep in mind these three important principles:

1. Keep the number of exercises low to ensure that maximal energy goes toward performing high-quality, powerful, and explosive actions. For the best power training benefit, keep the number of exercises low, but the number of sets high.

PLYOMETRIC TRAINING FOR THE DEVELOPMENT OF POWER

Plyometric training is an effective method for developing jumping power, elasticity, and reactivity, thus it aids the improvement of strength and power for young athletes.

Plyometric training results in the following:

- Quick mobilization and greater innervation activities
- Recruitment of most (if not all) motor units and their corresponding muscle fibers
- An increase in the firing rate of motor neurons
- The transformation of muscle strength into explosive power

Plyometric training develops the nervous system so that it will react with maximal speed to the lengthening of muscle. In turn, it will develop the ability to shorten rapidly and maximally.

When doing this type of training, keep in mind the following:

- Learning correct technique of plyometric exercises is essential.
- A muscle contracts more forcefully and quickly from a prestretch position (i.e., a slightly flexed joint).
- The more rapid the prestretch, the more forceful the concentric contraction.
- Repeated relative training induces fatigue, which affects both the eccentric, but more noticeably, the concentric work capacity. Fatigue is characterized by increases in the duration of contact phase time (Turner and Jeffreys, 2010; Taylor and Beneke, 2012, Laffaye and Wagner, 2013).

2. If athletes' speed of contraction or explosiveness begins to decline visibly, it is a definite sign that fatigue is beginning to set in. If fatigue occurs, athletes should stop the exercise, take a rest interval, and continue with the planned program of the day. When exercises are no longer performed explosively, athletes are actually beginning to train power endurance instead of training purely for power.

3. To ensure that FT muscle fibers are conditioned to increase their discharge rate, power exercises must involve acceleration through the entire range of motion, and the fastest acceleration should be reached at the end of an action. If maximum acceleration is not achieved during an exercise, FT fibers are not recruited maximally, which means power training objectives are not achieved either.

Power-Endurance Training

Power endurance requires a different type of power training. Specific parts of a game rely on the capacity of an athlete to repeat aggressive, energetic moves several times fast. To achieve these necessities, athletes have to duplicate many reps and sets during a training session. Consider the sample workout in table 9.9 only as a guideline; adapt the program to your athletes' needs, potential, and training environment. Again, to enhance the development of power endurance, the number of exercises is low, but the number of repetitions and sets high. Make sure the exercises you select address the needs of your athletes and the prime movers used in your sport.

The demand of a power-endurance workout as outlined in table 9.9 is very high. It is applicable only to athletes with a good background in strength and power training, particularly to U21-U23 athletes. If you want to apply these guidelines to U19 or state-level athletes, significantly reduce the amount of work, especially the number of sets and reps.

Table 9.9 Sample Workout for Training Power Endurance for Advanced Athletes

#	Exercise	Week 1	Week 2	Week 3	Week 4	
Training demand		L	M	H	H	RI (min)
1	Drop jump* followed by 10 bounding steps	6 reps × 4 sets	7 reps × 6 sets	8 reps × 6 sets	8 reps × 6 sets	2-3
2	MB side throw**	15 reps × 4 sets	15 reps × 6 sets	20 reps × 6 sets	25 reps × 6-7 sets	3
3	10 cone or low-hurdle jumps	12 reps × 4 sets	15 reps × 5 sets	20 reps × 5-6 sets	25 reps × 6 sets	3
4	Between-legs power ball/ MB forward throw**	15 reps × 5 sets	18 reps × 5 sets	20 reps × 7 sets	20 reps × 8 sets	3

Drop jumps: Athletes may use a barbell (30% of 1RM) or a 10-kilogram (25 lb) dumbbell in each hand. Maintaining correct technique and posture is crucial. Athletes should (1) land flatfooted, with the heel touching the ground, without allowing the barbell to bounce on the shoulders, and (2) keep the trunk vertical while decelerating the action to absorb the shock of landing (leg flexion) as quickly as possible. Once the athlete has landed, a coach or partner should immediately take the barbell off the shoulders in preparation for a series of jumping (bounding) exercises. The height of the box for the drop jump should be 20 to 30 inches (50 to 75 cm) at the most.

**MB throws: Use a weight of 5 to 10 pounds (3-4 kg). Starting from a half-squat position, athletes swing the ball forward and upward, with an accelerated knee extension; they follow through with a powerful forward and upward jump.

Training demand: L = low; M = medium; H = high.

When planning power-endurance training, follow these principles:

- Plan this type of program for the last five weeks of the preparatory phase, just before official contests in the selected sport begin.
- Continually monitor the level of fatigue of each athlete. Remember: Sloppy contacts on the floor are a sign of neuromuscular fatigue.
- If athletes cannot follow the program, it means they are not yet ready for such a demanding training program; in this case, you need to change the program by reducing the sets and, if necessary, also the number of reps. High number of sets represents one of the highest physiological challenges for most athletes, particularly for the young ones.

Running Stairs for Power Training

Power endurance in the legs can also be trained by running stairs (in a gym or stadium). As athletes run up the stairs, the triple extensors contract concentrically, while the same muscles contract eccentrically as the athletes run down the stairs. Consider the following progression and training options for running stairs:

- Running up and down from step to step
- Running up and down over one step at a time
- Running up and down over two steps
- Hopping upward over one or two steps
- Hopping downward over two steps
- Hopping up and down with a two-foot takeoff
- Hopping with a two-foot takeoff with a 180-degree rotation in one direction and then the other
- Performing crossover steps up and down the stairs over one or two steps (alternate leading with the right and left foot)
- Performing stutter jumps (land and immediately push off again for another jump) over one step
- Performing stutter jumps over two steps
- Performing a side shuffle over one and eventually (with practice) two steps
- Performing a quick-feet drill
  - The athlete places one foot on one step and the other foot on the next higher or lower step.
  - The task is to switch the position of the feet as quickly as possible; the right foot steps to where the left foot was, and the left foot steps to where the right foot was.
  - The athlete tries to maintain balance; the vertical projection of the center of gravity must remain inside the base of support.

Guidelines for running stairs include the following:

- Always maintain good body posture and body control.
- Follow a sensible long-term progression, such as run; run and hop over one step; run and hop over two steps; cross over; side shuffle; quick-feet drill; and hops with rotations.
- It may take younger athletes two to four years before they can perform more complicated run and hop combinations.
- Please remember: The more complex exercises are only possible when athletes have developed adequate leg power.
- Do not hurry! Give your athletes time to grow and mature. This is a sign of professional maturity on your side.

Phase 4: Maintenance of MxS and Power

The next phase of training occurs during the competitive phase, when athletes take part in league games. It should be obvious that if athletes do not maintain MxS and power training during this phase, many of the neuromuscular benefits gained in earlier training will fade away, resulting in **detraining** (Bompa, 1993; McInnis et al., 1995; Bompa and Buzzichelli, 2021). The detraining process occurs as follows:

- A failure to maintain MxS results in protein degradation (catabolism) or breakdown, because muscles are no longer needed to contract powerfully and less protein is required for tissue repair (Thomson and Buckley, 2011; Dasuri et al., 2013).

- Protein degradation results in a decrease in muscle cross-sectional area and a reduction in the recruitment pattern of working muscles (Appel, 1990; Clarkson and Hubal, 2002; Trauth et al., 2019).
- As protein degradation continues, gains in strength and power are reversed (McInnis et al., 1995). As MxS decreases, power, speed, and agility quickly follow suit.

Consider the following chain reaction:

$$\text{loss of MxS} \rightarrow \text{loss of power} \rightarrow \text{loss of speed, agility, and reaction time}$$

When the capacity to recruit FT fibers decreases, so does the neuromuscular ability to maintain a high discharge rate of the FT fibers. Furthermore, as the ability of motor units to recruit FT fibers decreases, the efficiency of nerve impulses to the working muscles also decreases. As a result, the quickness, power, and frequency of nerve impulses are diminished (McInnis et al., 1995; Turner and Buckley, 2012; Hensley 2019). Because a loss of power results in a loss of speed and agility, athletes have a difficult time performing at the same level as before despite equally strong levels of desire and motivation. Stated simply, athletes can perform only at levels the neuromuscular system is conditioned to perform.

Phase 5: Transition

During the transition phase, strength training (AA training) should continue at a lower intensity, with two workouts each week. This training is particularly important for athletes who have longer transition phases of five to eight weeks. Transition phases beyond the standard four to five weeks, especially totally inactive transitions, result in greater detraining or even a total loss of previous gains. Every time athletes start a new preparatory phase, they start from a low level of physiological readiness and potential. Therefore, the rate of improvement from year to year is very low because the first month of training is dedicated to regaining a decent training potential. Table 9.10 illustrates general guidelines for a five-week transition phase.

Table 9.10 Sample of a Five-Week Transition Phase

Weeks 1 and 2	Weeks 3 to 5

• Recovery from fatigue
• Physical therapy (if necessary)
• Relaxation
• Vacation
	• Aerobic training, low intensity: 1 or 2 times a week for 30 min
	• Strength training (injury prevention type): 2 times a week for 1 hr
	  • Low, stressless loads
	  • Compensation training for the antagonist muscles
	  • Training of stabilizing muscles

Note: Athletes can perform aerobic and strength training exercises on the same day, allowing them to train only twice a week.

PERIODIZATION OF LONG-TERM TRAINING

Parents, coaches, and fitness trainers are enthusiastic contributors to sports, fitness, and wellness—all activities that children love. They have the chance to witness how children develop into teenagers and then into successful adults. Over time, they directly participate in transforming young athletes into top performers in their selected sports. However, best results are not possible without a long-term vision, a long-term periodization. When properly applied, this concept represents a guarantee of a progression that enhances crude qualities into high-class athletic abilities (table 9.11).

The following sections include specific suggestions for strength training at every stage of development based on table 9.11.

U12

U12 represents the early years when young athletes are initiated into strength training. They are the years of building the foundations for overall, well-developed strength while preventing injury for the future. This base will positively influence the future development of the sport-specific abilities that are directly dependent on strength, namely, power, speed, and agility. A well-rounded, multilateral training program should consider the development of all the muscles of all the joints of the body. Most exercises should use body weight. Progressively you can also introduce low-weight MB throws, exercises with elastic cords, relays carrying heavier MBs, lateral rolls holding an MB, climbing on stall bars or rope, simple skipping-rope drills, game play, and relays. Children enjoy variety. A sport-specific training session can be followed by 15 to 20 minutes of basic exercises previously suggested. You can also plan a fitness training session in a gym setting, separate from the specific sport. Choose exercises that require simple equipment. If an exercise has a specific technique, always request to adhere to proper technique.

Flexibility training for U12 is mostly for the ankles, knees, hips, trunk, and shoulders.

U15

U15 strength training should be considered as a transition from low loads (mostly body weight exercises) to a training stage when other means of training could be introduced. Consequently, injury prevention and multilateral training must be continued, but still with

Table 9.11 Progression of Strength Training From U12 Through U23

Stages of development	U12	U15	U17	U19	U21-23
Scope of strength training	Initiation in the fundamentals of strength training Injury prevention using exercises that address most muscle groups	AA type of strength training Injury prevention Introduction of simple A/Q courses and P	AA P A/Q	AA MxS with low loads P PE A/Q	AA MxS P A/Q ME

AA = anatomical adaptation; A/Q = agility and quickness; P = power, PE = power endurance, ME = muscular endurance.

low loads, such as 3- to 5-kilogram (~6-11 lb) dumbbells, 3- to 4-kilogram (~4-9 lb) MB, the use of *training machines* with lower loads (40% of 1RM), elastic cords, climbs, rolls, and the like. The duration of fitness training can increase to 20 to 25 minutes, including the rest interval. The number of repetitions and the number of sets could increase slightly, yet the RI must be long enough (2-3 min) to allow children to recover fully between sets. At this stage of development, low-load power training can be introduced, along with agility and quickness courses and relays children usually enjoy. Be sure to constantly ask children to adhere to good technical norms for every exercise used in training and beware of gym instructors who constantly promote weightlifting moves (barbells). Parents and coaches should be aware that some exercises are difficult technically, and that the muscles (particularly the intervertebral muscles and knee ligaments of young children) are not ready yet for weightlifting.

For U15, a constant concern for flexibility training exists, particularly flexibility in the ankles and hips.

U17

At the U17 stage, strength training can become more specific, addressing the triple extensors (ankle, knees, and hips) and core area of the body and strengthening the intervertebral muscles to prevent the young athletes from future injuries. Once again, the duration of a fitness training session can be around 30 minutes. Training loads, number of reps, and number of sets have to be increased. Continue to observe good technique in both the strength, power, MB throws, simple plyometrics, and agility and quickness courses. Most exercises have to clearly switch to sport- and position-specific actions, while training demand can be increased again to the potential of U17 athletes. Many aspects of training have to follow the specifics of energy systems, particularly the oxidative (aerobic), phosphagen (alactic), and occasionally also to target the glycolytic (lactic) system.

Flexibility training for U17 is good overall flexibility with special attention to ankle and hips, where most injuries occur.

U19

Most athletes at the U19 stage of development have a determining factor; they can either make themselves visible to be selected for college or university teams, or they can become amateur athletes. Therefore, now is the time to specialize your athletes so that they can become highly fit physically and reach their highest levels of strength, power, speed, and agility. The motor abilities required in the selected exercises must be trained sport- and position-specific. AA training has to be maintained, but you have to also focus on MxS with medium loads (60%-80% of 1RM), power, power endurance, and agility and quickness. As usual, training programs addressing the specific needs of team sports have to be created based on the physiological concept of energy systems. Therefore, while you will employ all three energy systems, you have to also expose your athletes to the glycolytic system, a type of training that has not been employed too often during the U17 stage.

Always remember to maintain a good flexibility for U19 athletes and higher. Increase of MxS might result in an undesirable joint rigidity and even injuries (Pozzi et al., 2020; Afonzo et al., 2021). As suggested in this book, flexibility training starts at a young age and should never be abandoned throughout the life of an athlete.

U21-U23

After many years of investing your time, talent, and effective training programs, your athletes have reached the U21-U23 stage of pre- or high performance. From now on your training must be very selective; direct it only to what will take your athletes to the height of athleticism. Therefore, focus training on what will make your athletes more powerful to transform strength and power into maximum speed and agility. Once again, the role of strength, particularly MxS, will be more necessary than ever.

Top athletes must spend their energy efficiently. Therefore, invest time and energy only on what is working. From U21 on, eliminate many activities requiring multilateral training. Training must become more intensive and specific. Be selective and concrete. Disregard fake exercises and methods. Finish your training, and go home to rest. Never forget that top athletes need time for recovery and regeneration. Any extra time you may have must be used for rest and recuperation before the next workout. The strength training you often plan at the end of a workout should also be very specific and short.

- *For strength training*: Focus on MxS and power. Introduce muscle-endurance training, and spend less time during the AA phase. Reduce the number of exercises to the minimum; the more exercises you use, the lower your training effectiveness. Increase the number of sets and reps.

- *For speed training*: Focus on specific and nonspecific maximum speed and long rest intervals (RI). Remember that complex training makes athletes the best they can possibly be. They can reach the height of athleticism using simple tumbling (from gymnastics) and bounding (drills resembling triple jump from track and field) exercises that improve leg power, particularly the push-off phase of the running step.

CONCLUSION

Only doing sport-specific training does not cut it. Sports are very complex activities, requiring training to improve the many abilities you need for a contest or game. Make sure you provide to your athlete the training programs he or she needs that target the development of strength, speed, agility, and flexibility. This is the best road to creating successful athletes.

Some coaches and strength and conditioning professionals believe that sport-specific training is adequate for developing the power-endurance needs of athletes in any team sport. While some might question the need to train power endurance outside of the gym, off the field, off the ice, or out of the pool, remember that strength training, particularly MxS, is needed to play a strong physiological role even during league games, top-level contests (please refer to the strength maintenance program earlier in this chapter). This means that the role of strength and power must match the physiological profile of the sport. Athletes and coaches must assess their strength training needs according to the dominant energy systems of the sport and the position-specific needs of each athlete on the team.

For example, during the preparatory phase, athletes must be conditioned to perform fast and powerful athletic actions repeatedly (MxS, power-endurance training). The same type of training must be maintained during the competitive phase: twice a week, 20 to 30 minutes per session. If MxS is not maintained, detraining will occur, along with all the negative consequences that accompany it (e.g., loss of power), which ultimately leads to a significant reduction in levels of speed and agility.

As sport-specific training starts, the athletes need to be physiologically ready to perform all planned technical and tactical tasks. For teams that choose to train technical and physical elements simultaneously, the objectives of power training do not change. The same periodization of strength approach shown in table 9.2 still applies. In this case, however, the head coach must plan off-field, gym, or pool training in collaboration with the fitness coach to ensure that all the physical attributes of the athletes are trained appropriately to prepare them for the start of the competitive season.

Keep in mind the following:

■ Quality, science-based training is always better than quantity training.

■ The higher the number of exercises you use, the lower the adaptation and training benefits for prime movers. It is effective for the AA phase but not for MxS and power.

■ The rate of leg motion directly depends on the rate of arm drive (in the direction of running). Therefore, you have to also train the arm drive using the front lats pull-down, which directly addresses the latissimus dorsi.

■ In training and in competition, goalkeepers in soccer hit the ground hard and often. Certainly, goalkeepers need to jump, dive, be agile, and react. However, coaches who specialize in training goalkeepers should also train the muscles performing these specific moves. If you want a goalkeeper to jump fast and high, make sure you also train the triple extensor muscles; these leg muscles initiate the actions that goalkeepers perform. Weak muscles are incapable of jumping high, far, or quickly. Also, do not forget to train goalkeepers' reaction and movement time. During the game, goalkeepers' reaction is often challenged. However, if your training does not address the reactivity of a goalkeeper, it is totally unfair to expect her to have these qualities.

■ Most gyms are well equipped with strength training machines, such as the calf and leg press. They are better than barbells for young athletes who typically have a poor background in strength training. However, if you want to also use a barbell for squats, make sure you prepare young athletes' (U12-U15) core area of the body and knees to cope with the strain of lifting a barbell. Particularly focus on the intervertebral and lumbar muscles, the pillars to support many strength training moves performed by arms and legs.

■ Sand training is ineffective for developing speed and power. Because sand is not a solid surface, it does not have a strong and firm base, so no ground reaction occurs. Your force applied against the ground dissipates and is absorbed into the sand; consequently, you cannot expect the benefits of ground reaction that is so important for speed, jumps, and agility. However, running in sand can be fun, and it is beneficial for general fitness and overall endurance (AA phase).

■ One-leg training may not be as effective as you think. Eliassen and colleagues (2018) found that muscle activation during bilateral squats was significantly greater (rectus femoris) compared with unilateral (single-leg) squats. Naturally, two legs offer better stability. More importantly, however, muscle activation is higher with two-leg squats; it recruits a higher number of FT muscle fibers, resulting in visible benefits for the improvement of strength, power, speed, and agility.

■ One-leg training might be necessary only in the case of leg force inequality and can be trained during the AA phase.

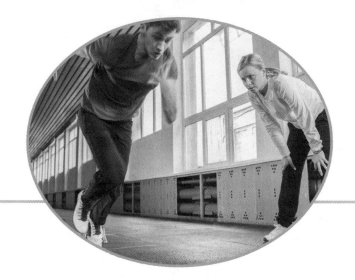

## chapter 10

Training Methods to Develop Speed

Speed is one of the most important motor abilities required in many sports. The ability to move very fast or cover a distance quickly is expressed as the ratio between space and time; it incorporates, among others, three major elements: reaction time, force applied by the legs against the ground (the push-off or propulsion phase of the running step), and frequency of movement per unit of time (**movement time**).

Speed is also multidirectional; running is performed in all directions during a game. In addition to running forward, athletes must often move sideways and backward (back-pedaling). They often have to pivot, zigzag, stop and go, cut, turn, and change direction in response to the dynamics of the game. Many researchers have studied the maximum speed athletes can generate during games or competitions.

- Average running (sprint) speed across all sports and levels: 15 mph (6.7 m/sec)
- Lionel Messi, soccer player: 20.2 mph (9 m/sec)
- Cristiano Ronaldo, soccer player: 20.8 mph (9.3 m/sec)
- Tyreek Hill, American football player (Miami Dolphins): 22.77 mph (10.2 m/sec)
- Usain Bolt, sprinter: 27.7 mph (12.4 m/sec)

Adapted from Mero, Komi, and Gregor (1992); Weyand, Sternlight, Bellizzi, and Wright (2000); Weyand, Sandell, Prime, and Bundle (2010); and Horsfield (2015).

For comparison, the average ball velocity in professional soccer is 59 mph (26.4 m/sec) for men and 49.2 mph (22 m/sec) for women.

WHAT MAKES AN ATHLETE FAST?

In a simple world, this question has only two answers:

1. Genetics
2. Maximum strength (MxS)

Genetics, which some call natural talent, refers to the proportion of fast-twitch (FT) and slow-twitch (ST) muscle fibers. If an athlete were lucky to inherit a higher percentage of FT fibers, they would naturally be faster. If an athlete were born with relatively few

FT fibers, they might be naturally suited for a number of sports that do not require high speeds. Given that you cannot alter your genetic code, the only option to become faster is to increase your MxS to the highest level possible.

High level of speed is achieved only when an athlete is capable of applying high force against the ground in the shortest time, particularly during the propulsion phase (the push-off against the ground). If you want to jump high to head, catch, or spike a ball, you have to apply high force against the ground to overcome the force of gravity. The same is true for speed; **the ability to generate high velocity is proportional to the force applied against the ground.** You have to apply the highest force in minimum time. Certainly, maximum force is a necessity, but equally important is to also apply it in the shortest time, meaning the shortest duration of the ground contact, or around 100 milliseconds. (The duration of ground contact for good sprinters is less than 150 milliseconds and for mediocre sprinters, it is greater than 200 milliseconds.)

FACTORS AFFECTING SPEED

Many factors influence speed development. Rather than treating the speed development as athletic action in its entirety, as a repetition of sprinting actions of various distances, you will be more successful if you address the development of its components (refer to the last part of this chapter), such as strength and power (propulsion force, duration of contact phase, reactivity, stiffness), psychomotor abilities, reaction time and movement time, and technique and concentration.

Unlike other motor abilities such as strength and endurance, where athletes can achieve significant improvements after sufficient training without possessing outstanding talent, speed is determined largely by one's own genetic code and requires a greater degree of natural talent.

Inherited factors such as the mobility of nervous processes, the quick alternation between excitation and inhibition, and the capacity to regulate neuromuscular coordination affect motor frequency and efficiency, which are both determinant factors in developing speed.

Strength and Power

Strength and power represent the capacity of an athlete to display force through muscular contraction. It is a major determining factor for performing fast movements in most sports. During training and games, external resistance to athletes' movements comes from a variety of sources, including gravity, the environment (water, wet field, snow, wind), and opponents. Athletes require power to overcome these opposing forces through enhanced muscular capabilities.

HORSEPOWER OR MxS

Consider this analogy: Why are some cars, such as sports cars, faster than most others? Simply put, it is not the shape of the car but rather the horsepower of the engine. Sports cars have very powerful engines. Do you see a similarity between cars and athletes?

Like a car with a powerful engine that can generate high velocity, an athlete with a powerful engine—a high level of MxS—can display high speed (run very fast) simply because he or she is very strong.

BEWARE OF PROGRESSION

Because the loads of strength training for young athletes have to be built progressively—reaching the highest loads at U21-U23—coaches must first prepare athletes to develop muscles for stability and core and back muscle strength prior to lifting heavy loads. Therefore, they need to strengthen the frame of the trunk, abdomen, lumbar, and intervertebral muscles in order to avoid discomfort and injuries.

Athletes must often perform a skill quickly and repeat it with the same quality many times during a game or race. As a result, athletes must complement the development of power with the development of power endurance during speed training, which will allow them to perform many fast and quick actions for the duration of a game.

Psychomotor Abilities

Reaction time, movement time (how fast you move a limb), wrist dexterity, and visual skills are other examples of largely inherited abilities that are important for successful performance in team sports. These skills are outwardly manifested in ball handling in basketball, handball, and water polo; precise receiving and passing in lacrosse; and passing and shooting in soccer and ice or field hockey.

Among the numerous psychomotor abilities, the capacity to react quickly is considered the most cherished ability in racket, contact, and team sports. It represents the time needed to initiate a response to a given stimulus, athletic action. Gaining control of the puck on face-offs in hockey or goalkeepers responding to the actions of offensive players in hockey, soccer, lacrosse, and handball are examples of the incredible importance of reaction time.

Technique and Concentration

When proper technique is used to perform skills, speed performance is improved by shortening the time of limb actions, correctly positioning the center of gravity, and using energy more efficiently. Proper form enables athletes to carry out skills effortlessly and with a high degree of accuracy, or coordination through the relaxation of antagonist muscles.

Strong concentration enables athletes to mobilize their nervous processes more effectively and maintain maximum alertness. Therefore, before any speed drill or exercise, athletes must be prepared to participate with maximum concentration as well as the will to go faster.

GUIDELINES FOR SPEED TRAINING

When planning speed training, you must consider the following methodological variables discussed in this section.

Intensity

Intensity refers to the qualitative aspect of work performed during training. Improvements in speed tend to occur when training intensities fall in a range from just below maximum to supermaximal levels. Athletes must always try to maintain good technique during high-intensity training to maximize efficiency. Whether running, skating, or swimming, skills should always be performed with as much technical proficiency as possible. The greatest training gains are usually made when fatigue from other activities does not hinder the development of maximum speed or quickness; this optimal time is usually immediately after a brief warm-up. Speed training is also more effective when it follows one or more days of rest or low-intensity training. Training for maximum speed is very demanding on both the body and the mind, so adequate rest is essential for optimal speed development.

For athletes in team sports, the appropriate intensity levels are determined by several factors:

- *Drill intensity.* Many drills used in team sports require powerful and explosive movements. Therefore, it is important to closely monitor the number and intensity of drills used during training sessions to avoid the potentially debilitating effects of fatigue and overtraining. To facilitate regeneration, energy systems can be alternated during a week (microcycle) of training. High intensity is suggested for U19 to U23 athletes, and lower and progressively increased intensity is suggested for U12 to U17 athletes.

- *Rhythm or pace of games and drills.* These factors can be physically and psychologically taxing on athletes. While it can be controlled during training, the pace of a game often depends on the dynamics of the game and the tactics of the opposing team. If your athletes are not well prepared to compete against teams that prefer an increased rhythm of play, your team is unlikely to be successful.

- *Number of games, matches, or races per week (microcycle).* Although you have very little influence over game schedules, model training can be used to help manage the stresses related to playing several games in one microcycle. It is generally not a good idea to plan exhibition games during the season unless you have only one game scheduled per week. Exhibition games should be limited to the preparatory phase or during a pause in league games (if you have one).

- *Minutes played by the best athletes on the team.* More is usually expected and demanded from the best athletes on a team during a game. For this reason, these athletes need to follow a more individualized and intense training schedule, employ unique postgame regeneration techniques, and reduce their training intensity during the first postgame training session. Fatigued athletes should never be exposed to vigorous training before the effects of fatigue have been eliminated from the body. The undesirable consequences may be exhaustion or even overtraining.

- *Athletes' rates of recovery.* Even among athletes with similar levels of aerobic conditioning, rates of recovery vary visibly. These variations need to be considered and monitored when developing individual and specific training schedules for each athlete. For athletes who regenerate slowly, the first postgame training session should be carried out at a lower intensity to allow for restoration of their energy levels.

- *Social and psychological stressors.* Many coaches successfully monitor and control the physiological sources of stress imposed on athletes through the volume and intensity of training sessions. However, coaches must be equally aware of the social and psychological stressors affecting their athletes (e.g., family, lifestyle, peer pressure). It is important to identify these external stressors and to discuss them privately with each athlete. Stress-free athletes are effective athletes.

Distance

The optimal duration of repetitions depends on the time needed by an athlete to **accelerate** (the ability to increase frequency of running or rate of motion), reach, and maintain maximum speed. The distance following acceleration is where athletes have to work on developing maximum speed. Therefore, you need to plan maximum speed sprints or drills for longer than 32 yards (30 m) for track sprinting and shorter than 32 yards for team sports, a distance dictated by the size of the field or court and the presence of opponents. If the distance is much shorter your athletes work only on the acceleration part and not on developing maximum speed.

If the ultimate objective of training is to attain maximum speed, quickness, or agility, training sessions should not be planned when athletes are in a state of fatigue because fatigue seriously hinders the development of maximum speed, quickness, and explosiveness.

Volume

The quantitative aspect of work performed during training is called **volume**, or the total amount of training during a training session or phase of training. Because speed training places a great strain on the central nervous system (CNS) and the neuromuscular system, training volume should remain low (20-30 min, depending on the duration of the drill and the rest interval allocated between repetitions).

Frequency

Compared to aerobic endurance training, the total amount of energy spent during speed training is relatively low. However, the energy expenditure per time unit is very high, which explains why fatigue sets in so quickly during speed training sessions. Therefore, athletes should repeat maximum intensities no more than six times per session, two or three times a week during the competitive phase.

Repetitions

Training to increase maximum speed in team sports, swimming, track and field, or speed skating is related to age and is best achieved by performing six to eight repetitions (reps) of 60 to 150 feet (20-50 m), with a rest interval of 3 or 4 minutes (lower number of repetitions and shorter distance for U12 and U15 athletes, and higher for U19-U23 athletes). By completing 8 to 12 or more repetitions at the same distance (mostly for U21-U23 athletes), you may also see improvements in athletes' speed endurance. This form of training is important for wide receivers in football; wings in handball; wingers in rugby; and midfielders and forwards in soccer, lacrosse, and field hockey, all of whom periodically require quick acceleration throughout a game.

Rest Interval

Between speed drills or high-intensity repetitions, athletes require a rest interval (RI) that ensures almost complete replenishment of the fuels used. Athletes should also relax mentally so that other repetitions of high intensity are possible. For drills using the phosphagen, also known as the alactic system (adenosine triphosphate and creatine phosphate, or ATP-CP), the RI should be around 2 to 3 minutes. However, the RI for glycolytic (lactic, anaerobic) system drills should facilitate optimal recovery (3-4 min), removing the lactates and restoring the oxygen debt almost completely. If the RI is not long enough, the athletes do not have the time to remove lactates from the system; consequently, lactates accumulate in quantities that may hinder performance during speed training. However, RIs should not be so long (5+ min) that the excitability of the CNS fades away. Active rest, such as light jogging or walking, and simple, relaxing ball handling or shooting are recommended for rest intervals.

TRAINING METHODS FOR DEVELOPING SPEED

Speed training is relatively simple, but it is very demanding with high energy expenditure. However, the only way to become fast is by repeating high-intensity speed drills, be they game-specific and position-specific drills, or nonspecific training methods.

Repetition Method

Repetition is the main method used to train speed. To achieve improvements in speed over a given distance, or the quickness and technical refinement of a movement pattern, a drill must be repeated several times at a high speed. Although the objective of the repetition method is to improve running speed, this approach may also be used to improve quickness in performing technical or tactical skills.

During repetition training, the athletes' concentration must be focused on performing each repetition at the described speed; in most cases, it is at maximum speed. Maximum concentration will help athletes reach superior speed and neuromuscular coordination. Finally, athletes must direct maximum attention and concentration to accomplishing a specific training task, such as the time to cover a given distance, but without rigidity (tightened muscles), with good form and arm–leg coordination.

Specific Training: Technical or Tactical Drill Method

In the case of game-specific drills, you have to create them while keeping in mind the specifics of position played and also the principles of energy systems.

To accomplish your objective to improve specific maximum speed, you have to employ drills with the ball or puck. In team sports, the ability to accelerate quickly is not sufficient. For many team sport athletes, **acceleration–deceleration coupling** (the ability to slow down quickly after running with maximum velocity) is as important as the ability to accelerate quickly. Because team sport athletes rarely accelerate in a straight line, they must become accustomed to executing many sport-specific actions and tactical maneuvers during training, including turns, direction changes, and stop-and-go movements.

The distance covered (see table 10.1) for such drills should be approximately 30 to 90 feet (10-30 m) and longer for wide receivers in football, wingers in rugby (90-150 ft; 30-50 m), and center fielders in baseball, and can be repeated 6 to 12 times, depending on age category. In basketball, lacrosse, team handball, ice or field hockey, and water polo, the distance is usually not longer than 45 to 60 feet (15-20 m), unless the athlete returns to her own basket or goal with the same speed.

RELAXED POSTURE IN MAXIMUM SPEED TRAINING

During repetitions of maximum speed ask your athletes to maintain a relaxed position, with the shoulders down and face relaxed. Facial grimace will tell you who runs in a relaxed manner and who does not. Rigidity in running is usually witnessed in facial expression and shoulders tightening, a posture that is not conducive to high-velocity sprinting.

Table 10.1 Selected Methods for Speed Training

Form of training	Distance of activity (m/yd)	Number of repetitions	Rest interval (min)	Number of weekly sessions
Nonspecific drills				
Maximum acceleration	10-30	6-10	3-4	1-2
Maximum speed	20-50	4-8	3-4	2
Sport-specific drills				
Acceleration	10-30	4-6	2	2-3
Deceleration	10-20	4-6	2	2
Stop and go	10-20	4-8	2	2-2
Acceleration or direction changes	10-30	4-8	2	2-3

Regardless of how far an athlete runs, skates, or swims with maximum speed, special sessions of speed training should be organized that incorporate elements of maximum acceleration and maximum speed. These types of training programs improve both acceleration and speed.

Other Nonspecific Training Methods

Originally, the nonspecific speed training methods were borrowed from track and field, but they were adjusted to the needs of a particular sport, and performed in three forms: accelerate from standing or walking to reach maximum speed, maintain maximum speed for a desired distance, and decelerate from maximum speed into walking or standing.

Maximum speed is always achieved after a previous acceleration. The more vigorous the athletes' acceleration, the more effective is their maximum speed. The purpose of training maximum speed is for your athletes to be faster than their opponents.

■ *Maximum acceleration* is the capacity to quickly move in the desired direction. It is not just a game necessity to be fast from a stationary position or walking; it often can have a tactical benefit to quickly explode away from an opponent toward a specific place to receive the ball.

■ *Increase arm drive and frequency.* To maximize speed or perform a speed break, athletes should emphasize a powerful arm drive, back and forth, in the direction of the run. As the arm drives forward quickly, it stimulates a subsequent knee drive of the opposite leg in the same direction. **Always remember: Arm drive dictates the leg frequency**. Do you want to increase leg frequency? You must first increase the force of arm drive and its frequency.

■ *Repetitions for improving maximum acceleration* must be performed from different positions, such as standing, walking, and backpedaling. For variety, you can use maximum acceleration drills by combining them with running in various directions (e.g., zigzag, slalom, sideways) or even combining them with specific action. Your imagination is the only limit. Acceleration drills can be repeated for 30 to 90 or more feet (10-30+ m), repeating the same action 6 to 8 times for U12-U15 athletes and 8 to 12 times for U19-U23 athletes. A rest interval of 3 to 4 minutes should include relaxation and easy stretching to maintain muscle elasticity.

For training maximum speed, you can also use the following training methods:

- *Handicap method.* This method of speed development allows athletes of different abilities to work together, provided they have similar training goals and levels of motivation. Before each repetition is performed, athletes are staggered depending on their speed potential to ensure that everyone reaches the finish line at approximately the same time.

- *Relays.* This method can be used extensively to improve speed, quickness, and agility, especially during the preparatory phase. This injection of fun into training not only breaks the monotony but also gives athletes needed variety during high-intensity training.

- *Anticipation practice.* Being a step ahead of the opponent always provides a huge advantage. The ability to read the game effectively and to anticipate what the opponent is going to do allows athletes to react and get into position quickly. Anticipation speed relies heavily on experiences, which allow athletes to quickly identify familiar signals and game cues that provide hints for how to respond quickly and most effectively. Experienced athletes have been there before; they have seen similar movements and actions executed in similar situations in previous games. It is also important to expose athletes to model training methodology, where all possible tactical situations are carried out in practice. Drills that attempt to replicate specific game situations enable athletes to improve their ability to anticipate the actions of opponents in similar situations in real games.

- *Decision-making practice.* The ability to make quick decisions is critical for all athletes. The faster the game, the shorter the time available to make decisions; therefore, the more important decision-making speed becomes. Athletes in team sports are exposed to a wide variety of stimuli, such as athlete movement and ball or puck movement. With all these stimuli to contend with, athletes must be always alert and attentive to be able to read the game effectively and to respond accordingly in a short period. As with anticipation speed, experience can have an enormous effect on enhancing decision-making speed and reducing decision-making times. Similarly, using the methodology of model training during practice brings the games to the athletes before they occur, preparing them for similar situations when they arise in an athletic contest.

Keep in mind that you do not need to use all forms of training in the same session. Because of its demanding characteristics, maximum speed is usually trained separately from other types of training, along with tactical training. However, if the number of repetitions is high, your athletes may also accumulate lactic acid. Therefore, be aware of the rest interval you prescribe for them and time it.

The suggestions outlined in table 10.1 may also be modified as follows:

- One or two days a week: Maximum-acceleration sprints, maximum-speed training, and acceleration with changes of direction
- Two days a week: Acceleration–deceleration and stop-and-go sprints

Speed training can be extremely taxing both mentally and physically, so it is important to monitor the amount and type of training used during each training session. A general guideline would be to incorporate two to four types of training for each session, two or three times a week, depending on the athletes' skill level and growth potential. The balance of training should focus on technical and tactical work.

Notice the suggested number of speed sessions a week in table 10.1. You can plan several of the suggested forms of training for the same day, setting aside only two or three days of highly taxing maximum-speed training each week. By using the concept of alternating energy systems in training, your athletes will be able to cope more effectively with the fatigue induced by high-intensity training.

REACTION- AND MOVEMENT-TIME TRAINING

The importance of reaction and movement speed is evident in all team sports. Various physiological processes are involved from the time the stimulus is observed, heard, or felt until the movement is initiated. The sensory organs must be aroused, the nerves must conduct the impulse to the brain (where decisions are made) and from the brain to the muscles, and the muscles must contract before an overt movement can begin. These processes involve time, and together they constitute reaction speed.

Components of Reaction Time

You can use different types of stimuli to improve reaction time training, including the following:

1. The appearance of a stimulus at the receptor level (visual, auditory, tactile)
2. The propagation of the stimulus to the central nervous system (CNS; afferent or sensory transmission)
3. The decision-making process in the CNS
4. The transmission of the signal from the CNS through nervous pathways to the muscle (efferent or motor transmission)
5. The stimulation of the muscle to contract and perform the movement

Common Types of Reaction Time

Goalkeepers, defenders, and offensive players must respond quickly to numerous stimuli throughout a game. Athletes are sometimes faced with a single stimulus, such as reacting to a dropped puck during a face-off in hockey or a jump ball in basketball. This describes a simple reaction-time or -speed situation. Simple reaction is thus a conscious response to a previously known stimulus performed unexpectedly (e.g., known movement or signal of a teammate, ball, or puck). These simple reaction-speed situations do not occur frequently in team sports because of the complex dynamics and interplay among athletes:

- *Choice reaction time or speed.* In most game situations, athletes encounter several stimuli or game-specific conditions, and they must choose from among them. Consider a football quarterback who must spot an open receiver and then begin the throwing action. This scenario describes a choice reaction-time or -speed situation because many possibilities for action are available to the quarterback. Depending on how the play unfolds, the quarterback may choose to throw to any one of the possible receivers or may even decide to run with the ball. How about a soccer goalkeeper who must defend against a shot on goal? He must contend with numerous stimulus–response alternatives regarding the speed, direction, and spin of the ball before responding appropriately.

- *Reaction time or speed.* When only one stimulus and one response are involved, reaction time is the fastest. As the number of possible alternative movements increases, a gradual increase occurs in the time required to respond to any one of them (an increase in choice reaction time). Thus, these situations provide you with information about the different decision-making processes in the nervous system of the brain.

- *Reflex time or speed.* Reaction speed, which reflects consciously controlled movements based on sensory information, must be clearly distinguished from reflex time or speed, which refers to stereotyped, involuntary rapid responses to stimuli that involve little or no conscious control; the knee-jerk reaction is a prime example. For example, when the body or limb of an athlete is subjected to unanticipated outside forces, such as body contact on a drive to the basket in basketball, modifications to control body or limb position in the air occur automatically to allow the athlete to get the shot off despite the contact. Similarly, when offensive linemen in American football encounter sudden external forces applied by opponents, the muscles and limbs of the linemen automatically adjust to the force with an appropriate amount of resistance. Sometimes these seemingly automatic responses can also be modified through conscious perceptions of sensory information (perhaps seeing a linebacker approaching from the outside) or because of learned responses that become automatic over time.

Developing Reaction and Movement Time

Possessing fast reaction time offers a great advantage for athletes in most team sports. Although the ability to react quickly is inherited at least to some degree, the good news is that it can be improved with proper training.

Reaction time to a visual stimulus, such as a ball in motion, is shorter for trained individuals (0.15-0.20 sec) than for untrained individuals (0.25-0.35 sec). This time is even shorter for elite athletes (Canadian Hockey Association, 1995). Several other sources indicate that reaction time to an auditory stimulus, such as a starting gun, is slightly shorter at 0.17 to 0.27 seconds for untrained individuals and 0.05 to 0.07 seconds for world-class athletes. Pain and Hibbs (2007) concurred with this conclusion, while Tonnessen and colleagues (2013) reported that top sprinters react extremely quickly to the sound of the starting gun (0.142 sec for male sprinters and 0.153 sec for female sprinters).

Improving reaction time depends largely on how well athletes understand the drills and exercises as well as how motivated and focused they are to perform the specific tasks. If an athlete's concentration is directed toward the drill to be performed rather than on how fast she hears the signal, reaction speed will be much faster. Reaction time is also faster if the athlete slightly preloads (contracts before stimulus) the relevant muscles.

Drills for reaction and movement time can be performed at the beginning of a training session when athletes are fresh. At least occasionally, however, these drills should be performed under conditions of fatigue to prepare athletes for similar conditions that arise during the later stages of a game. Use your imagination to create new and interesting drills to prevent monotony and boredom in training.

Audiovisual Training

The audiovisual training method is based on the relationship between reaction time and the ability to distinguish minor lapses (micro intervals) of one-tenth of a second. It is assumed that those who can perceive small time differences between various repetitions will develop good reaction time.

The standard training method involves repetitions in which the athlete reacts to both auditory and visual signals, such as a whistle, hand clapping, or any stimulating sound. Consider the following examples:

1. *Drill 1*: The athlete runs, swims, or skates backward toward the coach. At the coach's signal, the athlete turns to face the coach, who uses an arm to indicate the direction in which the athlete must move as quickly as possible.

2. *Drill 2*: The athlete runs backward toward the coach. At the coach's signal, the athlete turns to face the coach, who throws a ball—in a different direction each time—that the athlete must quickly control.

3. *Drill 3*: The coach stands to one side of the goal. The athlete backpedals or shuffles sideways away from the coach. At the sound of the whistle, the coach passes a ball in a given direction, forcing the athlete to change direction quickly, control the ball, and shoot on goal. The athlete can also be given the intermediate task of controlling the ball while running around a cone before shooting to score.

4. *Drill 4*: The athlete performs a reaction drill from lying on the field, court, or ice in various positions. At the coach's signal, the athlete stands up as quickly as possible and performs the action or task the coach previously indicated. Alternatively, the coach has two athletes push each other with equal resistance. At the coach's signal, they must perform a predetermined technical or reaction drill. Combine this exercise with various ball actions while slaloming between cones, zigzagging, and so on.

5. *Drill 5*: The athlete moves in a specified direction. At the coach's signal, the athlete performs a reaction or technical task. If shooting or attacking is involved, the coach will indicate at which part of the goal or court to shoot or attack.

Reaction-Ball Training

Because of its shape and bumpy texture, a reaction or agility ball (figure 10.1) thrown against the floor or wall always bounces in an unpredictable direction, so it challenges athletes to quickly react and catch. In addition to the traditional drills used to train movement time or speed for goaltenders and other athletes, a reaction ball is useful for improving agility and performing the following exercises:

- *Drill 1*: Athletes throw the ball against the wall and catch it as quickly as possible.
- *Drill 2*: Same as drill 1, but athletes kick or hit the ball in a predetermined direction.
- *Drill 3*: Athletes stand around 10 feet (3 or 4 m) away from a wall. They throw the ball against the floor and wall and try to catch it as quickly as it rebounds off the wall.
- *Drill 4*: Same as drill 3, but athletes use a foot to stop and control the ball.
- *Drill 5*: The coach throws the ball onto the floor and has two to four athletes battle to gain control of the ball with their arms, legs, or sticks.

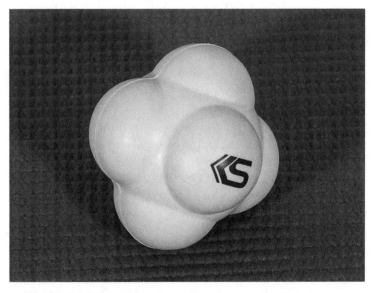

Figure 10.1 A reaction or agility ball.

- *Drill 6*: Throw the ball against the wall, let it bounce, and have two to four athletes battle to gain control of the ball and immediately attempt to throw it at a given target.
- *Drill 7*: The coach distracts the athlete's concentration (e.g., points to the ceiling), then quickly throws the ball in a given direction. The athlete has to gain control of the ball and throw or shoot toward a predetermined goal.

PRINCIPLES OF RUNNING TECHNIQUE

For practical purposes, speed training for team sports has three phases:

1. Acceleration
2. Maximum speed
3. Deceleration (into walking and rest)

During acceleration (30-45 ft; 10-15 m), athletes must reach maximum speed progressively and very quickly. After that point, athletes have to maintain maximum speed for the duration of the drill.

To achieve maximum speed, the ankles, hips, and knees must be fully extended; full knee extension can be achieved only if the quadriceps muscles are very strong. This triple joint extension demonstrates not only good leg, hip, and core power but also optimal technique. A strong body leads to good form, and good form leads to faster performances.

Although sprinting in track and field may differ from sprinting in team sports, the general mechanics of running are the same. Athletes in team sports are not always the most effective runners because training for team sports seldom works on the correct mechanics of running. As a result, many athletes use inefficient running technique.

Components of Effective Running Technique

To improve running efficiency, athletes should constantly be aware of correct running form. For example, a strong arm drive and leg driving frequency are crucial for achieving optimal running technique.

The thigh of the driving leg (the left leg in figure 10.2) should swing up to the horizontal; from this point, the foot of the same leg is projected forward and downward, toward the ground. The position of the body remains vertical, and the eyes focus ahead as the ball of the foot contacts the ground with a brushing action. The foot strikes the ground quickly, coming underneath the body as the body moves forward. While the body moves forward, the other leg (right) is driven forward; the left leg now pushes against the ground, projecting the body forward.

These actions are repeated if the sprint lasts in an unbroken, rhythmic cycle. During this cycle, both legs have alternately supportive and driving functions, while the rhythmic movements of the bent arms assist the stride rhythm.

The height of the center of gravity (COG) changes constantly for athletes in team sports depending on their pattern of movement. When an athlete decelerates and then accelerates in another direction, the COG lowers progressively during deceleration (the lowest point occurring when the athlete stops), while the COG rises progressively during acceleration (the highest point occurring during maximum acceleration). The COG will also adjust sideways, forward, and backward depending on the athlete's running pattern.

Team sports tend to be very dynamic and interactive. Therefore, athletes rarely run with a pure sprinting style except in situations where they run in a relatively straight line or along a slightly curvilinear path.

When analyzing running technique, look for the following components:

■ During maximum-speed sprinting, athletes should run on the balls and toes of the feet.

■ The contact phase of the supporting leg remains as short as possible. Prolonging the contact phase demonstrates a lack of power and reactivity. The fastest athletes generally have a contact phase lasting between 180 and 210 milliseconds. Elite sprinters come closer to 90 to 120 milliseconds (Bompa and Francis, 1995; Weyand et al., 2000; Udofa et al., 2017; Pandy et al., 2021).

■ The torso remains erect.

■ The hand of the driving arm lifts to the level of the face.

■ The shoulder and facial muscles are relaxed. Any tension of these muscles reflects unnecessary contraction, rigidity, and energy expenditure.

■ The hips are high to demonstrate that the propulsion (push-off) leg is fully extended. If they are not visibly high, the push-off leg did not complete the forceful action that is necessary during maximum speed.

Remember that an athlete achieves maximum speed only after accelerating for at least 30 feet (10 m). To reach maximum velocity, athletes must react quickly and apply maximum force against the ground to achieve a strong push-off. Stronger athletes achieve their maximum speed faster than their weaker counterparts.

Phases of Running

Proper running technique contains the following four phases:

1. *Propulsion phase*: The athlete pushes against the ground powerfully to drive the body forward quickly (see figure 10.2). To increase the propulsion (also called push-off) phase of the running step, you must increase the strength of the triple extensor muscles (calf, knee, and hip extensors). Compared to other muscles, the gastrocnemius and soleus contribute more than 50 percent to athletes' maximum speed, the quadriceps group contributes 18 percent, and the hamstrings and gluteus maximus contribute the balance of 32 percent. Together, all these muscles apply a force that is equivalent to three to five times the athlete's body weight (Sasaki and Neptune, 2006; Hemner et al., 2010).

2. *Drive phase*: The nonsupporting leg drives forward, with the thigh swinging up almost parallel to the ground. The forward-swinging arm also drives along the body; the hand is at shoulder height (arms remain bent at 90 degrees). Keep in mind that the frequency of leg movement directly depends on the frequency of the arm drive. (This concept does not apply on some artificial, fake drills, such as fast running on the spot). In addition, the more powerful and quicker the application of force against the ground (complete plantar flexion), the higher the maximum velocity.

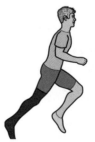

Figure 10.2 The propulsion (push-off) phase of the running step.

3. *Landing phase*: As the foot (or ball of the foot) strikes the ground, it quickly moves underneath the body in an action similar to a brushing of the ball of the foot on the ground surface. It is essential to keep the ankle locked stiff during the landing phase. Ankle stiffness, in particular, and leg stiffness, in general, are essential to sprinting ability (or the ability to resist to give to the force of gravity). To ensure that the calf muscles do not collapse at the instant of landing (when the ball of the foot touches the ground), you have to strengthen the reactive force of those muscles via MxS training. The best analogy to describe leg and vertical stiffness is a bouncing ball. When a well-inflated ball hits the ground, the ball immediately reacts and bounces upward. This is similar to leg spring when the foot hits the ground and reacts when running.

If the heel touches the ground, it is a sign of weak calf or leg muscles. If the calf and leg muscles are not strong enough to keep the ankle stiff during landing, it means a prolongation of the duration of the contact phase. Longer duration of the contact phase always slows down the speed of the athlete (Rumpf et al., 2015; Meyers et al., 2019). Therefore, calf stiffness increases as a result of MxS training. If you neglect to develop MxS, your athletes will need a miracle to increase leg stiffness, to shorten ground reaction, and, as a consequence, to become a fast sprinter. High vertical stiffness differentiates elite sprinters from lesser performing athletes (Meyers et al., 2019; Struzik et al., 2021). Elite sprinting with increased calf stiffness is proportional to the MxS of the gastrocnemius, soleus, and tibialis anterior. Remember that the landing action is performed eccentrically by the calf muscles, whereas the reactive action (push-off, jumps) is done by the same muscles but concentrically.

4. *Recovery phase*: As the heel of the driving leg moves toward the buttocks, the opposing arm is quickly driven forward. Maximum speed is achieved not only by the propulsion force but also by the quickness of contraction of the knee flexors of the recovery leg (hamstring muscles). Hamstring muscles have an important contribution for the forward ground reaction (Morin et al., 2015; Rumpf et al., 2015; Pandy et al., 2021). These muscles also have a higher innervation per square centimeter than the quadriceps muscles (Enoka, 2015). That proportion is why hamstrings tend to have high reactivity and speed of contraction and, as such, higher incidents of injuries, mostly at the upper junction of the hamstrings. Therefore, if you want to decrease the likelihood of injury to the hamstrings, you should increase their strength. An efficient exercise is the reverse leg press. This exercise effectively targets the upper part of the hamstring muscles. The quickness of an athlete relies not only on the force of the propulsion phase but also the quickness of knee flexion (the recovery phase of the running step) through the improved strength of the hamstrings. Strength of the gluteal sulcus, or fold (the junction where the upper hamstrings meet the gluteal muscles), is essential for the so-called pawing or brushing phase of the running step. Most injuries to the hamstrings are localized near the upper hamstrings at the muscle–tendon junction. The reverse leg press is a more effective exercise than the leg curl for strengthening the upper hamstrings.

TRADITIONAL SPEED TRAINING VERSUS MxS

In many aspects of speed training some traditions are still visible. Many coaches, from swimming to track and many team sports, are still repeating many short sprints in the hope of increasing athletes' maximum speed. However, science and methodology are telling us that best improvements in athletes' speed are directly dependent on propulsion force (see figure 10.3), leg stiffness, duration of contact phase with good running form (see figure 10.4), and muscle reactivity. All these abilities are directly depending on MxS. If you do not train it, how do you expect to produce faster athletes? Specific training improves your performance a lot. MxS takes it beyond that.

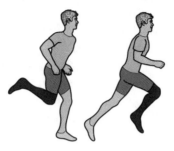

Figure 10.3 The landing (left) and the transition from landing toward the propulsion phase (right) of the running step. Note that the heel of the foot does not touch the ground.

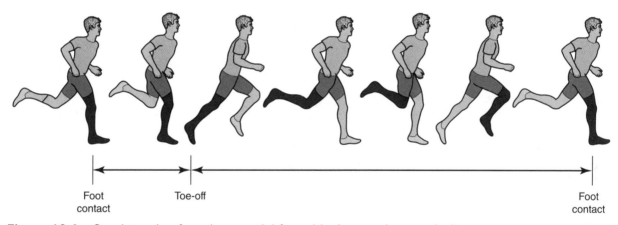

Foot contact   Toe-off   Foot contact

Figure 10.4 Good running form is essential for achieving maximum velocity.

PERIODIZATION OF SPEED TRAINING

The periodization of speed training depends on the characteristics of the sport, the athletes' performance levels, and the game schedule. Table 10.2 provides a general guideline for the periodization of speed training in team sports.

Annual Plan

Sport-specific methods and drills are essential for developing sport-specific speed and for refining related abilities, such as agility and speed of reaction. During the competitive phase, training intensity increases as you introduce more specific training methods and as more games are played. Although exercises specific to the sport are prevalent, you should also incorporate general training such as games for fun, relaxation, and active rest. Maintaining a balance between these two exercise categories lowers training stress and strain. Many athletes in team sports are prone to injuries because of high-intensity training. Therefore, alternating various means and intensities of training is both a deterrent to eventual training problems and an important methodological requirement.

Planning a Microcycle

Table 10.3 presents an example of a microcycle (week) of training for speed combined with technical and tactical training. When planning these types of training sessions, it is important to alternate the energy systems on different days and to include days for recovery and regeneration. In other words, to ensure an optimal training and recovery schedule, only one of the three major energy systems should be trained on any given day.

Long-Term Periodization

Development of all physical attributes needed for training in team sports, including speed training, should also evolve progressively. Long-term speed training should be viewed as a constant progression from U12 to U23. This progression is outlined in table 10.4.

Table 10.2 Guideline for Periodization of Speed Training—Annual Plan*

Preparatory phase			Competitive phase		Transition phase
General preparatory	Specific preparatory		Exhibition games	League games	Transition
2-3 wk	2-6 wk		2 wk	Entire duration of league games	4 wk
Nonspecific aerobic and anaerobic endurance	All 3 energy systems, with and without the ball/puck (if applicable)	Sport-specific speed Alactic and lactic endurance Agility Reaction time Speed endurance	Sport-specific speed Alactic and lactic endurance Agility Sport-specific endurance (ergogenesis)	Sport-specific speed (ergogenesis) Agility Reaction time	Other activities

*Duration of the plan depends on the calendar of competitions or games.

Table 10.3 Sample Microcycle for Athletes of Team Sports Combining Technical and Tactical Training

Monday	Tuesday	Wednesday	Thursday	Friday	Saturday	Sunday
Warm-up	Warm-up	Warm-up	Off	Warm-up	Warm-up	Off
TA drills	TA drills with direction changes, stop and go: 8-10 reps × 30 m	T drills		T/TA drills for speed and agility: 12 reps × 30 m	Acceleration with turns and direction changes: 6 reps × 30 m	
Acceleration–deceleration: 10 reps × 30 m	Scrimmage	Maximum acceleration: 6 reps × 15 m 6 reps × 30 m		RI = 4 min	Acceleration–deceleration: 8 reps × 30 m	
T drills with turns/direction changes: 12 reps × 30 m		RI = 2 min		T/TA drills with turns, stop and go: 8-10 reps × 1 min	Stop and go: 10 reps × 15 m	
Scrimmage		TA drills: 8 reps × 1 min		Scrimmage	RI = 2 min	
RI = 2 min		RI = 2 min		Power training		
Power training		Power training				

T = Technical; TA = Tactical; m= meters, RI = rest interval.

Table 10.4 Progression for Development of Speed for U12 to U23 Athletes

Stage of development	U12	U15	U17	U19	U21-U23
Energy system	Oxidative (aerobic), phosphagen (alactic, ATP-CP)	All three energy systems	All three energy systems	All three energy systems	All three energy systems
Types of training	Learning all types of running skills; specific and nonspecific	All forms of alactic accelerations; Alactic maximum speed	All forms of maximum acceleration/deceleration	All forms of maximum acceleration/deceleration with increased intensity	All forms of maximum acceleration/deceleration with further increased intensity

For a better comprehension of long-term speed training, consider the following information for each age group:

U12

- Teach children the technique and form of every type of running used in your sport.
- In the early parts of training, use lower-intensity speed, predominantly taxing the oxidative (aerobic) energy system.
- Progressively introduce simple technical drills with higher speed but short duration (6-12 sec).

SPEED TRAINING

When conducting speed training, you can use a variety of diagrams and represent all possible positions an athlete experiences during a game. Figure 10.5 depicts some of the common symbols used to represent various movements incorpo- rated into speed and quickness drills. Many possibilities exist for developing speed and quickness drills, especially because they can be performed with or without a ball or puck and can be designed to be specific to the sport and position.

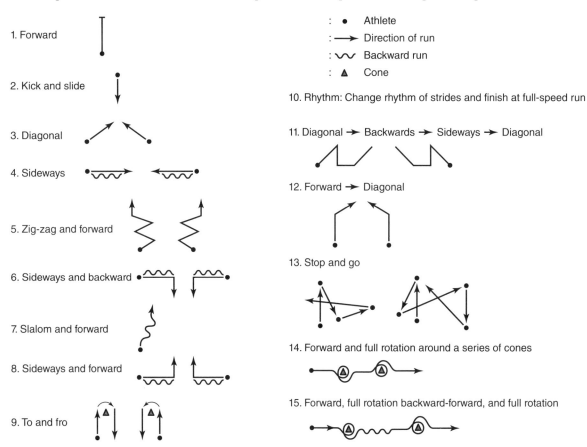

Figure 10.5 Selected running or skating patterns for developing specific speed. Running or skating may be initiated from standing, kneeling, or lying down, or from any other position an athlete may experience during a game. Use markers on the floor, field, or arena to suggest your selected pattern.

- Introduce children to simple, nonspecific running drills.
- Remember, U12 children can tolerate oxidative (aerobic) types of activities (slightly longer duration but with low intensity) and faster drills but of short duration, 6 to 12 seconds (phosphagen system).
- U12 athletes have a difficult time tolerating high-speed drills, 30 to 90 seconds (gly-colytic system). These athletes are not yet adapted to high-intensity work fueled by the lactic acid system; if you decide to use these drills with this age group, slowly introduce the drills and have patience with athletes as they build their stamina.
- Always allow children regular rest intervals in order to rest and rehydrate.

U15

- Continue to stress good running form in all directions.
- Use technical and simple tactical combinations with high speed (6-12 sec).
- Introduce more complex running drills; add changes of direction, acceleration–deceleration, stop and go, all possible situations encountered during a game, and so on.
- Expose children to a reduced number of repetitions of tactical drills taxing the lactic acid system: 20 to 30 seconds, but with longer rest intervals (2-3 min).
- Expand nonspecific speed training to ensure improvement of maximum acceleration and maximum speed.
- Hydration should be a constant concern.

U17-U19

- While maintaining high-quality work for technical and tactical training, taxing the oxidative and phosphagen systems, start exposing athletes to increased training demand: 20 to 90 seconds (glycolytic system).
- Create complex tactical drills with constant concern for higher velocity.
- Continue nonspecific training methods to improve maximum acceleration and maximum speed.

U21-U23

- Emphasize technical and tactical drills with maximum velocity, taxing all three energy systems.
- Focus extensively on drills taxing the phosphagen and glycolytic energy systems. These types of training will improve the quality of the game.
- Create tactical drills of longer duration (2-3 min), taxing the oxidative system.

Remember the following:

- Always observe good technique based on principles of biomechanics.
- Strength training is essential to the improvement of speed. Pay attention to long-term strength development, including the needs for developing torso (core) strength (abdominal, intervertebral, and lumbar muscles) before starting to lift heavy weights. These muscles ensure good body stability and support for many exercises.
- Beware of programs, exercises, and equipment based on unproven theories; use only those that are based on sound scientific research.

SPEED TRAINING: WHAT WORKS AND WHAT DOES NOT

Many drills and pieces of equipment are advertised as improving speed, but they often are ineffective. Examples include the following:

- *Fast running on the spot.* This drill does not improve speed. Increased velocity is achieved by improving force; it is not achieved with more rapid leg movement (Weyand et al., 2000; Clark and Weyand, 2014; Seitz et al., 2014). Fast running on the spot is the result of good leg muscle coordination, when muscles learn to work together quite efficiently. The claim that fast running on the spot increases speed or leg frequency is false. Leg frequency relies on the ability of the calf muscles to push forcefully and quickly against gravity.

- *Stride length.* Some coaches use markers on the ground to force athletes to increase stride length. However, stride length depends on the push-off force of calf muscles and not on jumping over artificial markers.

- *Stride height.* Some coaches use low hurdles for athletes to stride over them. They create the impression that this routine will increase the height of the stride and increase speed. However, stride height is far from being a determinant factor in improving speed. On the contrary, higher stride means prolonging the time necessary to complete a stride, consequently reducing speed.

- *Speed sled.* This exercise is promoted as a training method for the development of power and speed. For athletes to pull forward a sled loaded with heavy weight, they must overcome drag, a long duration of friction of the sled on the ground. The heavier the load, the higher the drag, and, as a result, the longer the duration of the leg–ground contact. By now you know that long duration of the contact phase is far from increasing speed; on the contrary, it decreases speed. *Improvement of speed is best achieved by using the MxS method.* Speed sled is not conducive to the development of speed that requires fast application of power, because the pull forward is slow, with a long duration of the contact phase. Quickness and high velocity are possible only when the duration of the contact phase is very short and the power application against the ground is very high. However, heavily loaded sleds may have some benefits in the early part of the preparatory phase, during the anatomical adaptation (AA) subphase. In addition, the speed sled can be used as a method to strengthen the Achilles tendon and to enlarge the size of this tendon's attachment on the calcaneus (heel bone). A sled loaded with lower loads can also be used as an interval-training method to develop glycolytic endurance (anaerobic or lactic energy system).

- *Speed training against elastic bands placed on the thigh.* It is a myth that the bands will increase the speed by recruitment of the FT muscle fibers. In addition, the following technical errors demonstrate the incomplete biomechanical and physiological knowledge of those who promote and those who use this technique.

  - *Technical error #1:* The band placed on the thighs is far too weak, and the resistance is very low to stimulate the recruitment of FT fibers. To generate high velocity, an athlete has to apply heavy loads very quickly; the bands do not provide enough resistance.

  - *Technical error #2:* The position of the band on the body (on the mid-thigh) is wrongly placed. The only muscle benefiting from this exercise is the iliopsoas, a small muscle of the hips that lifts the knees up by flexing the hip. This muscle has nothing to do with speed development; uplifting the knees is not a limiting factor for the improvement of speed. In addition, lifting the knees up to hip level is far from being a training challenge. If you want to increase speed, you have to direct the exercise to recruit the calf muscles, gastrocnemius, and soleus, not the iliopsoas. This approach is consistent with MxS methodology.

- *Lateral speed.* Lateral speed drills to improve speed are yet another myth. In several team sports (basketball, handball, volleyball, lacrosse, field hockey), quick lateral moves are used during both defensive and offensive tactical actions. The intention of lateral speed exercises is to increase the strength of the legs to move faster laterally during competition. An elastic cord is placed above the knees of both legs with the intention of applying force against the cord and stretching it to improve leg strength. The lead leg initiates the lateral motion while the trail leg (the push-off leg) exerts the propulsion force against the ground to move laterally. Unfortunately, proponents of this misjudge the role and activity of the two legs. During a lateral action, the lead leg does not encounter any resistance; it simply moves through the air. To move sideways, the push-off leg, not the lead leg, has the determinant role. This leg is the engine of lateral moves since it must overcome gravity and the athlete's own body weight. In other words, this exercise loads the wrong leg. To increase the force of the push-off leg, increase the strength of the triple extensor muscles instead.

CONCLUSION

Speed is a highly regarded athletic ability in both individual and team sports. Quickness and reactivity are also determinant factors in martial arts, racket, and contact sports. Have you seen lately how aggressive and fast Nordic skiing is? Incredible! This is also a form of speed, particularly the skating style of Nordic skiing, but for longer distances. Yet, these athletes can still benefit from strength training.

Many tactical maneuvers in team and racket sports heavily rely on quick action and reactions during the game. However, as mentioned in this chapter, improvements in speed come from good skills, but also from good and effective improvements in MxS. Sports are very complex activities, so ensure that your training plans also address the complexity of training all physical abilities.

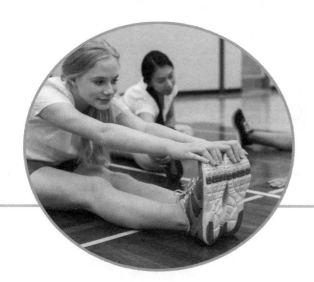

chapter 11

Training Methods to Develop Agility and Flexibility

Most information in this book is presented in condensed form. Agility and flexibility are presented together in this chapter because there is a close relationship between agility and flexibility in the ankles, knees, and hips. If, for instance, ankle flexibility is inadequate, the effectiveness of agility drills that involve the ankle may not be performed as efficiently as possible. A similar situation may happen in the case of the Achilles tendon. If the tendon is rigid, it may affect the mobility of the ankle that, in turn, might restrict a proper execution of some agility drills involving this joint.

AGILITY TRAINING

Traditionally, agility is viewed as the ability to swiftly accelerate and decelerate movement, quickly change direction, and rapidly vary movement patterns. High-frequency footwork or quick feet, speed of reaction, dynamic flexibility, and the rhythm of timing of athletes' movements are important intrinsic elements of agility. It is important to recognize that agility does not exist independently as an ability; rather, it relies on the development of a host of other abilities, where power is determinant.

To better understand what high-frequency footwork means, watch how quickly basketball and handball players move their legs on defense to stay in front of the opponents they are guarding. Their legs are always moving—and moving quickly—to be ready to react to any game situation that will arise. Quickness, quick feet, and high-frequency footwork depend directly on the power of the calf muscles.

THE RELATIONSHIP BETWEEN QUICKNESS AND POWER

A high level of quickness and agility can be developed by improving the strength of the major leg muscles (gastrocnemius, soleus, and tibialis anterior) and major thigh muscles (quadriceps). Nobody can be fast, be agile, or have quick feet with insufficient strength. Many coaches view agility as evolving from speed. However, they should remember that speed itself depends directly on athletes' leg power. Therefore, one can certainly say that only a powerful athlete can be a fast athlete. This concept also applies to agility: Only powerful athletes can be agile.

Deceleration–Acceleration: The Key to Agility and Quickness Training

To rapidly change directions during a game, athletes must first slow down (decelerate) before moving quickly in another direction (accelerate). In other words, the action is performed in two phases:

1. *Deceleration phase*: This phase, where the athlete slows down almost to a stop, results from the eccentric loading (lengthening) of the quadriceps muscles.

2. *Acceleration phase*: In this phase, elastic energy stored in the muscles during deceleration is then used so that the athlete can begin to run quickly again. The ability to rapidly change directions relies on two main muscle groups: the calf muscles (gastrocnemius and soleus) and the muscles on the front of the thighs (quadriceps). During the deceleration phase, the quadriceps muscles contract eccentrically (lengthen); during acceleration, they perform a **concentric contraction** (shorten) along with the gastrocnemius and soleus.

Therefore, the ability to decelerate and accelerate quickly relies heavily on the ability of these muscles to contract powerfully, both eccentrically and concentrically. Deceleration appears to be the determinant and limiting factor for agility. If power is not trained adequately, deceleration–acceleration coupling will be slow. All actions requiring agility or quick feet rely on leg power. In order to defend against offensive opponents, you need strong legs. At the same time, to elude a defender you need to rely on two elements: a skillful first step and a strong push-off against the ground. They are described as follows:

3. *Technique of the first step*: Performing the first step quickly depends on how quickly the athlete moves the opposite arm. For example, if an athlete initiates a forward step or crossover with the left leg, the quickness of that step will depend on how fast the athlete moves the right arm forward. In both sprinting and agility runs, the arms and legs should move in perfect alternating synchrony and coordination. The arm–leg coupling is performed in the following sequence: (a) the arm action and (b) the leg reaction. The second part is a *re*action because it reacts to the arm motion. However, the interval between the arm action and the leg reaction is just a fraction of a second.

4. *Force applied against the ground*: The stronger the push-off against the ground, the more powerful the ground reaction works in the opposite direction. As the eccentric action is performed (flexion of ankle, knees, and hips), the leg muscles are loaded eccentrically. The explosiveness of the push-off (propulsion phase) during the first step depends on the amount of force load during the eccentric muscle action. The higher the eccentric loading, the more explosive the propulsion.

AGILITY LADDERS

Agility ladders are used to train agility in athletes aged 6 years to adulthood and beyond. Perhaps because it is a common modality, people rarely question how effective this exercise is. Teenagers can improve agility by learning the technical aspects of a drill, from repeating various exercises used on agility ladders, but what about mature athletes?

Do you think that agility for mature athletes can be improved by the types of training discussed above? It certainly can, but the road to the highest level of agility can be found in constantly improving strength and power (Sonoda et al., 2018; Hornikova and Zemkova, 2020).

Guidelines for Agility Training

For best results in your quest to improve agility, you should consider the following suggestions.

Maintain Intensity and Movement Quality

Athletes must perform most (if not all) agility and quickness exercises at a very high intensity (90%-95%). At a much lower intensity you may be training something, but it isn't agility. The quality of agility exercises is very much dependent on the neural responses and reactivity of the neuromuscular system, and elevated intensity levels tax that system. Therefore, this type of training is often referred to as **neuromuscular training**. The ability of the central nervous system (CNS) to send fast, powerful, and high-frequency impulses to the fast-twitch (FT) muscle fibers involved in performing agility exercises directly influences the discharge rate of FT fibers. To improve your athletes' agility and quickness, apply agility drills of high intensity and high quality only.

Monitor Duration

The duration of agility exercises is dictated by the energy system being trained. Allow 4 to 12 seconds for exercises taxing the phosphagen (alactic, ATP-CP) energy system and 20 to 90 seconds for drills relying on the energy supplied by the glycolytic (lactic) system. To avoid the potentially detrimental effects of fatigue on the performance of high-intensity agility exercises, the total time per training session dedicated to agility should be between 5 and 10 minutes. When rest intervals between repetitions of a drill are also considered (often lasting 2-3 min), the total time of agility training per training session can be as high as 30 minutes. It is the coach's responsibility to gauge the progression and intensity according to athletes' background and physical potential.

Watch Foot Contact

To maximize the effect of the **myotatic stretch reflex**, foot contact with the ground should always occur on the balls of the feet. (*Myotatic stretch reflex* refers to the reflex of the muscle spindles, which causes a muscle to contract as a reaction to passive stretching.) This approach is called having light feet; it is characterized by springy actions generated by muscle elasticity. In contrast, hard landing on the soles constitutes having heavy feet. Any lengthening of the duration of the contact phase (between the foot and the ground) results in a significantly slower, sloppy movement. Therefore, athletes must perform agility exercises quickly by emphasizing light feet, maximizing the elasticity of the muscles, and reducing the duration of the contact phase.

TRADITIONS AND EFFECTIVENESS IN AGILITY TRAINING

The duration of most agility drills in soccer and other sports is 4 to 8 or 10 seconds. Yet, coaches of top soccer players comment that many of their athletes have difficulty keeping control of the ball for a longer time and that they can rapidly fatigue. Obviously, there is a contradiction between what they train and the energy demand during the game. The energy for agility drills in soccer is supplied by the phosphagen system, also called the alactic energy system. Yet, the dominant energy system in this sport is aerobic! Player fatigue is not surprising when coaches train the completely opposite energy system needed in soccer. The answer to this obvious contradiction is quite simple; train your players to fit the energy needs of the sport that they play (see more on this topic in chapter 6).

Listen to the Sound of the Step

Listening to the sound of the athlete's step provides important feedback regarding the quality of exercise. It is just as important to listen to athletes performing agility exercises as it is to watch them. A sloppy and noisy or clapping sound is an indication that the feet are landing on the sole rather than on the ball of the foot, which significantly reduces the effectiveness of performing speed, quickness, and agility drills. The quieter the contact phase with the ground, the more fluid and elastic the movement, which usually results in improved levels of power. Be aware of clapping or noisy feet, especially toward the end of a workout; it can be the first indication that athletes are experiencing neuromuscular fatigue.

Observe the Height of Step

An athlete's steps should remain as low in height as possible so that the athlete can get the foot in contact with the ground quickly for another push-off. For fastest agility actions, athletes should consider the following:

- Try to step below the height of the ankles. Upward movements are inefficient and lead to loss of time and quickness.
- Try to move as quickly as possible between the two points of the agility step (the propulsion and landing phases). The dynamic elements of movement requiring speed and quickness are in the propulsion phase; the more frequently an athlete pushes against the ground, the faster the body moves.

Examine Body Mechanics

It is important that athletes maintain the correct body posture or stance whenever possible: Feet are shoulder-width apart, feet are pointing forward, and body weight is equally distributed on both legs. The vertical projection of the center of gravity (COG) should fall within the base of support (between the feet). However, to improve dynamic body mechanics that more closely reflect game situations, some agility drills should start from an unbalanced position, where the athlete's COG falls outside the base of support.

Maximize the Power of the Push-Off (Propulsion Phase)

Although agility is often characterized by light feet, sometimes it is beneficial to have the heels of the feet in contact with the ground, such as at the start of an agility drill or when changing directions. Having the heels in contact with the ground allows for a more powerful push-off by taking advantage of the acute angle between the calf and the foot and, as a result, exerting a powerful calf muscle. If the heels are raised, propulsion power can decrease by as much as 30 percent of maximum force (Bompa, 2006). In other words, the power produced during the push-off phase is angle specific. Many athletes find it difficult to maintain this acute angle because of a lack of ankle flexibility (dorsiflexion). Unfortunately, ankle flexibility is one of the most neglected factors in sports training.

Detect Athlete Fatigue

During drills for agility and quickness training, the neuromuscular system is the first to experience fatigue as the neural reactivity of the FT muscle fibers and the effectiveness of the myotatic stretch reflex diminish.

Fatigue manifests itself in the visible deterioration of technique—when you can see athletes struggle to perform the agility drill effectively. In these situations, athletes look sloppy, and foot contact becomes noisy and of longer duration (as the heel of the foot touches the ground). These responses clearly demonstrate a high level of neuromuscular fatigue. Under these conditions, coaches should stop the drill and provide a longer rest interval (4-5 min), or terminate the training session.

Execute in an Effective Order

High-intensity training should occur immediately after the warm-up, when the CNS is still fresh, well rested, and capable to respond quickly to various stimuli. However, if the goal of a specific training session is to train quickness and reaction time under the conditions of fatigue, agility exercises should be performed toward the end of the session. Although fatigue interferes with the reactivity of the CNS, athletes can adapt progressively to high levels of fatigue and still perform fast and quick movements.

Considering this training objective, drills must remain short (5-10 sec) and must be performed as quickly as possible. This approach must be employed if athletes are expected to be as sharp, fast, and explosive as at the beginning of the game.

Periodization of Agility Training

For best athletic efficiency, agility, like all other motor abilities, has to be well planned, organized, and periodized; you should create specific training phases that lead to best adaptation and performance improvement. The periodization models seen in tables 11.1 and 11.2 may be used as adequate guidelines for you and can help you create your specific agility models for both the annual and the long-term plan. Note that in both cases, the level of strength development is essential for any substantial increase of agility. Remember the adage *Nobody can be agile before being strong* (see chapter 10).

DESIGNING THE AGILITY AND QUICKNESS COURSE

During the preparatory phase, coaches should design agility courses for each energy system starting with the MxS phase. Agility and quickness courses should be based on the energy systems:

- Phosphagen (alactic, ATP-CP): 4 to 12 seconds
- Glycolytic (lactic): 20 to 90 seconds
- Oxidative (aerobic): 2 to 3 minutes

Table 11.1 Sample Periodization of Agility and Quickness Training for an Annual Plan for U19-U23 Athletes

Preparatory		Exhibition games	League games
AA	MxS A/Q PE	P A/Q/ PE	Maintenance of A/Q

AA = anatomical adaptation; MxS = maximum strength; A/Q = agility and quickness; P = power; PE = power endurance (see chapter 10).

Table 11.2 Sample Long-Term Periodization of Agility and Quickness Training

Stage of development	U12	U15	U17	U19	U21	U23
Type of strength	AA	AA/P	AA/P; MxS (50%-60%)	MxS (60%-70%); P	MxS (60%-80%); P/PE	MxS (70%-90%); P/PE
A/Q and energy systems	A/Q: Learn simple drills; lactic energy system.	A/Q: Slightly increase the difficulty; alactic energy system; introduce simple lactic drills.	A/Q: Use difficult drills; alactic and lactic energy systems; low to medium intensity. Introduce simple aerobic drills.	A/Q: Use difficult agility drills; for the alactic and lactic acid energy systems Increase the duration of aerobic drills.	A/Q: Use all 3 energy systems; increase load; medium to high intensity.	Combine A/Q drills; use all 3 energy systems combined with plyometrics, bounding, and high athleticism.

AA = anatomical adaptation; P=power; A/Q = agility and quickness; MxS = maximum strength; PE = power endurance (see chapter 10).

Annual Plan

For maximum benefit in your athletes' progress in the area of agility and quickness, parts of your annual plan have to be dedicated to the development of strength (table 11.1). As exemplified in chapter 10, the annual plan starts with developing the foundation of strength (anatomical adaptation) followed by maximum strength (MxS). High capabilities in MxS will visibly reflect in the improvement of power as well as agility and quickness.

Long-Term Periodization

Table 11.2 sheds a better light on the progression of strength and the development of agility and quickness for long-term training. Note that strength and agility and quickness training are periodized in such a way that they ensure a clear progression throughout the stages of athletic development. While in the case of strength training, the load is suggested in percentage of one-repetition maximum (1RM), the agility and quickness drills are instead organized according to the principles of the involved energy systems and the difficulty of the drill. For instance:

- *U12:* Agility and quickness training for this stage implies simple agility drills using the phosphagen (alactic, ATP-CP) system, such as slalom running and simple steps for ladder training.
- *U15:* Slightly increase the rate and difficulty for most agility and quickness drills, using the phosphagen (alactic, ATP-CP) and glycolytic (lactic) systems.

- *U17:* Increase the difficulty of some drills by carrying a 4- to 6-pound (about 2-3 kg) medicine ball, and use medium-weight belts and vests while performing agility and quickness drills. Plan to use the phosphagen (alactic, ATP-CP) and glycolytic (lactic) systems, and introduce simple drills using the oxidative (aerobic) system.

- *U19:* Increase the loads by using belts, medicine ball (6-9 lb; 3-4 kg), and heavier vests during the agility and quickness drills. Plan agility drills involving all three energy systems.

- *U21-U23:* Use complex drills combined with plyometrics and simple tumbling to reach high athleticism; employ all three energy systems. *Improvement of athleticism* means to combine series of complex athletic exercises with power and quickness, such as bounding and different types of jumps (on and off low benches or boxes), medicine ball throws, and any other implements available in a gym.

FLEXIBILITY TRAINING

As a physical ability, **flexibility** refers to the range of motion around a joint. Good flexibility enables a person to improve the scale of athletic moves and helps prevent injuries. When training flexibility, an athlete should be mindful that flexibility of a joint must be greater than what the specific skills or athletic moves of the sport require. For instance, for a soccer athlete to be able to control a ball that is approaching at chest height with his or her foot, he or she has to be able to lift a leg up to that level. However, for optimal performance, the athlete's flexibility training goal should be to be able to easily lift a leg up *higher* than chest height (e.g., to head level).

To be successful, flexibility training should be planned in every training session; the session should begin immediately after the warm-up, when muscles are warm and ready, and it should last 5 to 10 minutes. The development of flexibility is more difficult to achieve during adulthood than in the early years of sport activities. Therefore, training to develop flexibility has to start from the childhood years of an athlete's involvement in sport. If flexibility is properly trained during childhood, the goal from this stage on is to simply maintain it. It is much easier to maintain flexibility that is well developed during childhood (U12) than after starting it at U17, especially if your athletes have also been exposed to strength training. Stronger muscles are more difficult to stretch if you begin at a later age, such as U17. You will need to spend more time overcoming flexibility deficit from what you neglected during U12-U15.

Most sports involve repetitive movements that are often through a limited range of motion, such as running or simply playing the game without any off-the-field activities. This routine can lead to muscle tightness and possibly muscle strains and tears. A careful and progressive increase in flexibility will comfortably allow the athlete to stretch the muscles, relieving tightness and helping prevent injury.

While inadequate level of flexibility development can lead to injury, so can a low level of fitness. The groin and adductor muscles do not outwardly appear to be directly engaged in running and sprinting, but soccer players need a tremendous amount of hip and groin flexibility when sliding and tackling. Thus, it is important that flexibility, like other attributes, can allow the muscles to adapt and enhance the quality and effort of play (Herbert and Gabriel, 2002; Ingraham, 2003). Flexibility needs to be multifaceted and include more than basic static stretching before a practice or game. It must be an ongoing training priority, which provides more than the necessary range of motion required by the basic skills of the sport. For instance, soccer athletes must spend time stretching their quadriceps muscles and hamstrings without neglecting their groin and adductor muscles.

In most cases, girls have better flexibility than boys, especially after puberty when boys begin to grow stronger muscles. Post puberty, the trend of sex differences continues. As girls approach adolescence, however, they seem to reach a plateau (Alaranta et al., 1994; Kohl and Cook, 2013), which might maintain or even decrease during maturity. Therefore, overall flexibility training should be a constant focus for everyone involved in sports.

Developing Flexibility

Children, particularly at the U12 level, are quite flexible. This reality tends to change during the U15-U17 years, especially in boys, presumably because of gains in strength and muscle size. For best athletic benefit, flexibility training has to be well developed throughout the stages of development of young athletes. Once an athlete achieves the desired degree of flexibility, the objective of the flexibility training program should be on maintenance throughout all stages of athletic development. This basic requirement of well-rounded development of all athletes is an athletic necessity. If neglected, athletes will quickly lose flexibility, making them more prone to injuries. Consequently, during U12 is the ideal time to start a good program to develop and maintain flexibility. In addition to overall flexibility development for all joints, specific flexibility training with a focus on ankle and hip flexibility is necessary.

Training Methodology

Athletes can perform stretching exercises in several different ways, including the following:

- *Static stretching* refers to stretching and holding the position at an acute angle for 5-10 seconds.
- *Dynamic stretching* involves bobbing or other active movements that reach the limits of motion.
- *Proprioceptive neuromuscular facilitation (PNF)* involves stretching the muscles to their limits, holding that position for 4 or 5 seconds, then stretching again to the limits. PNF can also be trained with a partner; when one athlete reaches the limit of flexibility, the partner can apply pressure to extend the degree of flexion or extension beyond that limit.

For many years, mostly during 1970-1990 particularly in the United States, most coaches and athletes preferred static stretching. In Europe, the preference was dynamic flexibility, particularly in the traditional sports of track and field and gymnastics. In more recent years, dynamic flexibility has gained recognition in the United States, and it is backed by many scientific publications (Kumar and Chakrabarty, 2010; Blackhurst et al., 2015; Stoddard, 2016). Furthermore, compared to static stretching, dynamic flexibility is regarded as more specific for preparing athletes' muscles for the dynamics of sports and games.

Periodization of Flexibility

Compared to other motor abilities, periodization of flexibility is much simpler. Therefore, this section refers only to long-term periodization. The general scope of periodization of flexibility is exemplified in table 11.3.

Long-term flexibility training (table 11.3) can be organized in two segments based on developmental stages:

1. *U12-U15*: The scope of training for this group is to develop the overall general flexibility of all joints of the body. Progressively, coaches should also start stretching the three most important joints of the body for athletes in team sports: ankles, knees, and hips.

Table 11.3 Sample Periodization of Long-Term Flexibility Training

Stages of development	U12	U15	U17-U23
Scope of flexibility training	Develop general flexibility. Introduce flexibility for ankle, knee, and hip joints.		Maintain general flexibility for upper body and arms. Emphasize sport-specific flexibility, particularly in ankle, knee, and hip joints.

2. *U17-U23*: The main scope of training during these stages of athletic development is to maintain the flexibility for the upper body and arms and to maximize specific flexibility (mostly for the ankles, knees, and hips—the most important joints for team sports performed on the ground).

CONCLUSION

Both agility and flexibility are important physical attributes that ready the athlete for the vigor and dynamism of athletic competitions. Agility helps athletes to perform quick motions with fast changes of direction, while well-trained flexibility ensures the mobility of major joints of the body, particularly the ankle, hips, and shoulders. Train them all to prevent athletic impediments.

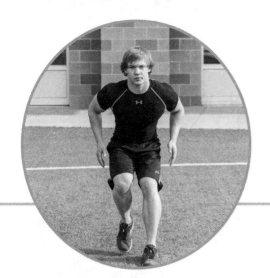

chapter 12

Training Methods to Develop Specific Endurance

For any continuous activity lasting over 2 minutes, endurance makes an important and significant contribution to athletes' performance. **Endurance** is the capacity to perform longer-duration work with a given resistance. Athletes are said to have endurance when they do not fatigue easily, or when they can cope with and continue to train or play in a state of fatigue. Athletes can perform under conditions of fatigue when they have adapted to the specifics of the work being performed.

CLASSIFICATION OF ENDURANCE

Considering the needs of training for different age groups, endurance can be classified in two basic categories:

1. *General endurance* (U12-U15) is the capacity to perform longer-duration activities that involve many muscle groups and physiological systems (neuromuscular, cardiorespiratory, and central nervous system).
2. *Specific endurance* (from U17 on), also known as *game- or sport-specific endurance*, refers to an athlete's ability to perform many repetitions of technical and tactical actions during training or competitions.

Specific endurance relies heavily on general endurance, indicating a strong relationship between the two. Every athlete needs general endurance because it helps athletes perform a high volume of work, overcome fatigue during training and competitions, and recover faster between training sessions and after games. In addition, the stronger an athlete's specific endurance, the more easily the athlete will overcome training and game stressors.

ENDURANCE AND THE ENERGY SYSTEMS

Based on the three energy systems presented in chapter 6, endurance is further classified into alactic, lactic, and aerobic endurance.

Alactic Endurance

Alactic endurance is the capacity of an athlete to repeat short-duration (5-12 sec) maximum-intensity activities or drills and to tolerate the fatigue induced by such activities. Performance relies to a great extent on strength and speed, so anaerobic processes supply up to 80 percent of the energy required for short athletic actions. The resultant high oxygen debt is repaid only during rest intervals (RIs).

Lactic Endurance

The ability to perform medium-duration work lasting 30 to 90 seconds is known as **lactic endurance**. The intensity is higher than for activities performed under the conditions of aerobic endurance (discussed in the next section), and the oxygen supply cannot totally meet the body's needs. Therefore, athletes develop an **oxygen debt** or **oxygen deficit** (the anaerobic contribution to the total energy cost of an activity), which must be repaid during rest intervals. The energy produced by the glycolytic (lactic) anaerobic energy system is proportional to the speed or pace of the activity or game. High-intensity drills that tax this system produce high amounts of lactate. If athletes are not trained to cope with the buildup of blood lactate, they must either slow down the pace of a drill or stop to recover.

Aerobic Endurance

Aerobic endurance is the capacity to perform work for a longer period and to cope with the specific fatigue induced by aerobic training. Energy is supplied mainly by the oxidative (aerobic) energy system, which involves the cardiovascular and respiratory systems. Aerobic endurance is intimately related to muscular endurance because the working muscles rely on the oxygen supply that is sent by the pumping heart, delivered through blood, and used by the muscles. Because oxygen supply is a determining factor for performance, the vital capacity of the lungs and the volume of the heart are limiting factors as well. They also reflect the athlete's adaptation to the stress of such long-lasting endurance activities.

Proper breathing technique plays an important role in endurance training. During longer periods of activity, athletes must learn to breathe deeply and rhythmically. Active inhalations and exhalations are critical for maintaining stamina for an entire workout or game. Most athletes need to learn to move as much air as possible in and out of the lungs. Of note, because oxygen will be quickly extracted from the air that is present in the lungs after it has been inhaled, incomplete exhalations of the oxygen-poor residual air will dilute the concentration of oxygen in the freshly inhaled air and performance will be adversely affected. Forceful and complete exhalations to empty the lungs of residual air and make room for oxygen-rich air are even more important during critical phases of a game when athletes are very tired.

FACTORS AFFECTING ENDURANCE

In the quest to improve team performance, it is important to be aware of several factors that may help or hinder the development of endurance. These factors are described as follows:

- *Central nervous system (CNS).* During endurance training, the CNS adapts to the specifics of training demand. As a result of training, the CNS increases its working capacity, which improves the nervous connections needed for well-coordinated functioning of the organs and systems. Fatigue, which often impairs training capacity, occurs at the CNS level. Therefore, a decrease in the working capacity of the CNS is a major cause of fatigue.

- *Athlete's willpower.* Willpower is an essential ingredient in endurance training. Athletes rely on willpower mainly when forced to perform under conditions of fatigue or when the level of fatigue increases because of prolonged training. The need for strong willpower and mental fortitude becomes even greater as intensity levels increase during training. Athletes cannot maintain required levels of intensity unless their will challenges the CNS to continue working at the same level or higher, particularly at the end of a game. Human beings possess a great capacity for endurance, which can be maximized by appealing to their will to overcome the weaknesses that often accompany fatigue.

- *Aerobic capacity.* Aerobic potential, the body's capacity to produce energy in the presence of oxygen, determines an athlete's endurance capacity. Aerobic power is limited by the ability to transport oxygen within the body. As a result, improving the delivery of oxygen to working muscles should be part of every program designed to improve aerobic or endurance capacity. High aerobic capacity also facilitates faster recovery between and after training sessions and games. A rapid recovery allows athletes to reduce their rest intervals and to perform work at higher intensities.

- *Anaerobic capacity.* The performance intensity of a particular tactical drill determines how much energy is contributed by the anaerobic system, which produces energy in the absence of oxygen. The body's anaerobic capacity is affected by CNS processes, which facilitate continuing intensive work or work under exhausting conditions. A high aerobic capacity transfers positively to anaerobic capacity. If an athlete improves aerobic capacity, anaerobic capacity will also improve. As a result, the athlete will be able to perform effectively for longer periods before levels of blood lactate increase or before incurring an oxygen debt. Furthermore, an athlete with high aerobic capacity recovers faster after building up an oxygen debt, which is important for most athletes.

GUIDELINES FOR ENDURANCE TRAINING

To improve endurance, athletes must develop the ability to overcome fatigue, a natural process that is the result of their ability to adapt to training demand. Successful adaptation is reflected in improved endurance, which is demonstrated during testing as well as during highly demanding training sessions and games.

Athletes must strive to develop all three types of endurance—alactic, lactic, and aerobic—according to the specifics of the sport and the position they play. The development of endurance depends on the volume and intensity of training planned by the coach.

Training Guidelines for Alactic and Lactic Endurance

Most of the methods used for developing alactic (phosphagen system) and lactic (glycolytic system) endurance involve high-intensity activity. The following guidelines may help you better understand the specifics of alactic and lactic endurance:

- Training intensity may range from submaximal to maximal levels. Although a variation of intensities is used during training, intensities around 90 percent to 95 percent of maximum should be emphasized for improving alactic endurance.

- The duration of work may last between 5 and 90 seconds, depending on the energy system the athlete is targeting; it is less than 12 seconds for the phosphagen (alactic) system and 20 to 90 seconds for the glycolytic (lactic) system.

- The RI following an activity of high intensity must be long enough to replenish the oxygen debt. Recuperation is a function of the intensity and duration of work and may take between 2 and 7 minutes. Plan the longest RI so that the accumulated lactic acid will have sufficient time to dissipate. Athletes can then start the next set almost fully recovered.

- Activity during RIs must be light and relaxing (e.g., jogging or low-intensity technical skills, such as passing) to facilitate recovery and energy replenishment. Total rest (i.e., lying down) is not advisable because it causes a drop in the excitability of the nervous system.

- Work designed to develop alactic capacity tends to be very intense, so the number of repetitions must remain at low (3-4) to medium (5-6), which supports training at high intensity.

- If the goal of training is to improve lactic endurance, the number of repetitions is higher; often it is 9 to 12.

Training Guidelines for Aerobic Endurance

The physiological effectiveness of various organs and systems involved in aerobic activity increases more efficiently when training consists of lower-intensity, longer-duration work. Poorly trained athletes have difficulty maintaining aerobic activity for extended periods and experience the effects of fatigue relatively quickly. Well-conditioned athletes, on the other hand, can maintain continuous activity under conditions of fatigue but are also capable of recovering faster.

The following points highlight the training principles that are significant for developing aerobic endurance:

- Training intensity must remain below 70 percent of maximum velocity. As a general standard to follow, intensity can be measured by the time of performance over a given distance, velocity in meters per second (m/s), or heart rate in beats per minute (bpm). Training stimuli that do not increase the heart rate above 130 bpm will have an insignificant effect on the improvement of aerobic capacity. Under normal conditions teenagers reach a heart rate of 200-208 bpm during maximal endurance training, depending on age and sex. Girls tend to have a higher heart rate (by 6-8 beats) than boys. As a general guideline, you can calculate your target heart rate for aerobic endurance work by taking 50 to 85 percent from your maximum heart rate attained during exercise and subtract it from your maximum heart rate, say 202 bpm. Your target heart rate for endurance training can be around 140 to 164 bpm.

- The duration of repetitions must vary within training sessions and from one training session to another. Although some repetitions should range between 60 and 90 seconds to improve lactic endurance, which is important at the beginning of a game, longer repetitions of 3 to 5 minutes are also needed to improve overall aerobic endurance through nonspecific or specific technical and tactical drills.

- For developing aerobic endurance, RI should fall between 90 seconds to 5 minutes. Longer rests can cause the capillaries (the blood vessels that connect arteries with veins) to constrict, thereby restricting blood flow for the first few minutes of work. Traditionally, coaches use a heart rate method to calculate the target heart rate during training, but also to calculate an appropriate RI. Usually, when the heart rate drops during a rest period to 120 bpm, work can resume without difficulty. However, always remember individual differences for both the duration of work and the duration of rest interval.

- Activity during the RI is usually of low intensity to facilitate natural biological recuperation. Walking and jogging are familiar activities for well-trained athletes, but easy passing or ball control exercises can also be performed during RIs.

DEVELOPING SPECIFIC ENDURANCE

Throughout the preparatory phase of the annual plan, coaches need to challenge their athletes' physiological limits by planning endurance sessions two or three times a week. Several training methods are designed for building a solid base of endurance during this stage.

Aerobic Endurance

One common characteristic of all long-distance training methods is that RIs do not interrupt work. The most used methods for team sports are the uniform (steady-state) method and the repetition method.

Uniform (Steady-State) Method

A high volume of work without any interruptions characterizes the uniform, or steady-state, method. The uniform method is most used during the first 2 to 4 weeks of the preparatory phase. The technique of running is a comfortable length of steps, performed with ease and uniform.

The main training goal is to improve athletes' aerobic capacities. Although the uniform training method is not very effective for top athletes, for those at U12 to U15, it is essential to build an aerobic base; to develop the lung capacity; and to develop and strengthen the leg muscles, ligaments, and tendons in a specific form of athletic activity.

The early part of the annual plan, particularly for U15 to U17, can start with uniform training, progressively increasing from shorter distances to 150 yards (or meters; this is just an approximate distance guideline) or longer, then decrease to shorter distances as the intensity increases. The last part of the program is geared toward specific training; distances remain short as specific speed training is stressed. Shorter distances (well under 100 m [9.3 yd]) should involve game-specific activities, such as slalom runs, shuttle runs, and different forms of running, with changes of direction and **stop-and-go drills** (athletes accelerate to maximum velocity, decelerate to a stationary stop, and again accelerate in another direction) performed in all directions.

Repetition Method

The base for aerobic and anaerobic endurance must be built during the preparatory phase. Many coaches believe this base is best developed by continuous, low-intensity activity, such as light jogging of longer duration (3-5 km [2-3 mi]). Those coaches are mistaken.

Jogging alone does not meet the needs of game- or sports-specific endurance (discussed later in this chapter) in team sports. Because jogging does not accurately reflect the intensity at which most team sports are played, it does little for the specific aerobic adaptation of the organs and related functions of most athletes. Another type of activity, repetition training, is more effective for athletes in team sports because it more closely reflects the dynamic nature and pace or rhythm of team sports. The aerobic benefit gained from this type of training is cumulative. A single repetition of 150 meters (164 yd) relies almost entirely on the glycolytic (lactic) anaerobic system, but several repetitions covering the same distance provide, cumulatively, ample aerobic benefits. As lactic acid builds up with each repetition, the energy system can no longer supply the necessary fuel (glycogen), so the body must tap the oxidative (aerobic) system for additional energy.

As a popular training method, repetition training refers to repeating specific distances, from 20 meters (21 yd) to 80 (87 yd) or longer, alternated with an RI. Distance for each repetition should depend on the needs of the sport and space of the gym or field. Shorter repetitions target the phosphagen energy system while the longer ones employ both the phosphagen and glycolytic systems. The suggested intensity is distance related; it is 80 percent for short repetitions and 60 percent for longer repetitions. Longer repetitions help develop game-specific endurance. Longer, steady repetitions (80-150 m [87-164 yd] or more) or drills place a stronger emphasis on the aerobic component of the game. Shorter, intensive repetitions (20-30 m [21-32 yd]) or tactical drills, on the other hand, are more game-specific because the speed more closely mimics game speed. By performing many such repetitions at a steady pace, athletes develop specific endurance and willpower, an important side effect of the repetition method. The total number of repetitions (5-8 or more) is distance related; more repetitions are performed for shorter distances. The volume of work may be 20 to 30 minutes, with an RI of 3 to 5 minutes depending on the distance and intensity of the repetition.

Variations in training plan should recognize the complexity of the technical, tactical, and physical characteristics of team sports that can specifically enhance the physiological and motor skills required during a game. Coaches can create their own plans or models to train the complexities of their respective sports by first making a list of the activities or actions athletes perform during a game. Keeping position-specific details in mind ensures that athletes will be trained according to the specific physiological demands and physical qualities necessary to excel at their positions.

Table 12.1 can be adapted to the specifics of any team sport (e.g., the size of the pool for water polo and the smaller court, field, or ice surfaces for volleyball, basketball, lacrosse, and ice hockey).

Game-Specific Endurance

Developing endurance is more complex than first meets the eye because most team sports involve a combination of aerobic and anaerobic components. As a result, several of the methods and variations presented in this chapter must be used to achieve the best adaptation. Physiological effects are not the only reason for selecting a particular training method; psychological benefits (e.g., willpower, perseverance, aggressiveness) are also essential considerations because they often have visible advantages for the athlete.

Aerobic training for team sports is complex in its own way. As soon as a team begins training as a unit, specific technical and tactical drills must be used for best aerobic training. To develop and maintain all three energy systems used in team sports, the following specific drills can be designed to enhance a given energy system:

- High-intensity drills of 5 to 12 seconds tax the phosphagen (alactic, ATP-CP) system.
- Intensive drills of 20 to 90 seconds tap the glycolytic (lactic) system.
- Continuous medium-intensity drills of 2 to 5 minutes or longer (up to 10 min) can be used to develop or maintain the aerobic needs of athletes (oxidative system).

Table 12.1   Endurance Training for Team Sports According to Type of Activity

Type of activity	Approximate distance (in m or yds)	Intensity (% of maximum)	*Rest interval (RI) between reps (min)
Sprinting	30	100	2-3
Striding	30-50	70	2
Cruising	20-40	50	1-2
Bending run or cuts	10-30	80-100	2-3
Acceleration – deceleration	10-20	90-100	2-3
Slalom run	20-30	70-90	2
Stop and go	10-20	80-100	2
Side shuffle	10-20	70-100	2
Forward run and back paddle	10-20	70-90	2-3
Repetitions	20-150	60-80	2-5 (Higher intensities require longer RI.)
Simple obstacle course	10 in each direction	70-85	2-3
T/TA drills	Depending on the taxed energy system	60-90	3

*If the suggested RI is not long enough to allow athletes to recover to a desired level, it may be extended by 1 or 2 minutes.

Technical and tactical drills should be organized and performed according to the specifics of repetition training: distance, intensity, number of repetitions, and RIs. Unfortunately, coaches rarely organize drills with the energy systems in mind. In most cases, particularly in soccer, technical and tactical drills are short and very intensive, lasting 5 to 8 seconds. Consequently, these drills tax primarily the phosphagen (alactic, ATP-CP) system and cumulatively the glycolytic (lactic) system. Game-specific drill combinations can include the following:

- Sprint, pivot, stride, side shuffle, bending run, stop and go, compensation activities (e.g., jogging)
- Acceleration–deceleration, slalom run, cruise, backpedal, and light jogging during rest intervals between activities
- Stride, side shuffle, change of direction, pivot, compensation jog between activities
- Sprint, stride, stop and go, backpedal, forward sprint, compensation jog between activities
- Slalom run, stop and go, bending run, acceleration–deceleration, leap over simple obstacles, compensation jog between activities
- Simple obstacle course, jump over obstacles (a cone, bench), jog, change of direction, jog, acceleration–deceleration, compensation jog between activities

To avoid exhaustion from high-intensity training and especially overtraining, workouts must be organized in such a way that energy systems are trained alternately, at times on separate days. Table 12.2 provides an example of this type of organization.

SPECIFIC TACTICAL DRILLS

Coaches can organize tactical drills specific for offense and defense, various game combinations, transition from defense to offense or offense to defense, counterattacks, and so on. They can involve small groups of athletes, lines, and offensive and defensive athletes. In addition, they can repeat parts of tactical schemes for the next game.

Table 12.2 Sample Microcycle (1 Week) of Training for U15-U17 Athletes: 1 Game/Week

Day	1	2	3	4	5	6	7
Activity	Game	Recovery	Training	Off	Training	Training	Game
Energy system(s)	All	Oxidative (aerobic)	Phosphagen (alactic, ATP-CP)/ glycolytic (lactic)		Glycolytic (lactic)/ Oxidative (aerobic)	Phosphagen (alactic, ATP-CP)/ glycolytic (lactic); small number of reps	All
Training demand	High	Low	High		High	Low	High
Training objectives	Apply game tactics and game objectives.	Recover using light activities with or without the ball.	Perform T/ TA drills.		Perform T/ TA drills based on the game plan set for the next game.	Perform TA drills based on the tactical plan set for the next game.	Apply game tactics and game objectives.

T = technical; TA = tactical.

Note: Observe the alternations of energy systems and training intensities.

Position-Specific Endurance

To accommodate the specifics of certain positions in team sports, training programs require some adjustments. In the case of volleyball, a power-dominant sport, model training must incorporate exercises that mimic athletes' positions (e.g., spiker or libero). Most athletes need programs for agility and quickness (e.g., simple tumbling, varied and continuous jumps, dives and rolls), reaction time, and movement time, and exercises that train game-specific actions and reactions.

Other positions in team sports, such as goalkeepers in soccer and hockey, sweepers in soccer, or outfielders in baseball or softball, require other types of position-specific activity combinations, such as the following:

- *Goalkeepers in soccer and hockey*: Simple tumbling, series of leaps, side shuffling, crossovers, spike jumps (athletes hold a medicine ball in both hands and throw the ball over the net), changes of direction (5-10 m [5.5-11 yd] in different directions), jogging, low-impact plyometrics, overhead and sideways medicine ball throws, compensation jogging

- *Sweepers in soccer*: Backpedaling, side rolls, dives with quick recovery to the feet, push-ups, acceleration–deceleration (5-10 m [5.5-11 yd] in various directions), jogging, simple plyometrics, medicine ball throws, compensation jogging

- *Outfielders in baseball or softball*: Skipping rope, overhead and sideways medicine ball throws, reactive jumps, jogging, changes of direction, acceleration–deceleration, side shuffling, dives, jogging, backpedaling, step-ups, compensation jogging

The game- and position-specific physiological requirements of most team sports differ, and coaches can take a very specific approach to power and endurance training. The dominant biomotor ability for many positions in team sports is not power but power endurance. To be able to repeat a high number of powerful and quick actions over an hour or two of play requires specific training in the form of game-specific and position-specific endurance.

The high intensity of high-volume formula can be planned for training all three energy systems. Preferably, this formula can be used for technical, but most importantly, for tactical drills:

- 12-15 reps × 12 sec for alactic endurance
- 8-12 reps × 30 sec for lactic endurance
- 5-8 reps × 3 min for aerobic endurance

PERIODIZATION OF ENDURANCE TRAINING

Periodization of endurance must be discussed from the point of view of the long-term plan and the annual plan. Long-term periodization has to represent a guideline for the several annual plans that coaches create for the childhood and the teen years. Consequently, these two types of plans have to be closely linked together to ensure a continuation of the development of endurance.

Annual Plan

For best game- and position-specific endurance, during an annual plan, endurance develops in a very systematic way throughout the three main training phases shown in table 12.3. Aerobic endurance should be developed throughout the transition and early preparatory phases, using the uniform, long-repetition, and short-repetition methods at moderate to medium intensities. Cardiorespiratory functions and the efficiency of oxygen utilization improve progressively by adhering to these methods. Workloads should also be increased progressively, especially total training volume as the training reaches its highest level during the specific preparatory phase of the annual plan.

The development of anaerobic and game-specific endurance is extremely important for achieving the goal of overall endurance training. During the transition from aerobic to anaerobic and game-specific endurance, it is essential to maintain aerobic endurance. High-intensity training, a hallmark of the competitive phase, may not produce the desired results unless a solid foundation of endurance is established during the preparatory phase. Depending on the specifics of the sport, the ergogenesis of each activity, and the position played by each athlete, elements of anaerobic activity are gradually introduced. The rhythm of activity and the pace of specific drills become progressively more intensive.

Game-specific endurance coincides with the precompetitive phase and continues during the competitive schedule. The utilization of appropriate training methods depends on the ergogenesis of the sport and the athletes' needs. For many sports, it is beneficial to emphasize a training intensity that exceeds the game's intensity. Alternating various intensities during training facilitates recovery between training sessions, leading to a strong peak during league games.

Table 12.3 suggests how to organize a periodization of endurance program for your team. Many team sports have specific periodization with specific duration dictated by climate or seasons, so you can adapt table 12.3 according to your specific conditions. However, try to follow the suggested sequence as closely as possible, but also adapt it to the specific traditions of some countries.

Long-Term Periodization

Table 12.4 illustrates a progression of endurance training throughout the stages of athletic development of young athletes as follows:

- *U12.* The scope of endurance training for U12 is to build the foundation of aerobic training, and, as a side benefit, to progressively strengthen the leg muscles, ligaments, and tendons. The specific and nonspecific training programs must be organized without any anatomical stress but with a large dose of patience; children need time to naturally grow and develop.

- *U15.* Training for U15 represents a transition from dominance in oxidative and phosphagen to all three energy systems:

  - Phosphagen (alactic, ATP-CP) training of short duration (5-12 sec) must precede the glycolytic (lactic) training for the simple reason that children enjoy fast but short-duration actions.
  - Glycolytic (lactic) training (20-90 sec) is far more stressful and difficult to tolerate at this age (taxing the children both physiologically and psychologically).
  - The oxidative system can be trained by using game- and position-specific training.

- *U17.* From U17 to the rest of their athletic career, athletes have to be exposed to all three energy systems with a position-specific emphasis. As athletes progress throughout the age categories, intensity and volume of training have to be increased to best adapt for the game and position played.

Table 12.3 Sample Periodization of Endurance Training: Annual Plan for Team Sports

Training phase	Preparatory		Competitive		Transition
Training subphase	General	Specific	Precompetitive	League games	Transition
Duration (wk)	2	2-4	2	Entire duration of league games	3-4, or for the duration of vacation
Periodization of endurance	Aerobic, uniform, endurance	Aerobic, lactic, and alactic endurance; striding; game and position-specific endurance (ergogenesis)	Game- and position-specific endurance (ergogenesis)	Game- and position-specific endurance (ergogenesis)	Aerobic (informal) endurance

Table 12.4 Long-Term Periodization of Endurance Training

	U12	U15	U17	U19	U21-U23
Scope of endurance training	Foundational development of aerobic endurance	Alactic endurance and aerobic endurance	All three energy systems; game- and position-specific endurance	All three energy systems; game- and position-specific endurance	All three energy systems; game- and position-specific endurance

CONCLUSION

The development of specific endurance is always very challenging. To be successful you have to consider the complexity of training the energy systems, but also adapt it to the needs of the sport and individual athlete.

This is why training is so challenging. It has captivated all of us. This is why we love sports and all the challenges we have encountered over the years. We did not just train athletes but real human beings, who, because of our work, we hope are better members of our society. Just love it.

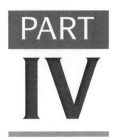

SELECTED EXERCISES FOR STRENGTH, POWER, AGILITY, SPEED, AND FLEXIBILITY

Most scientific experiments and testing of athletes occurred at the biomechanics laboratories at Polytechnic University in Timisoara, Romania.

Exercise Finder

U19

U21

U23

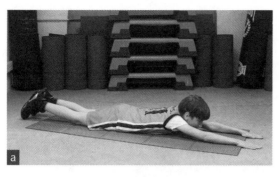 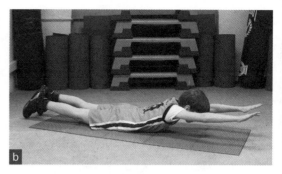

Back extension with arms raised.

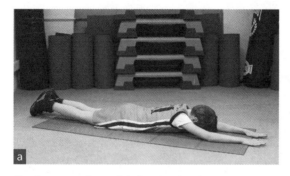 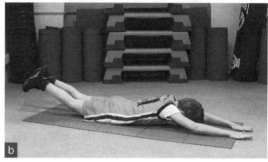

Back extension with legs raised.

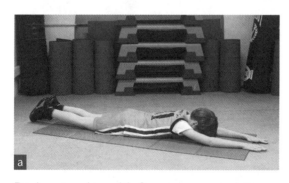

Back extension with Superman pose.

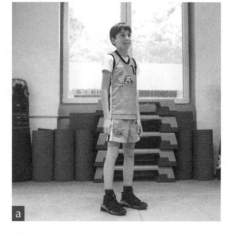 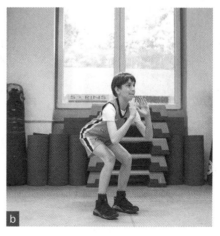

Bodyweight squat.

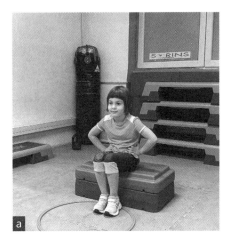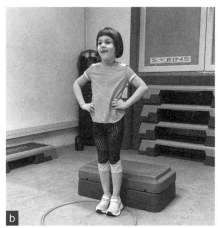

Box squat.

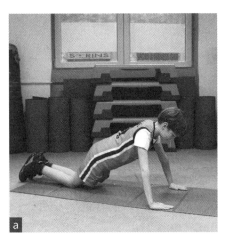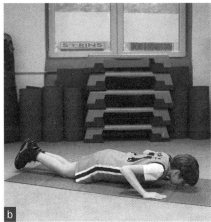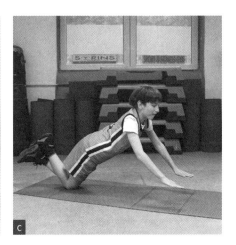

Explosive kneeling push-up.

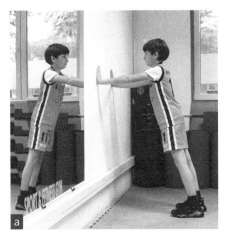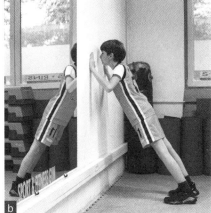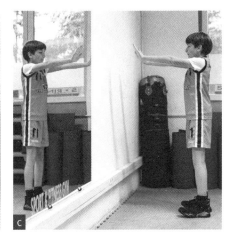

Explosive wall push-up.

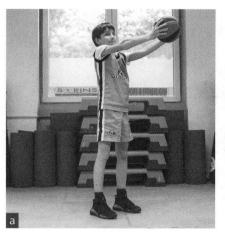 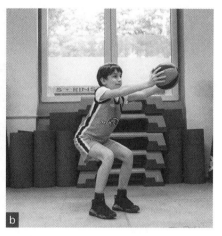

Front squat with medicine ball.

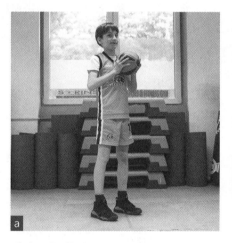 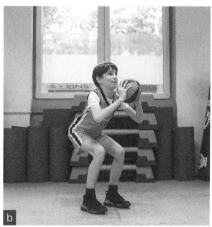

Front squat with medicine ball chest press.

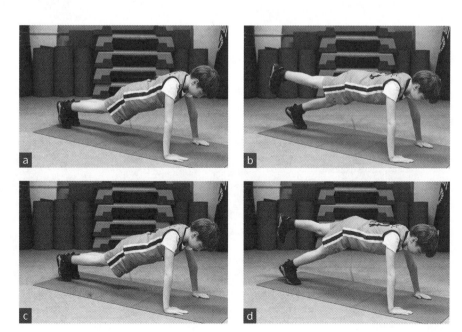

Full plank with leg lift.

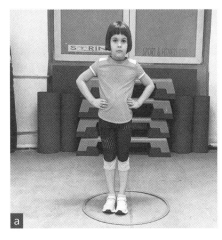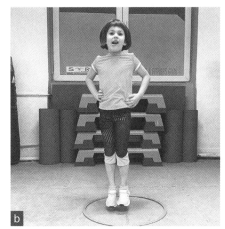

Jump in the circle.

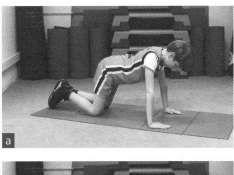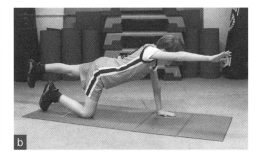

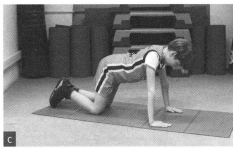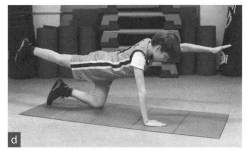

Kneeling arm and leg reach.

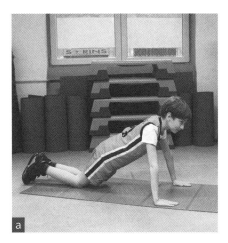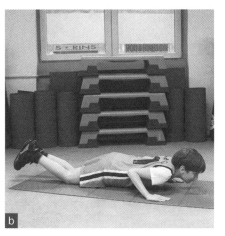

Kneeling push-up.

186

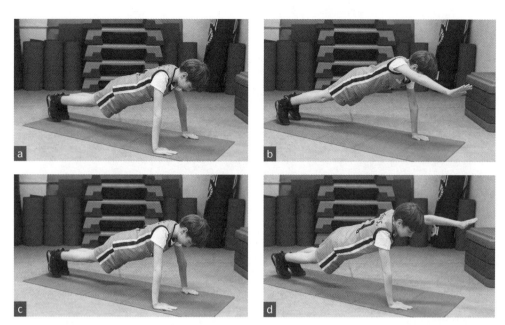

Plank with forward reach.

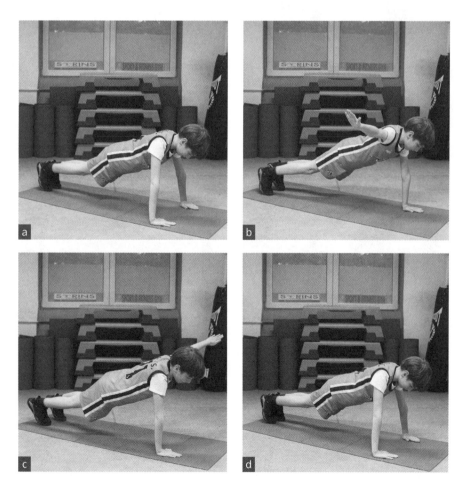

Plank with lateral arm raise.

187

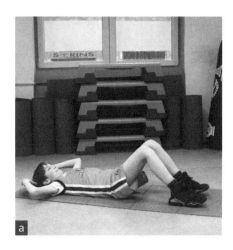 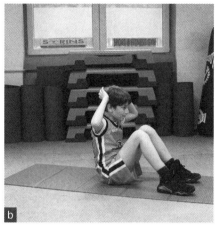

Sit-up.

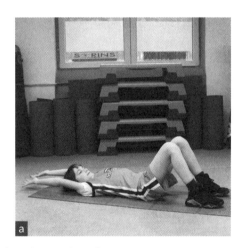 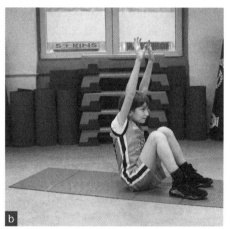

Sit-up with hands overhead.

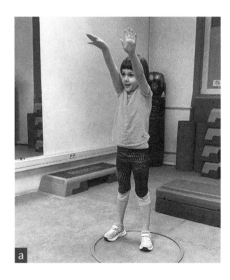 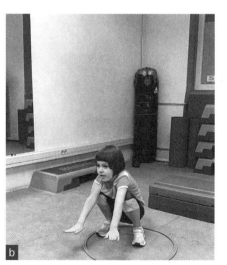

Squat.

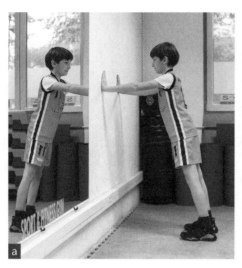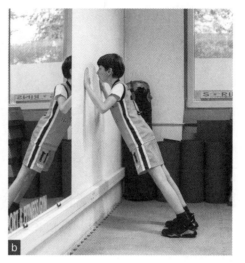

Wall push-up.

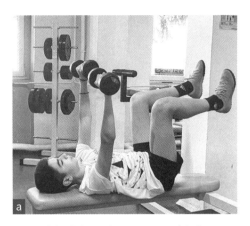 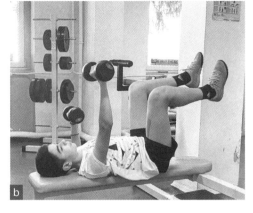

Alternating dumbbell bench presses with legs up.

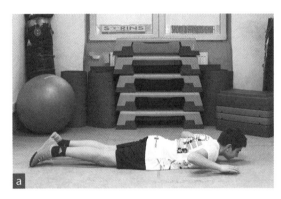 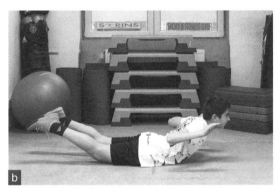

Back extension.

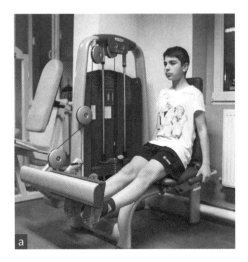 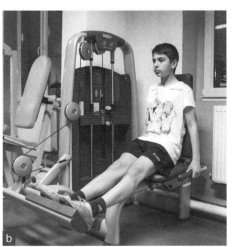

Calf press.

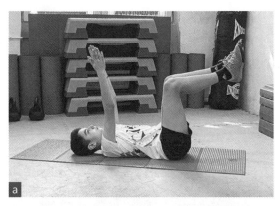
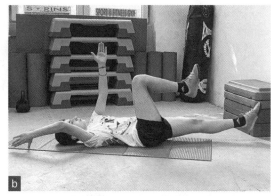
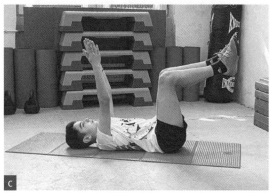
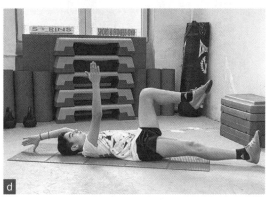

Dead bug pose.

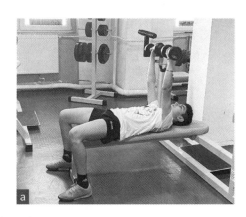
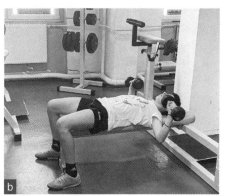

Dumbbell bench press.

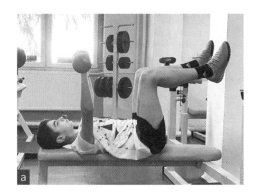
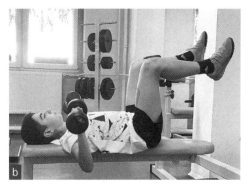

Dumbbell bench press with legs up.

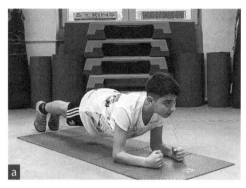

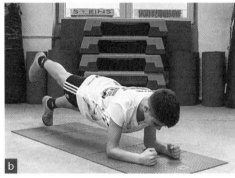

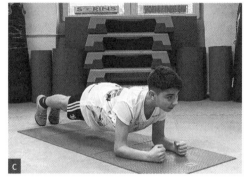

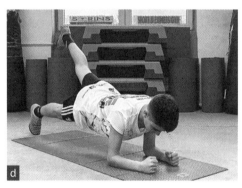

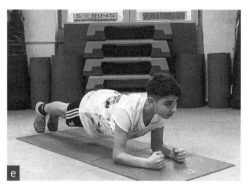

Forearm plank with leg lift.

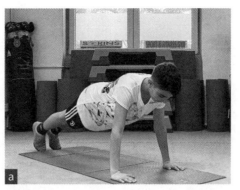

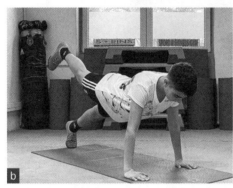
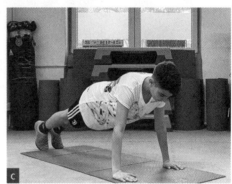

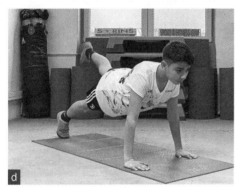
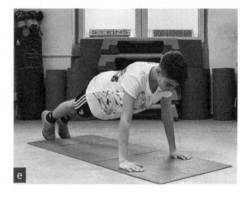

Full plank with leg lift.

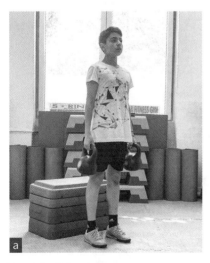
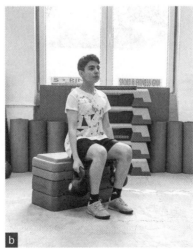
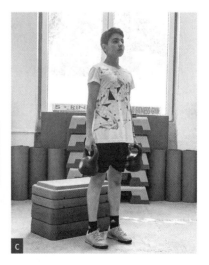

Kettlebell box squat.

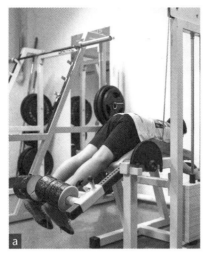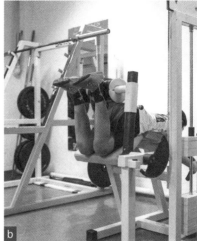

Leg curl.

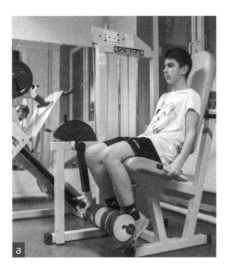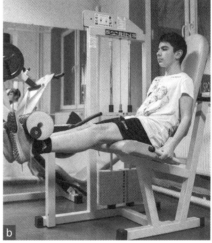

Leg extension.

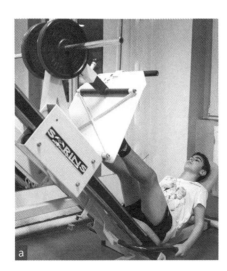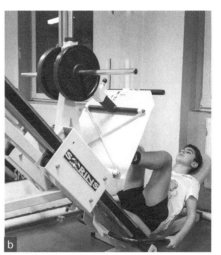

Leg press.

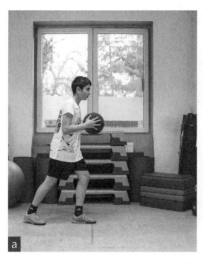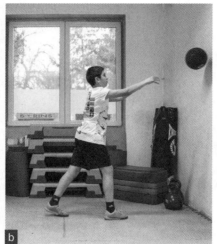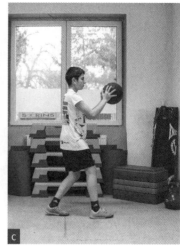

Medicine ball chest pass to wall.

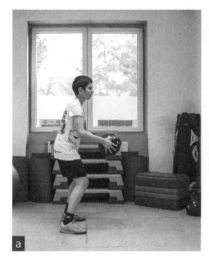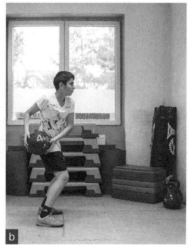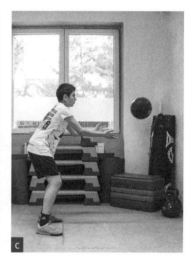

Medicine ball parallel rotational throw.

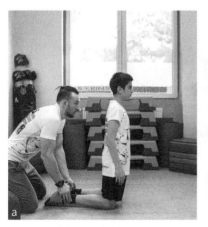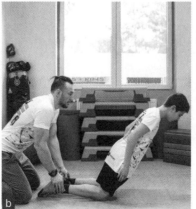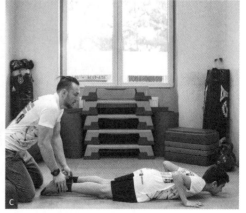

Nordic hamstring curl.

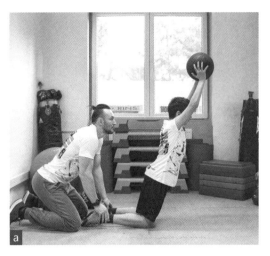 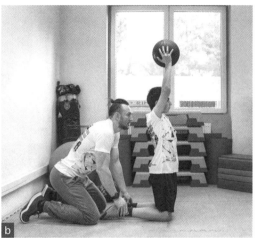

Nordic hamstring curl with medicine ball.

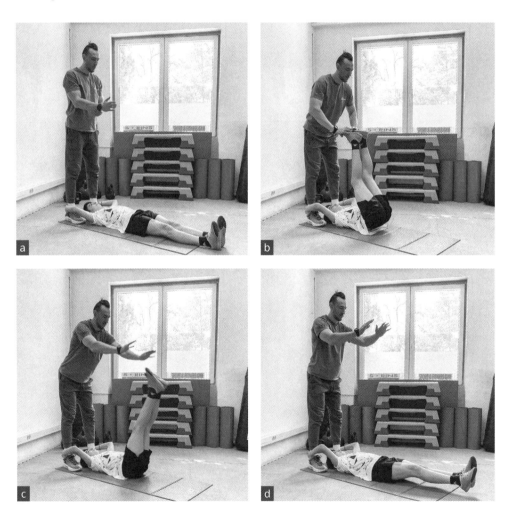

Partner lying leg raise with throw down.

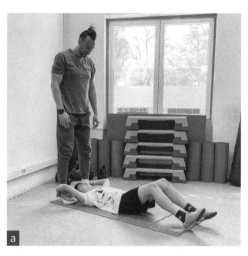 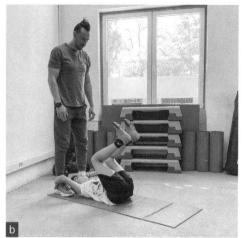

Partner reverse crunch.

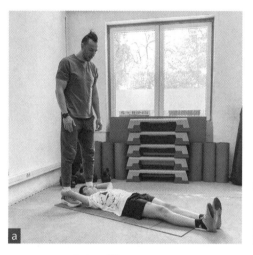 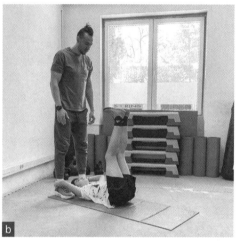

Partner reverse crunch leg lift.

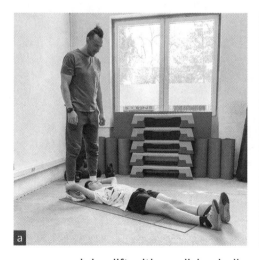 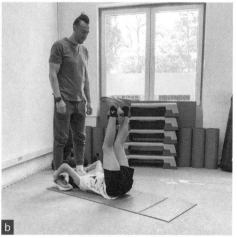

Partner reverse crunch leg lift with medicine ball.

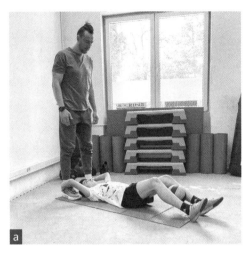 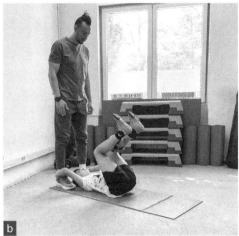

Partner reverse crunch with medicine ball.

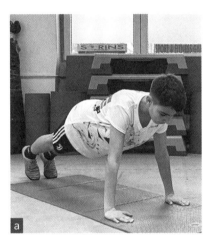 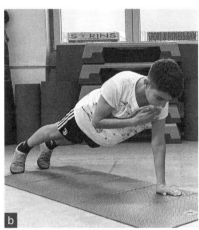

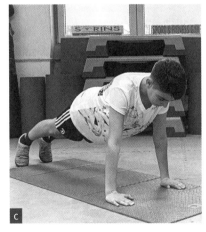 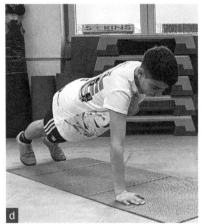 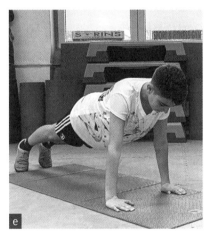

Plank tap.

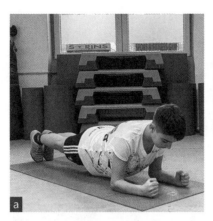 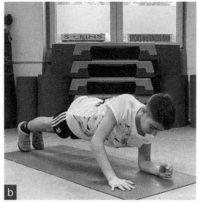

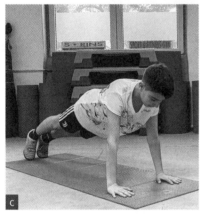 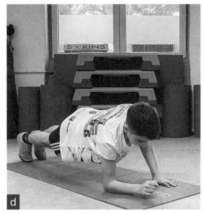 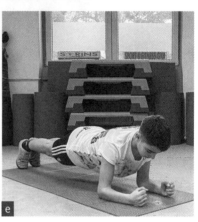

Plank-up.

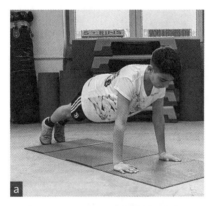 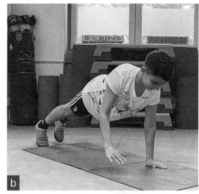

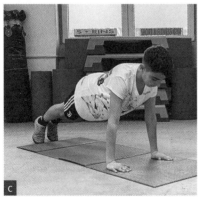 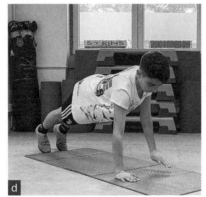 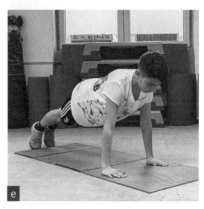

Plank with hand lift.

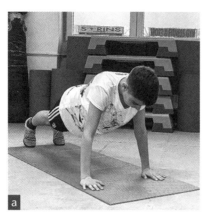
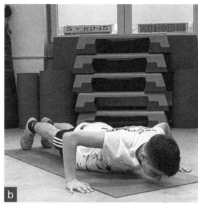

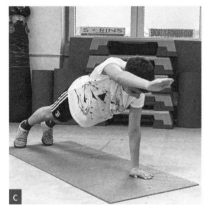
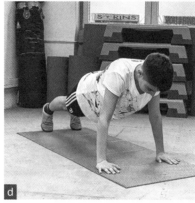
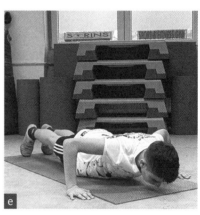

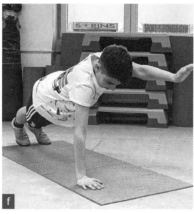
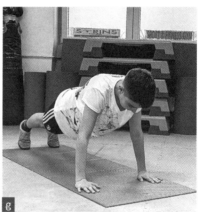

Push-up with forward arm raise.

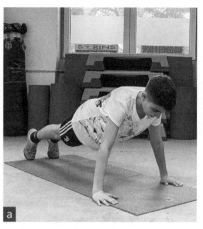
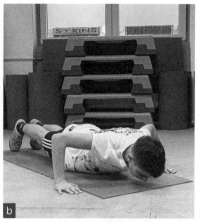

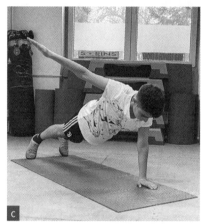
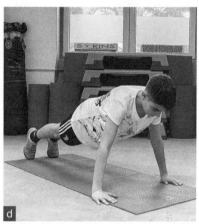
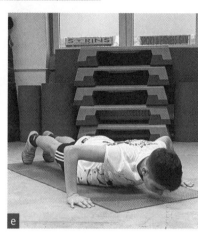

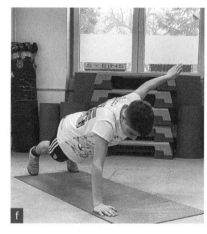
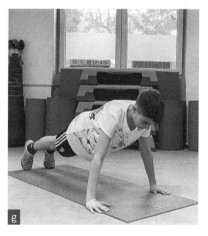

Push-up with lateral arm raise.

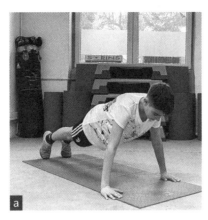 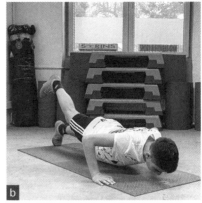

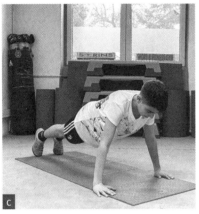 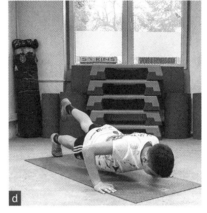 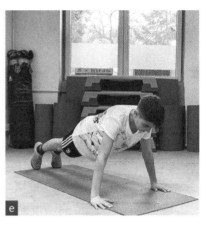

Push-up with single-raised leg.

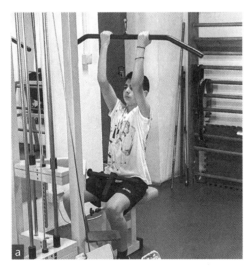 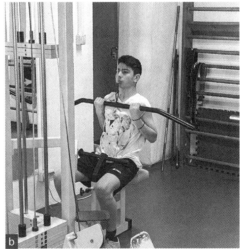

Reverse close-grip lat pull-down.

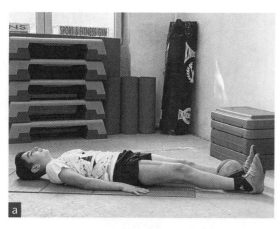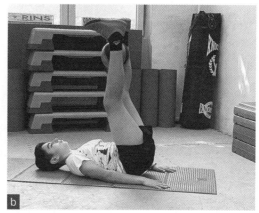

Reverse crunch leg lift with medicine ball.

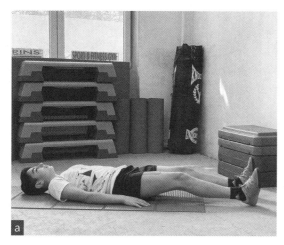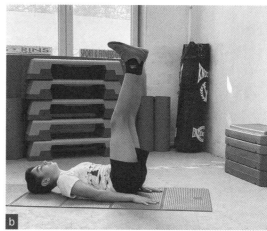

Reverse crunch leg lift.

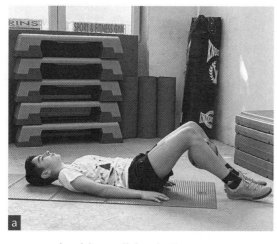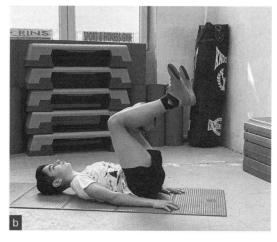

Reverse crunch with medicine ball.

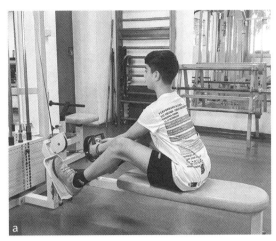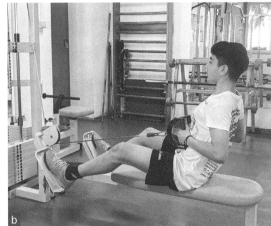

Seated cable row.

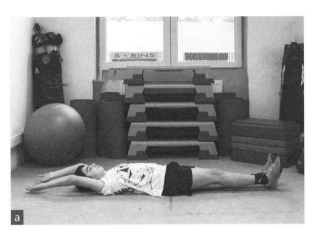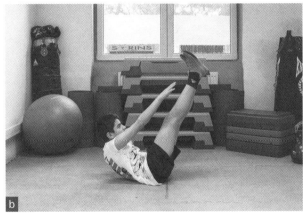

V-up.

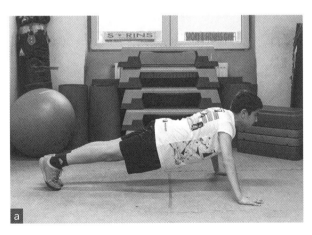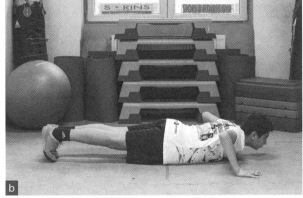

Wide-arm push-up.

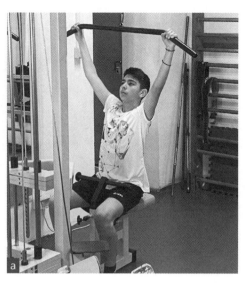 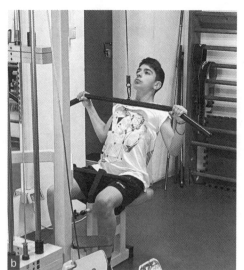

Wide-grip lat pull-down.

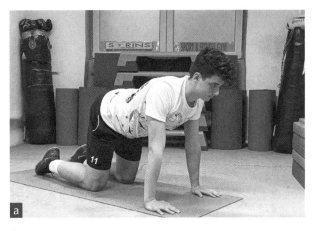 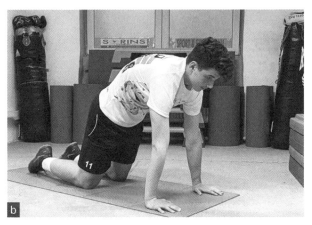

Arch.

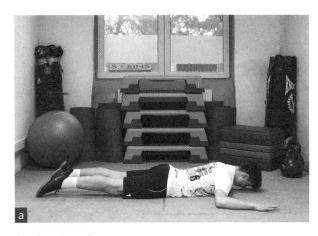 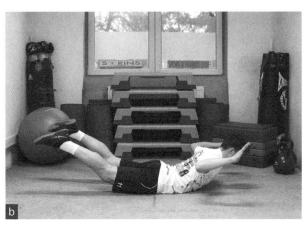

Back extension.

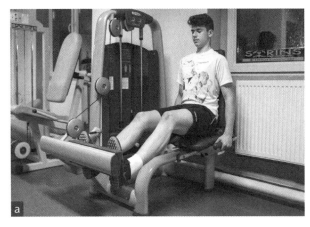

Calf press.

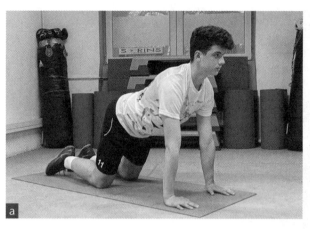 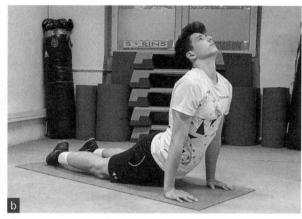

Cobra pose.

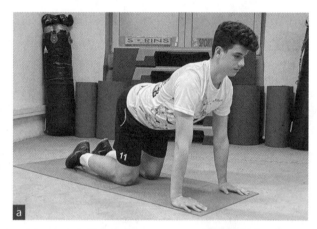

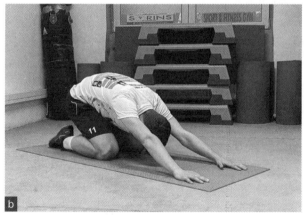 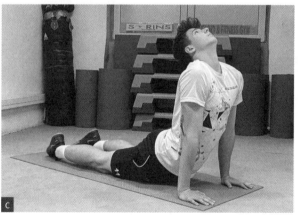

Cobra pose with back emphasis.

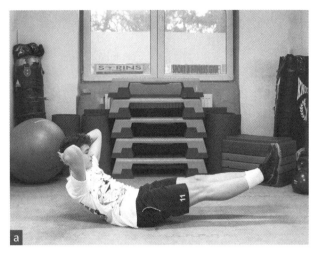

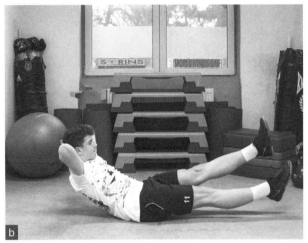

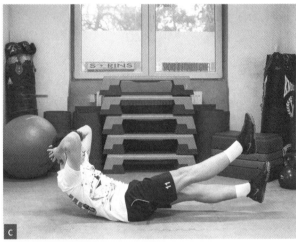

Flutter kick.

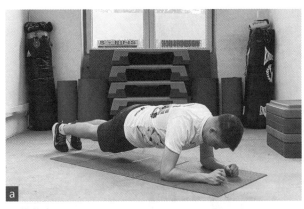
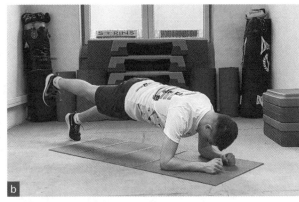
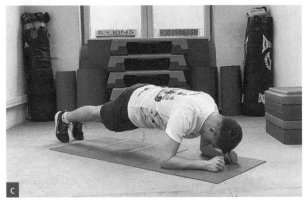
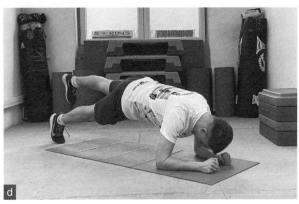

Forearm plank with leg lift.

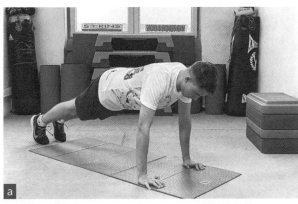
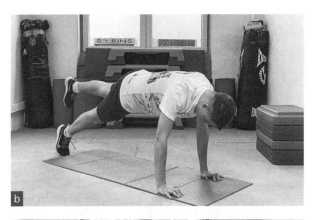
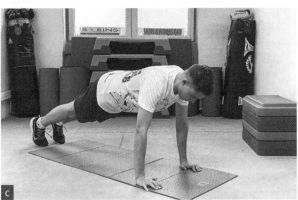
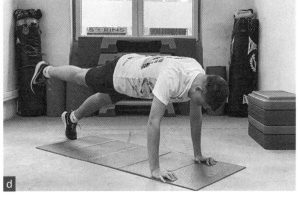

Full plank with leg lift.

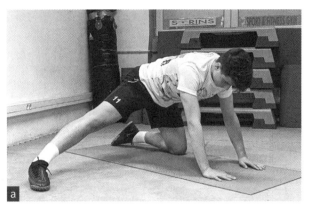

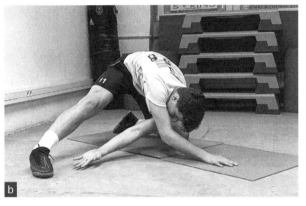

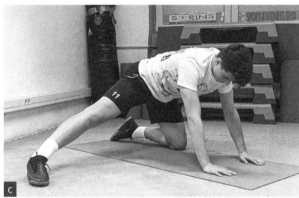

Gate pose with thread the needle pose.

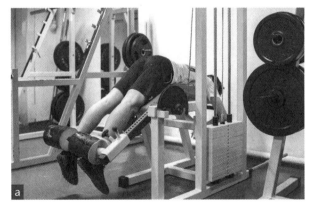

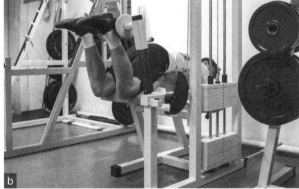

Leg curl.

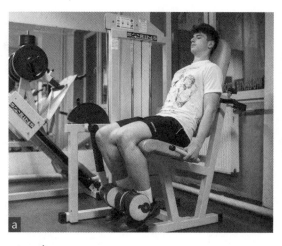 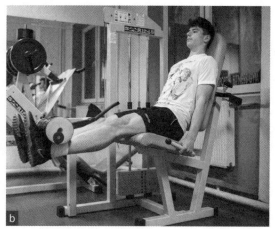

Leg extension.

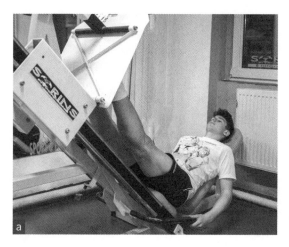 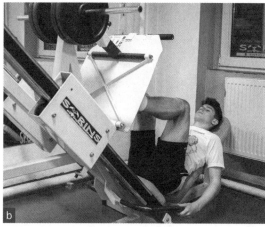

Leg press.

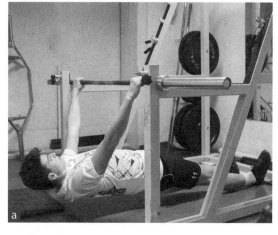 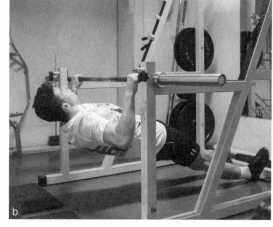

Lying pull-up.

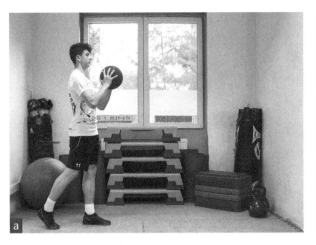
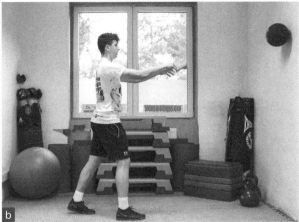

Medicine ball chest pass to wall.

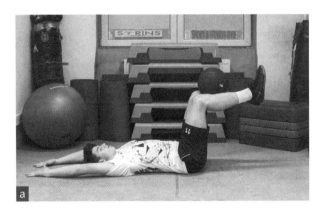
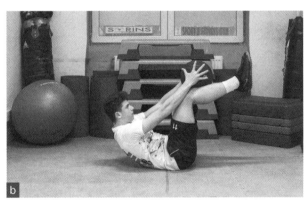
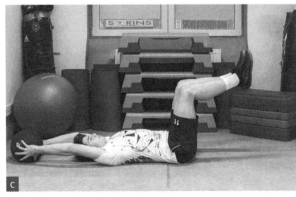
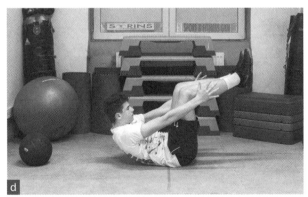

Medicine ball leg crunch.

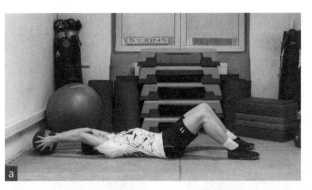

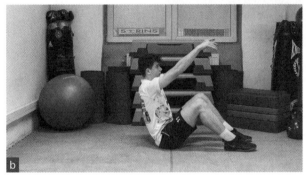

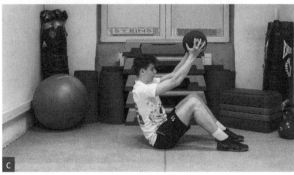

Medicine ball overhead sit-up throw.

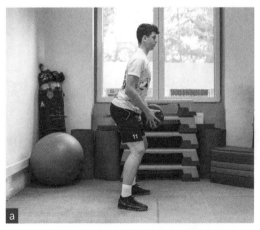

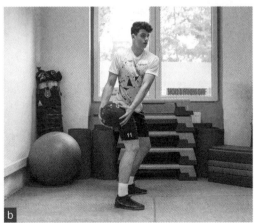

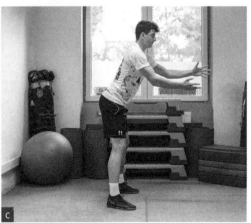

Medicine ball parallel rotational throw.

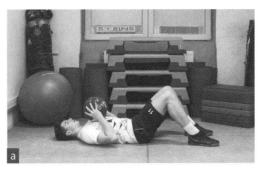

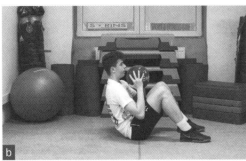

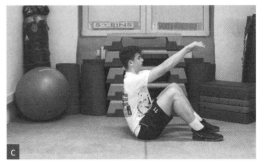

Medicine ball sit-up chest throw.

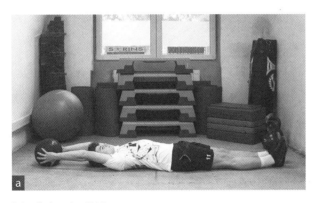

Medicine ball V-up.

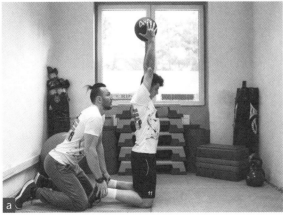

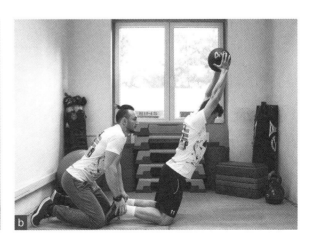

Nordic hamstring curl with medicine ball.

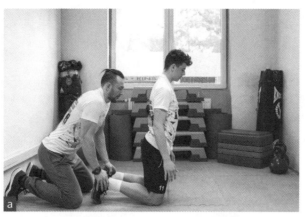

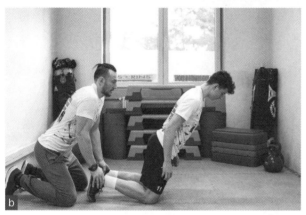

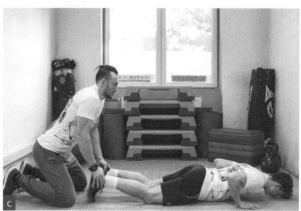

Nordic hamstring curl.

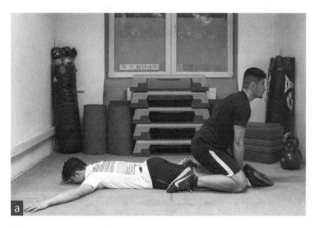

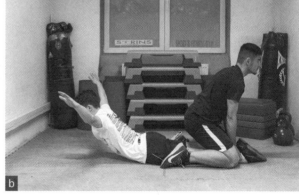

Partner back extension.

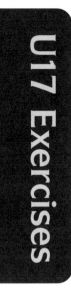

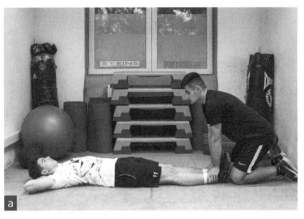

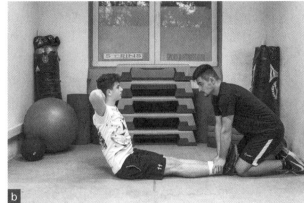

Partner sit-up.

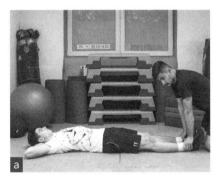

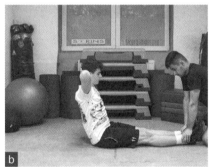

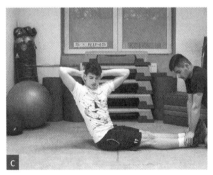

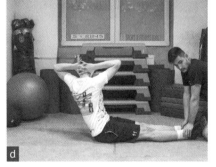

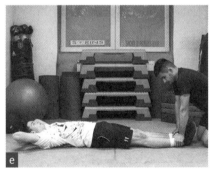

Partner sit-up with double twist.

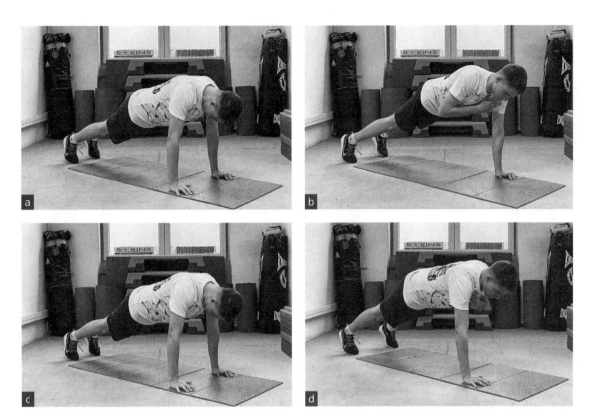

Plank tap.

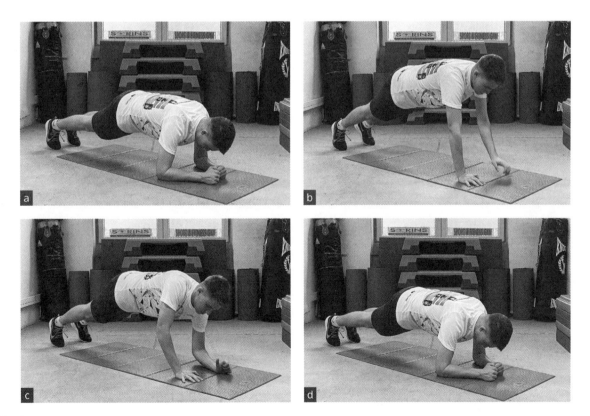

Plank-up.

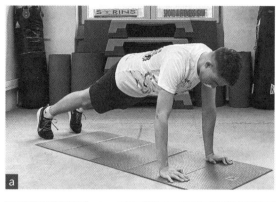 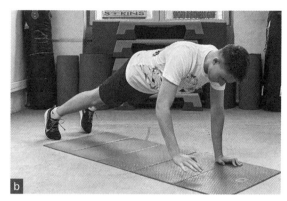

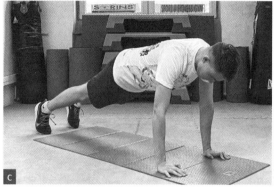 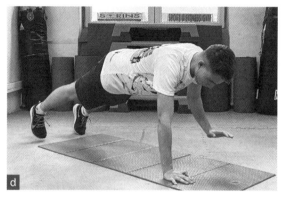

Plank with hand lift.

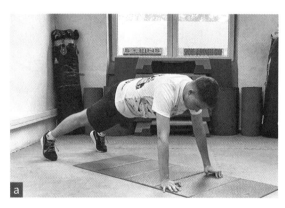 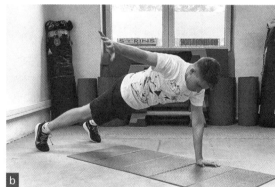

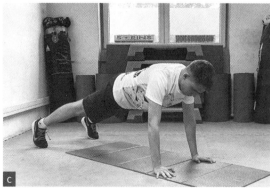 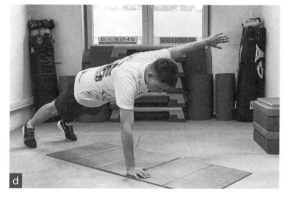

Plank with lateral arm raise.

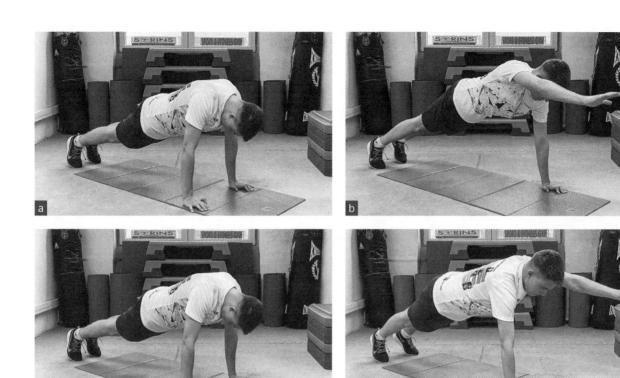

Plank with forward reach.

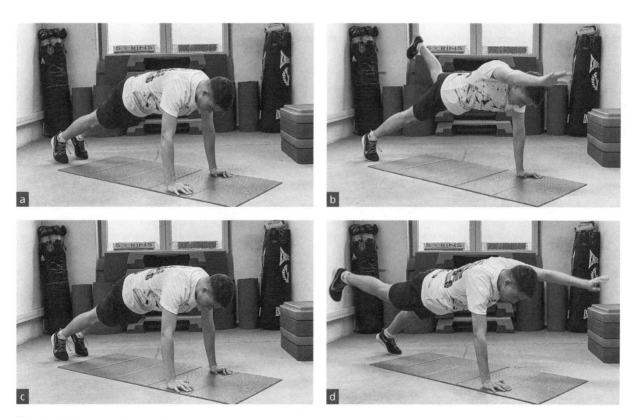

Plank with opposite reach.

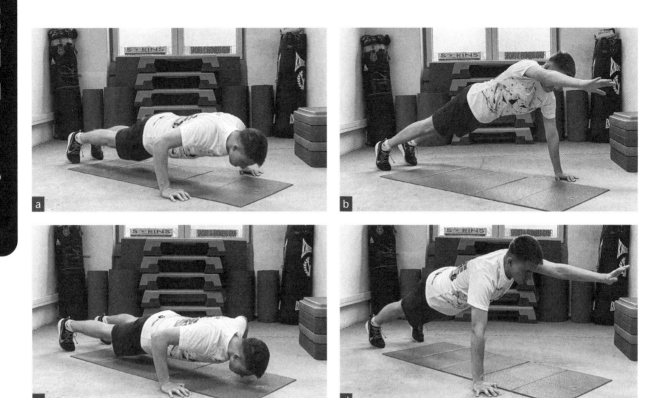

Push-up with forward arm raise.

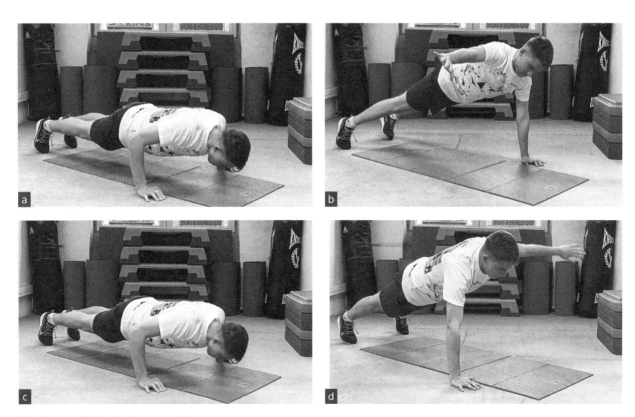

Push-up with lateral arm raise.

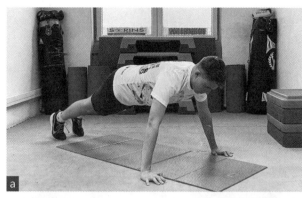 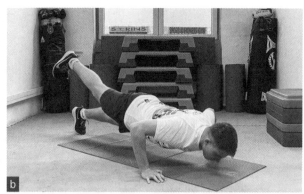

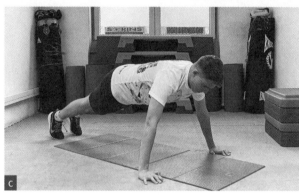 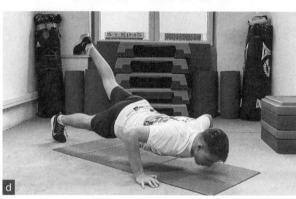

Push-up with raised leg.

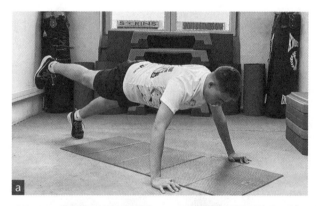

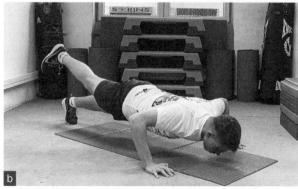 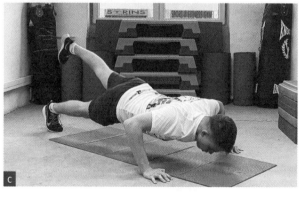

Push-up with single leg.

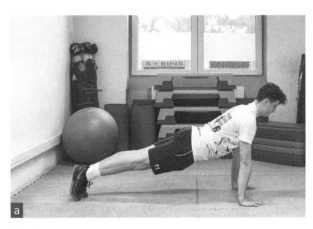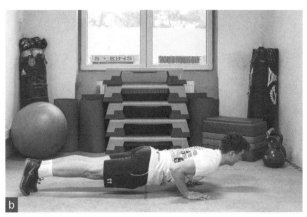

Push-up.

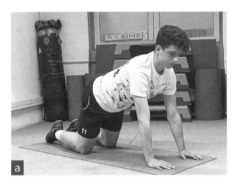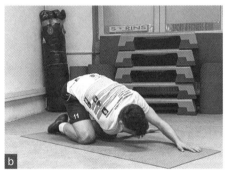

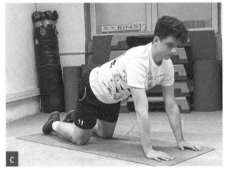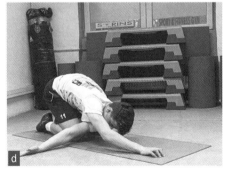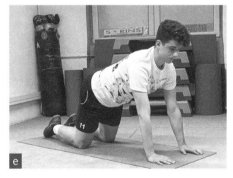

Thread the needle pose.

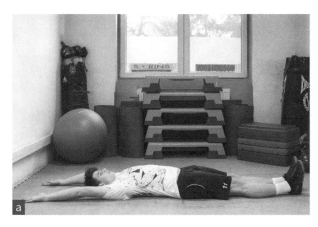
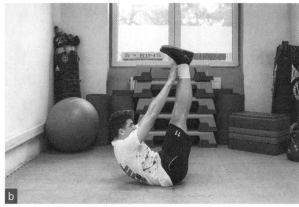

V-up.

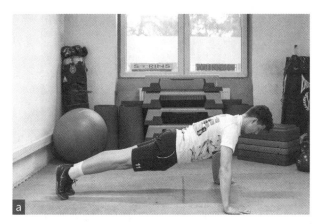
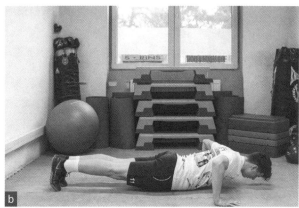

Wide-arm push-up.

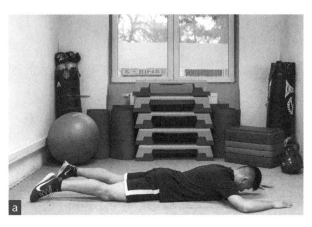 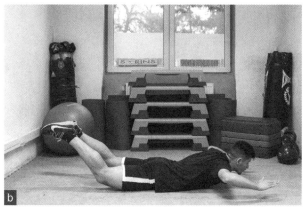

Back extension.

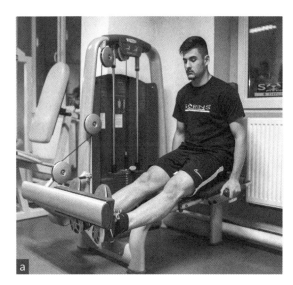 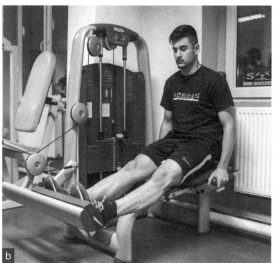

Calf press.

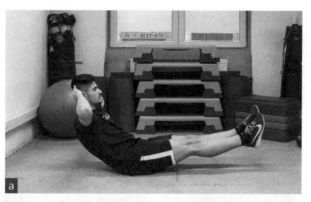

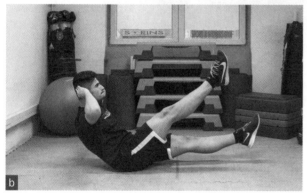

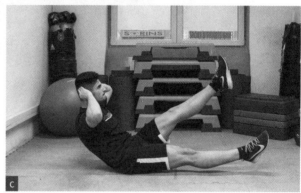

Flutter kick.

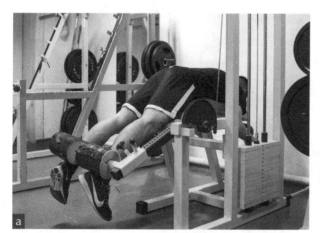

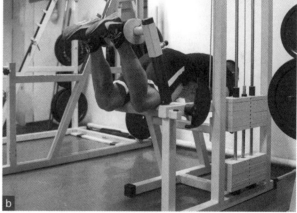

Leg curl.

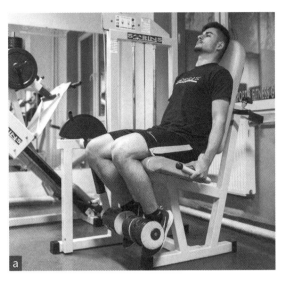 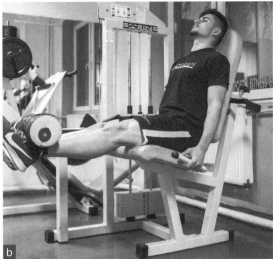

Leg extension.

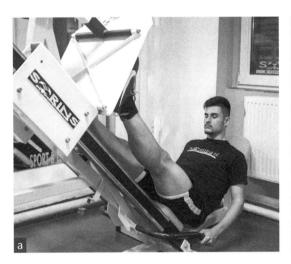 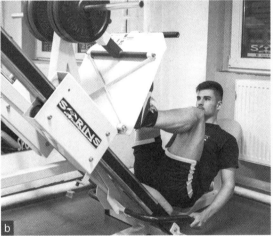

Leg press.

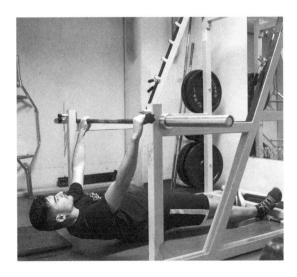

Lying pull-up.

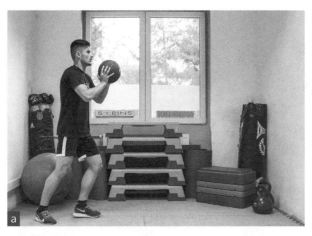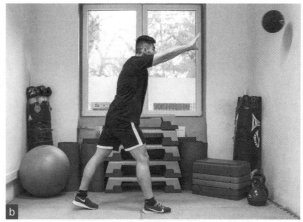

Medicine ball chest pass to wall.

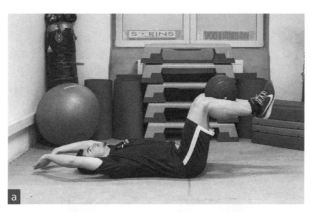

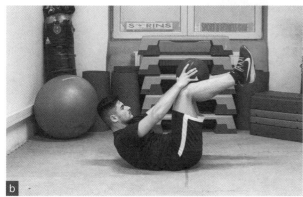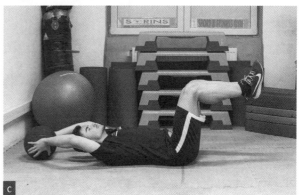

Medicine ball leg crunch.

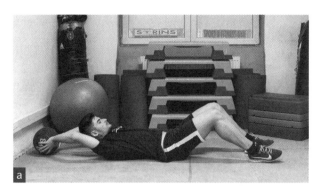

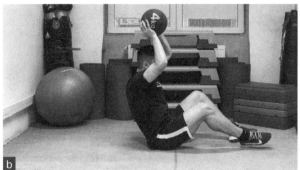

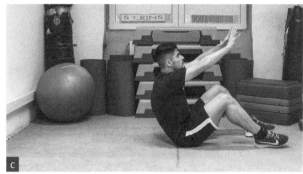

Medicine ball overhead sit-up throw.

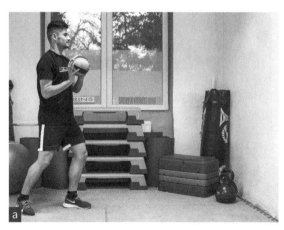

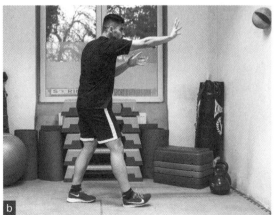

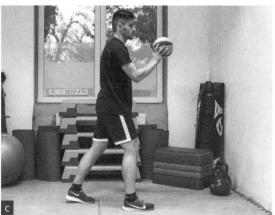

Medicine ball shot-put throw.

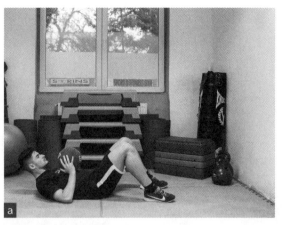

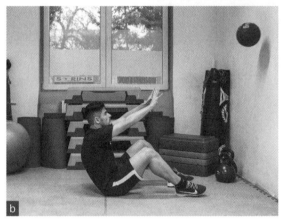

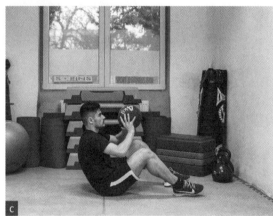

Medicine ball sit-up with chest throw.

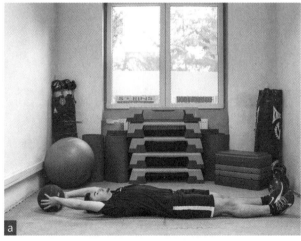

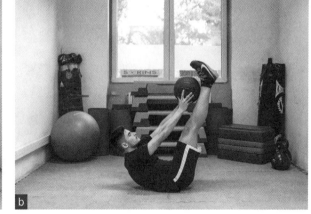

Medicine ball V-up.

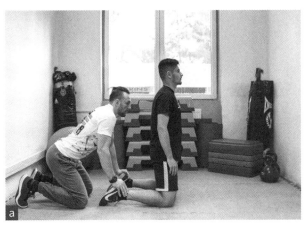

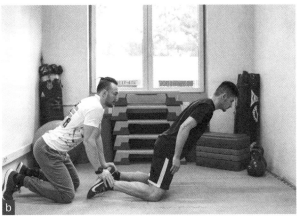
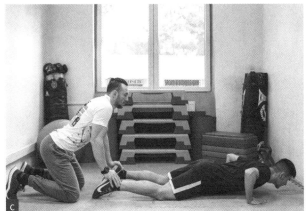

Nordic hamstring curl.

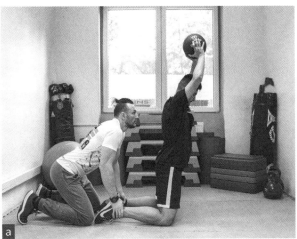
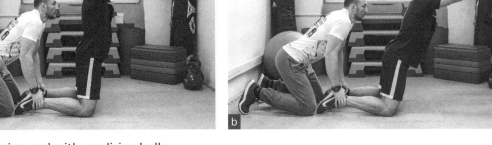

Nordic hamstring curl with medicine ball.

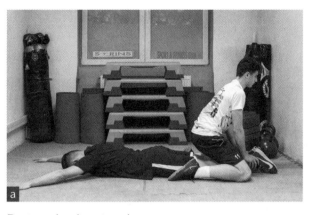 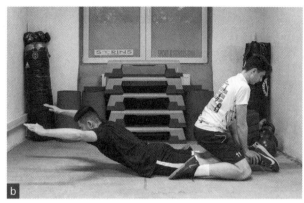

Partner back extension.

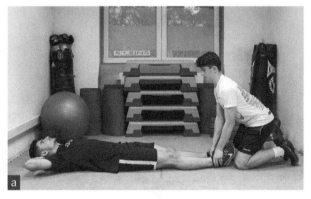 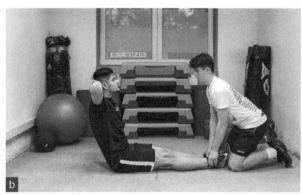

Partner sit-up.

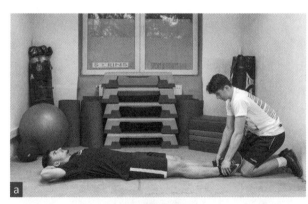 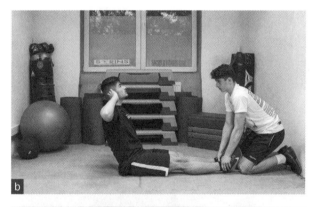

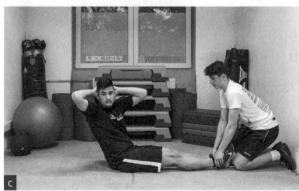 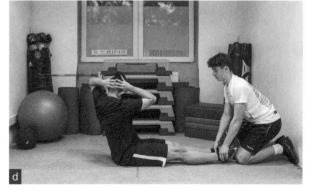

Partner sit-up with double twist.

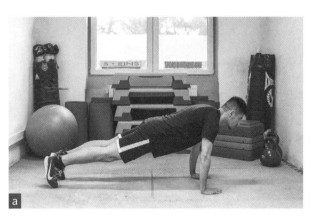 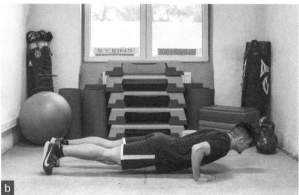

Push-up.

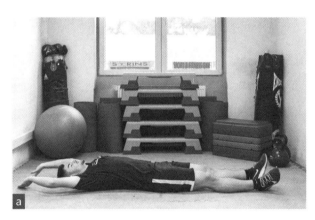 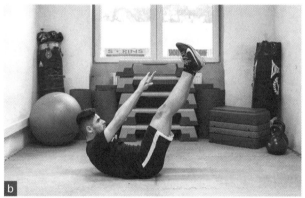

V-up.

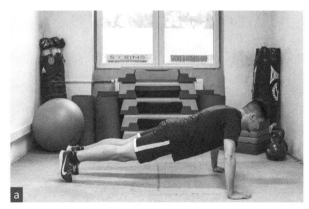 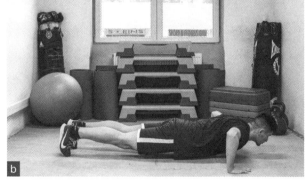

Wide-arm push-up.

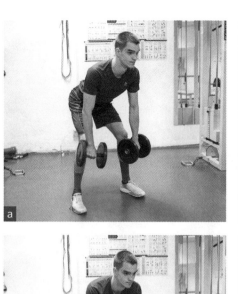
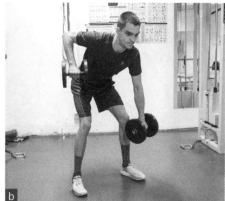
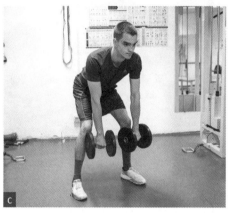
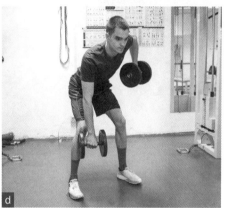

Alternating bent-over rows.

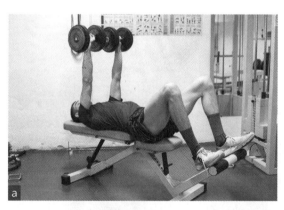
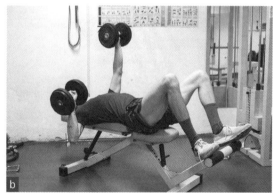
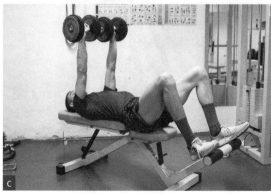
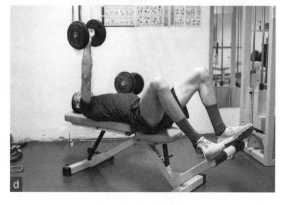

Alternating dumbbell chest presses.

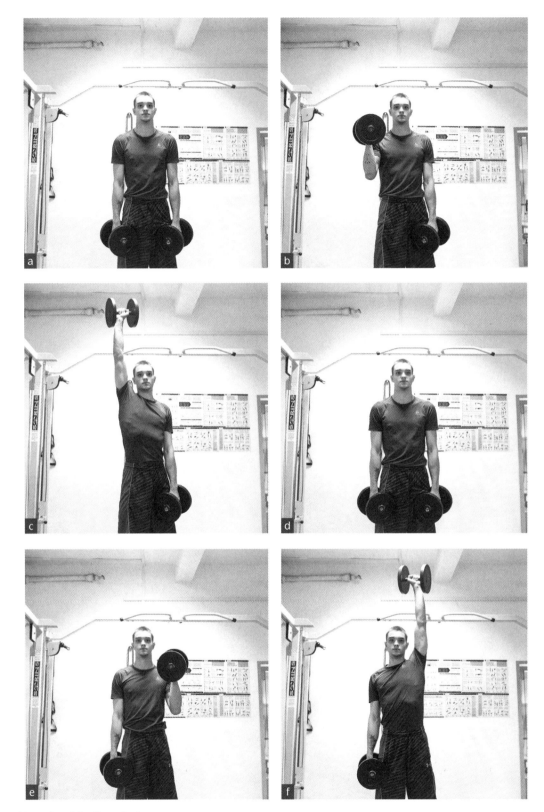

Alternating dumbbell curls to presses.

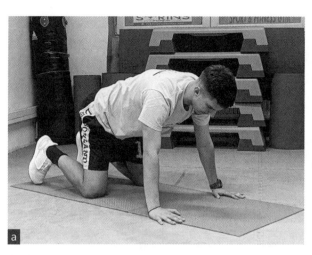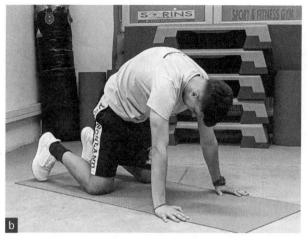

Arch.

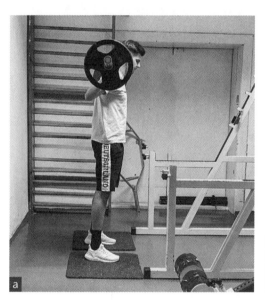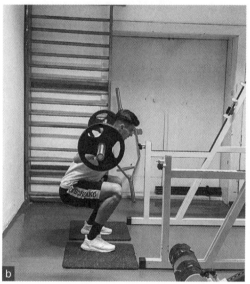

Barbell back squat.

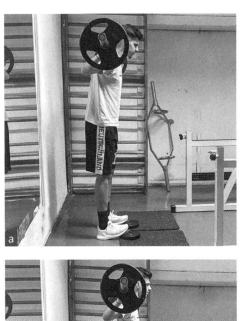
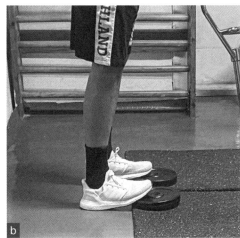
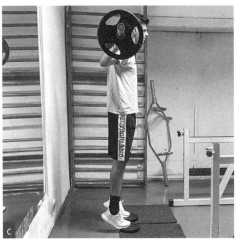
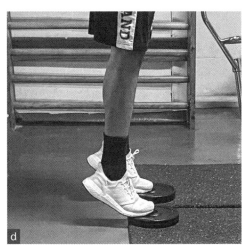

Barbell calf raise.

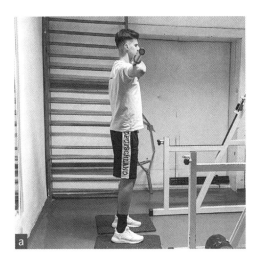
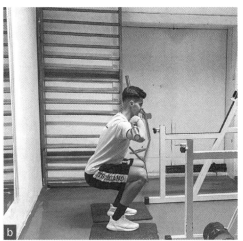

Barbell front squat.

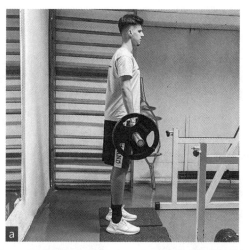

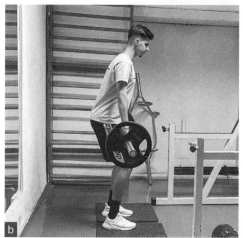
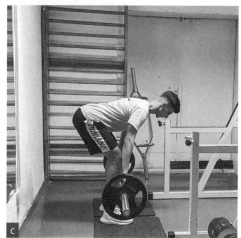

Barbell Romanian deadlift.

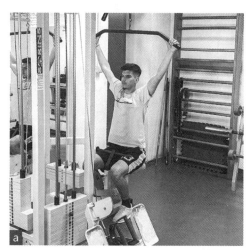
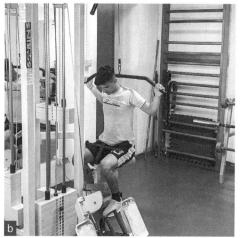

Behind the neck lat pull-down.

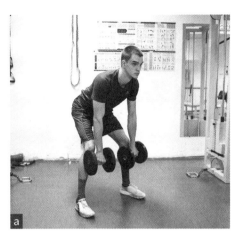 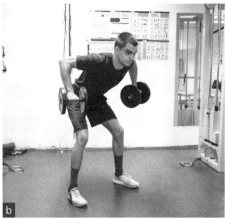

Bent-over dumbbell row.

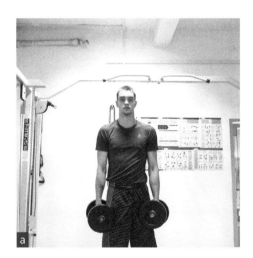

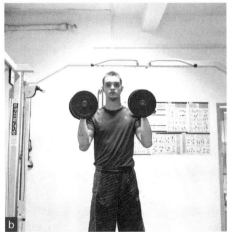 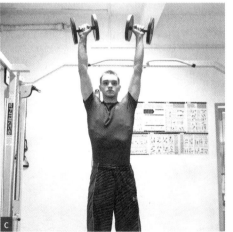

Biceps curl to overhead press.

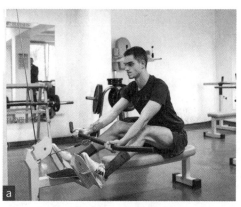

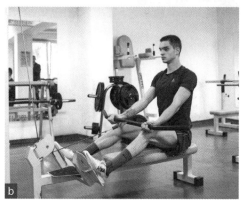

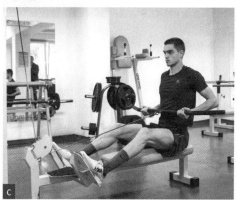

Cable reverse-grip seated row.

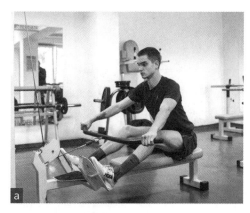

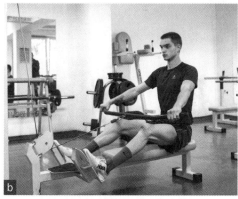

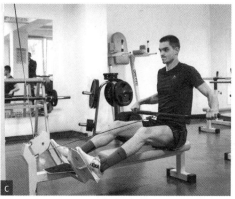

Cable wide-grip seated row.

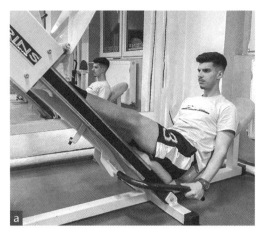 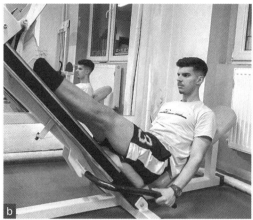

Calf press.

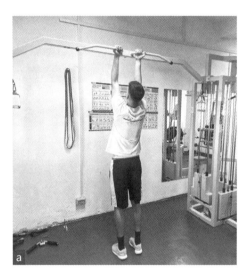 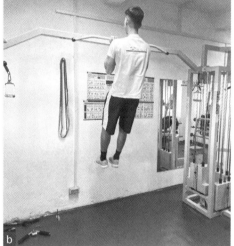

Chin-up.

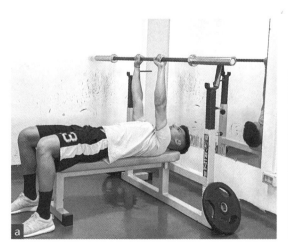

Close-grip flat bench press.

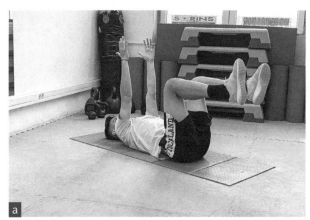
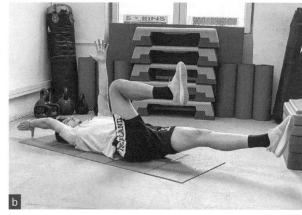
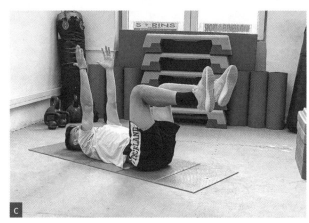
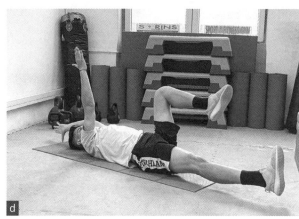

Dead bug pose.

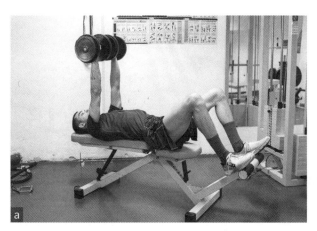
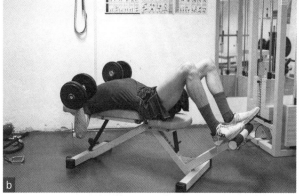

Dumbbell flat bench press.

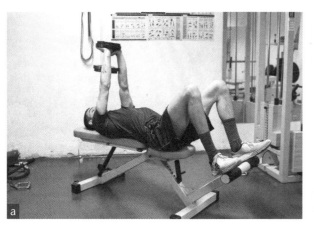 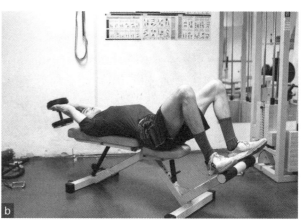

Dumbbell pullover.

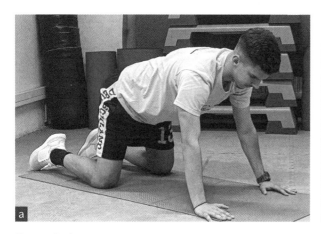 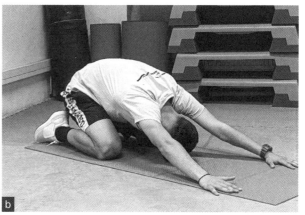

Extended puppy pose.

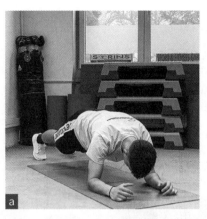
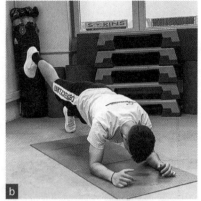
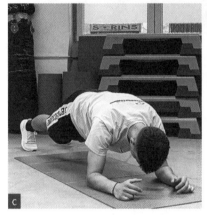
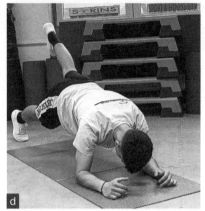
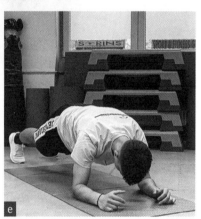

Forearm plank leg lift.

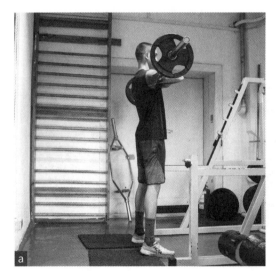
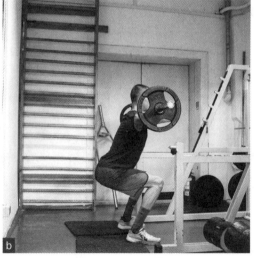

Front squat.

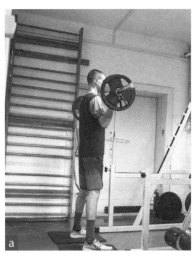 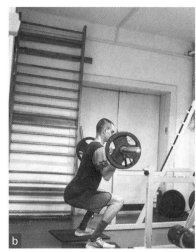 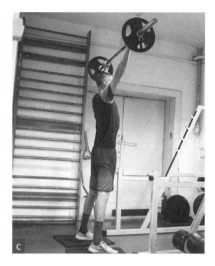

Front squat to push press.

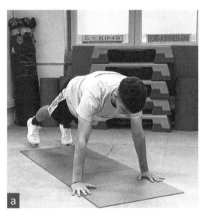 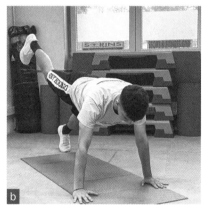

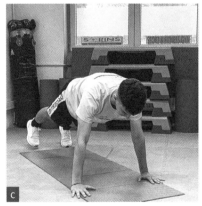 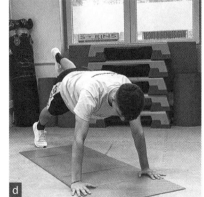 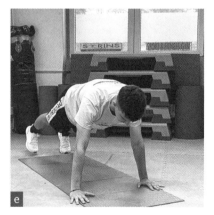

Full plank with leg lift.

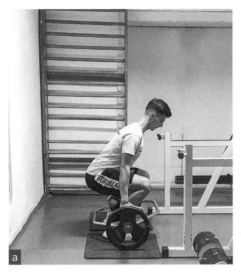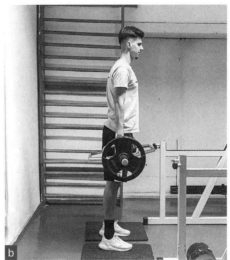

Hex-bar squat.

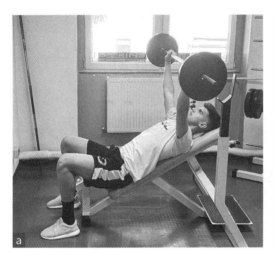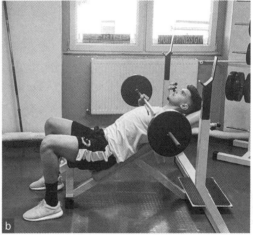

Incline barbell bench press.

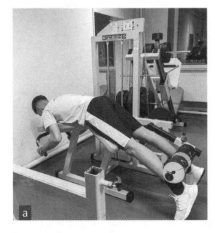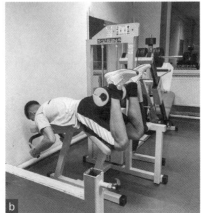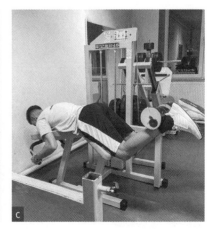

Leg curl.

245

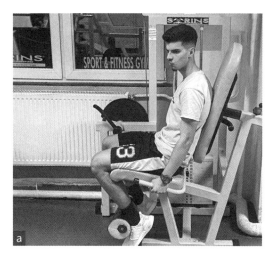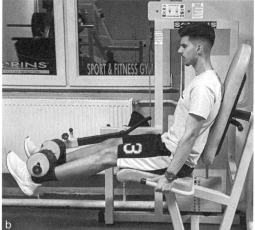

Leg extension.

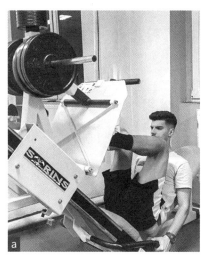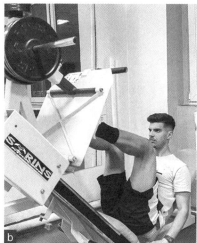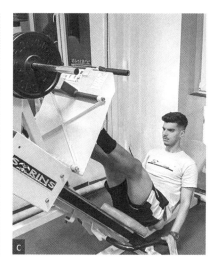

Leg press.

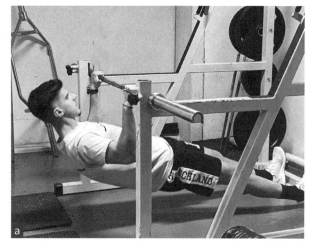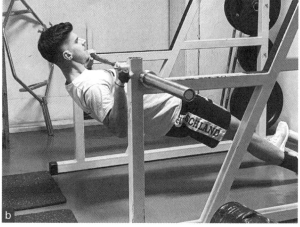

Lying pull-up.

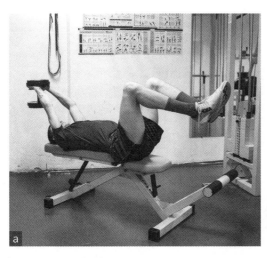 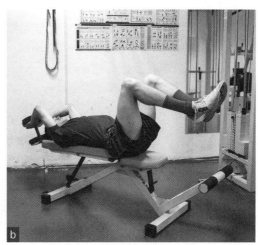

Lying triceps extension.

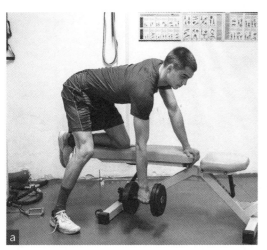 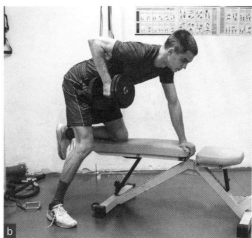

One-arm dumbbell row.

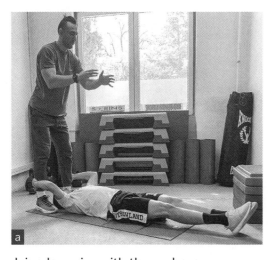 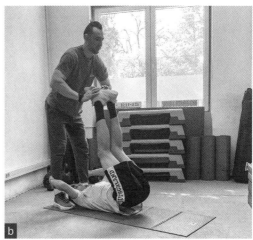

Partner lying leg raise with throw down.

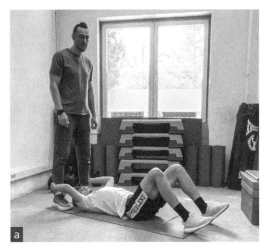 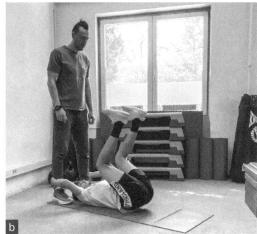

Partner reverse crunch.

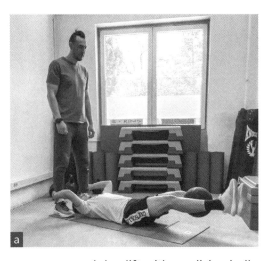 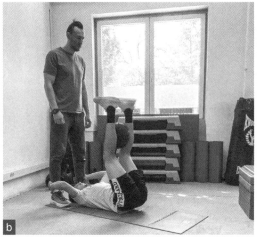

Partner reverse crunch leg lift with medicine ball.

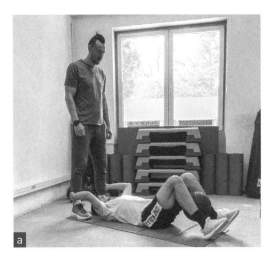 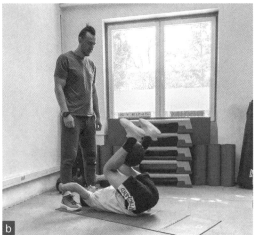

Partner reverse crunch with medicine ball.

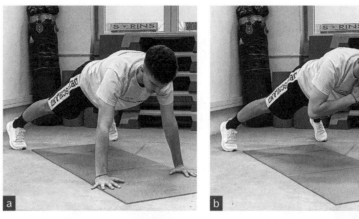

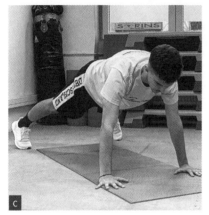
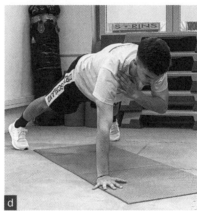
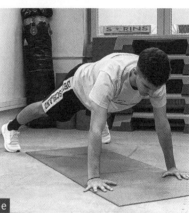

Plank tap.

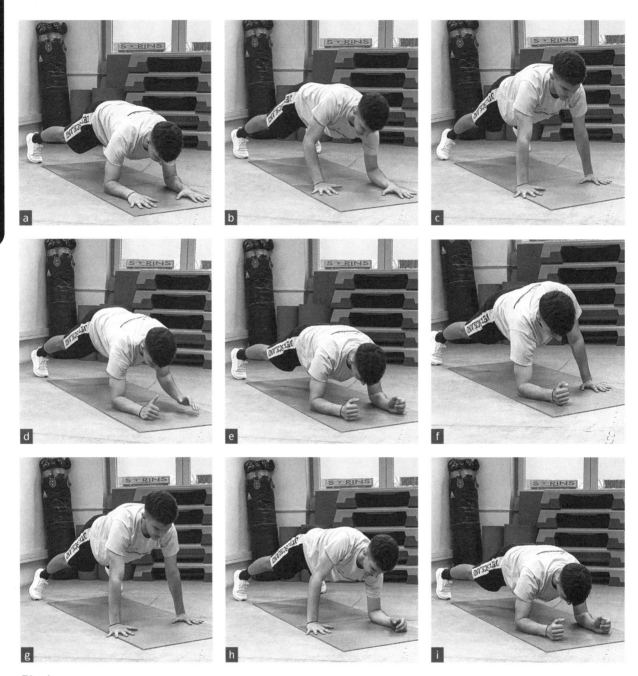

Plank-up.

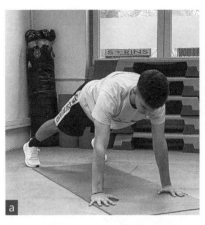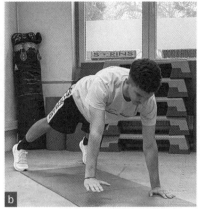

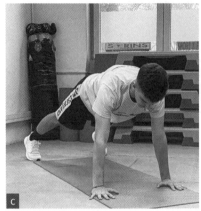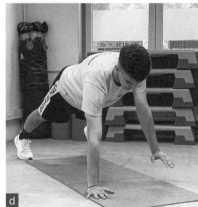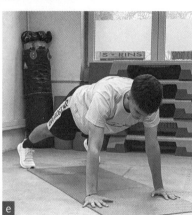

Plank with hand lift.

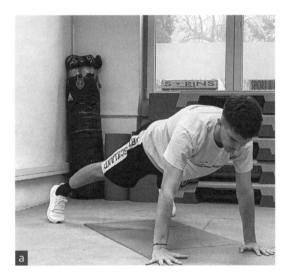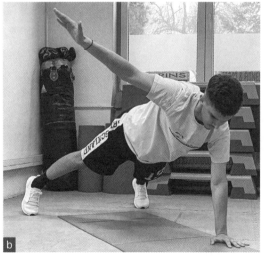

Plank with lateral arm raise.

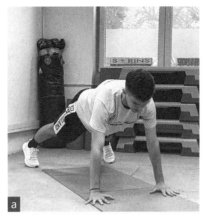 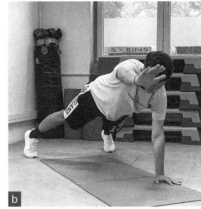

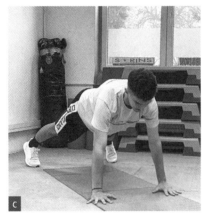 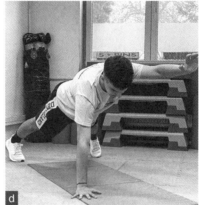 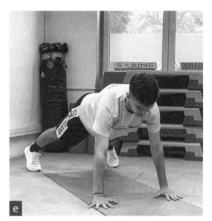

Plank with forward reach.

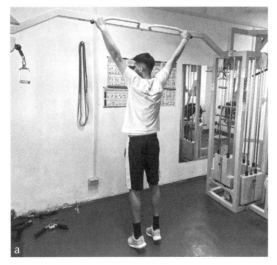 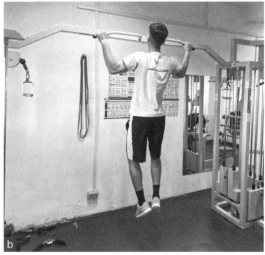

Pull-up.

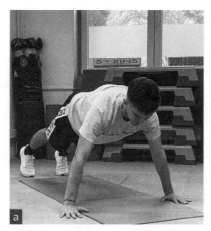 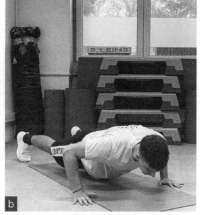

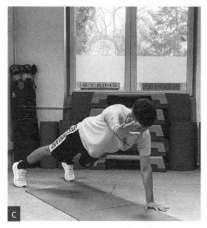 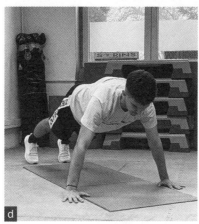 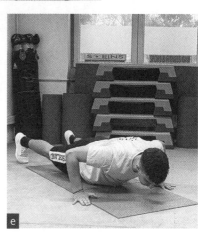

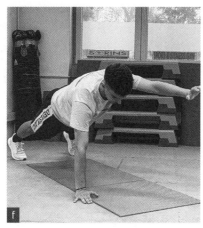 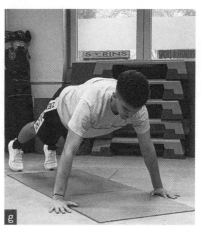

Push-up with opposite reach.

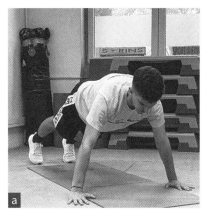 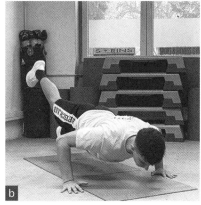

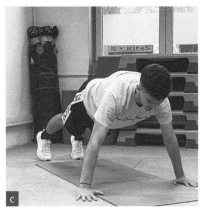 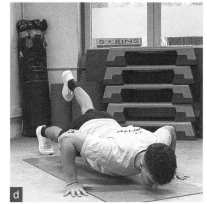 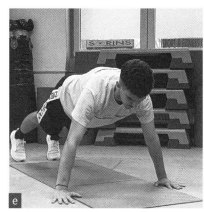

Push-up with raised leg.

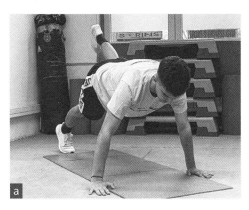 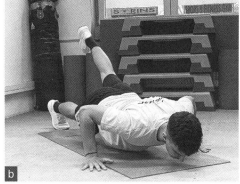

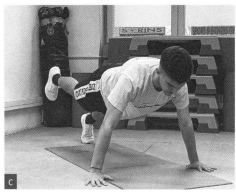 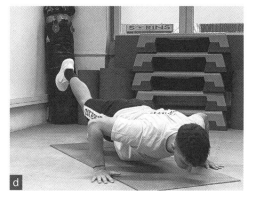

Push-up with single leg.

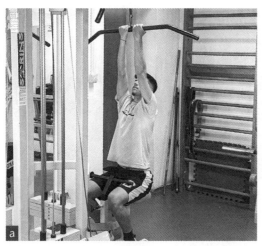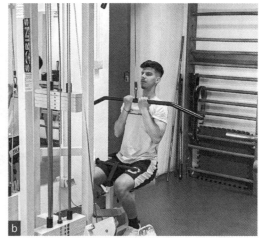

Reverse close-grip lat pull-down.

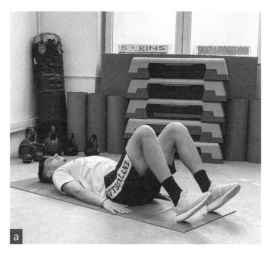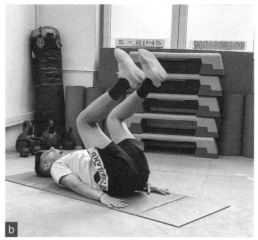

Reverse crunch.

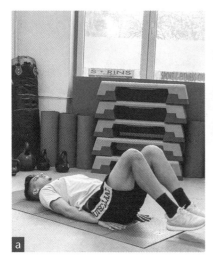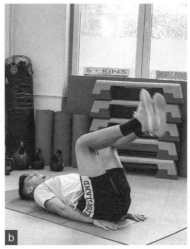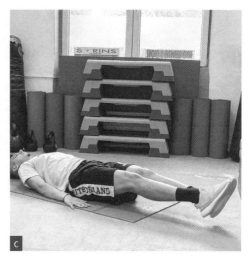

Reverse crunch leg extension.

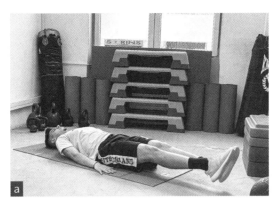

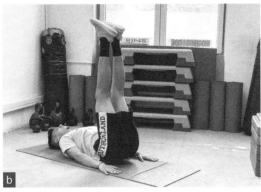

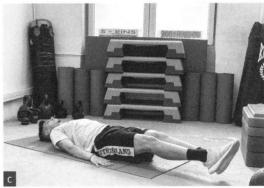

Reverse crunch leg lift.

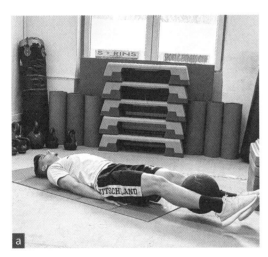

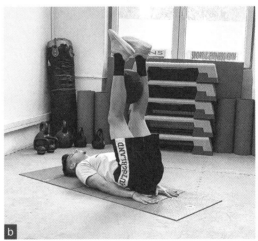

Reverse crunch leg lift with medicine ball.

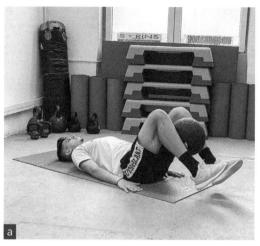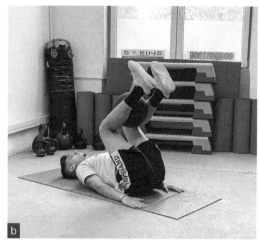

Reverse crunch with medicine ball.

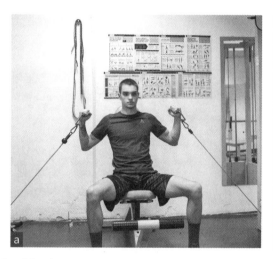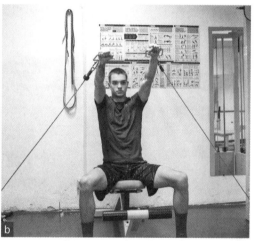

Seated cable chest press.

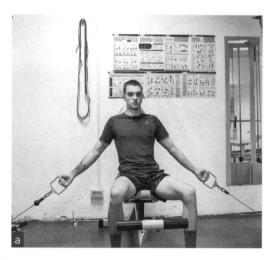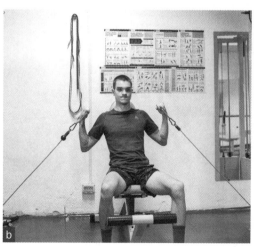

Seated cable curl.

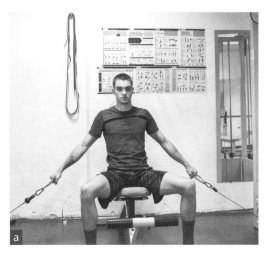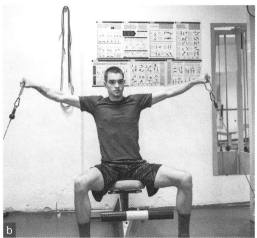

Seated cable lateral raise.

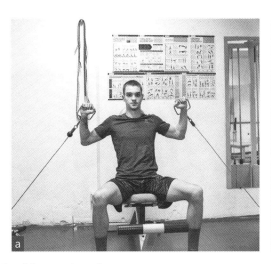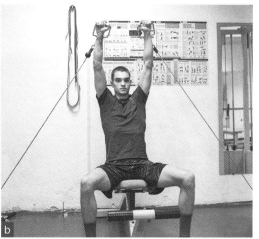

Seated cable overhead press.

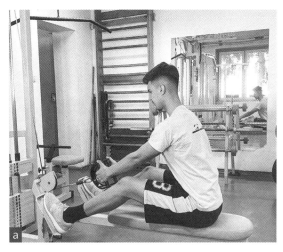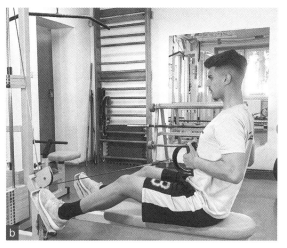

Seated cable row.

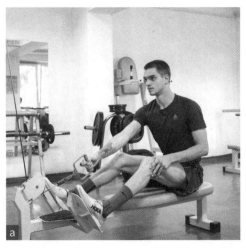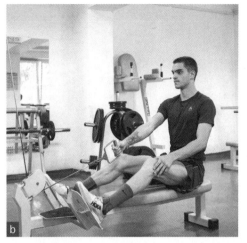

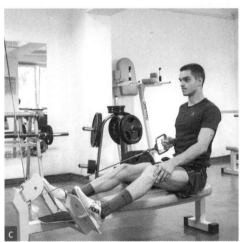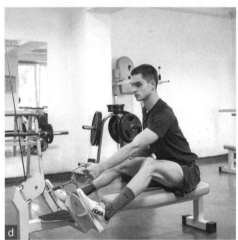

Seated one-arm cable row.

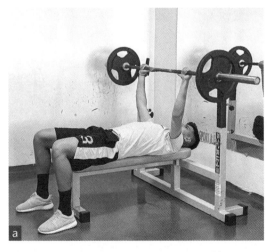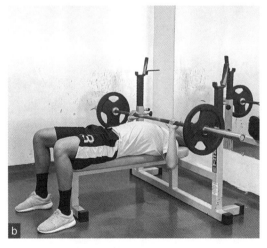

Wide-grip flat bench press.

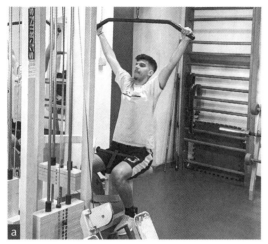 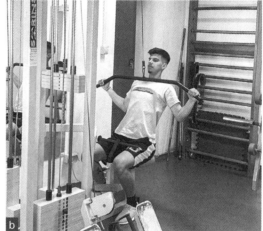

Wide-grip lat pull-down.

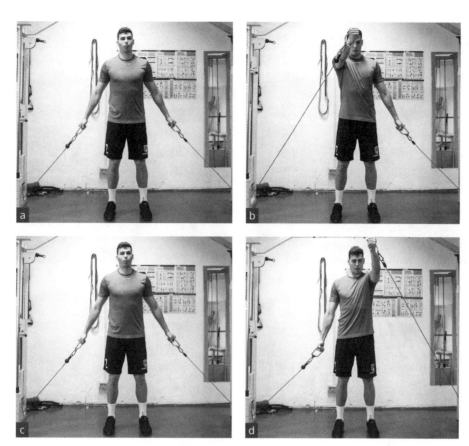

Alternating cable front raises.

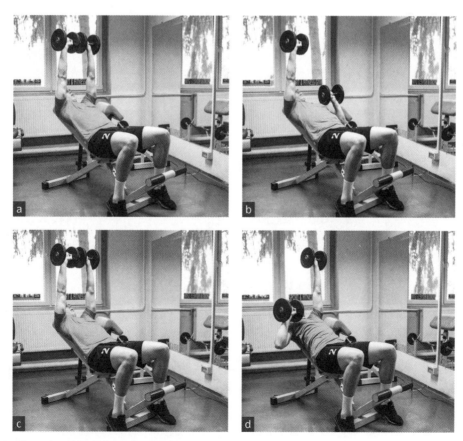

Alternating incline dumbbell bench presses.

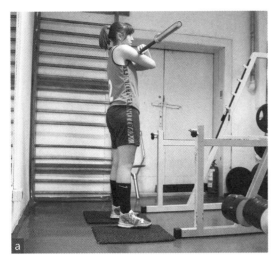 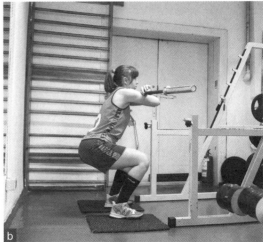

Barbell front squat.

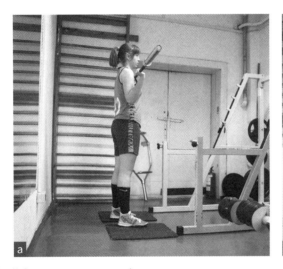 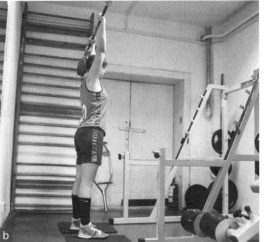

Barbell front squat to push press.

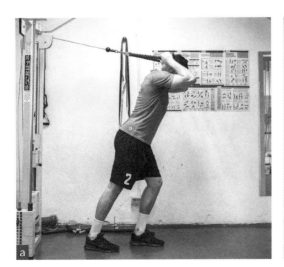 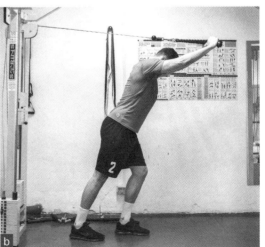

Cable overhead triceps extension.

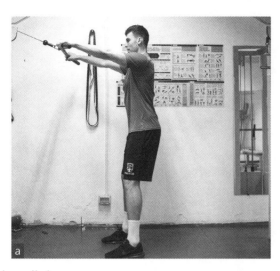 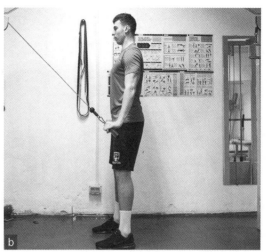

Cable pull-down.

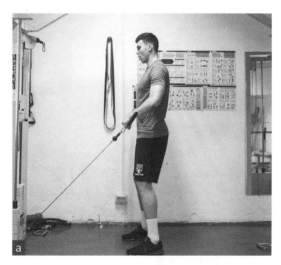 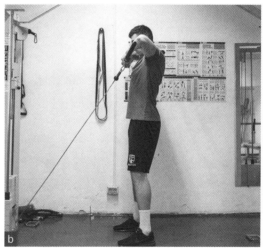

Cable upright row.

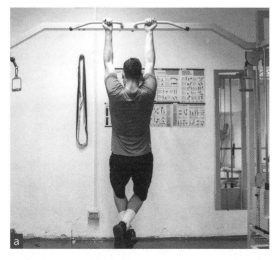 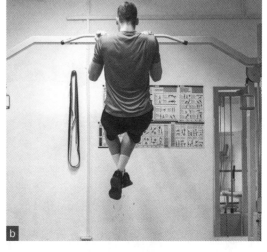

Chin-up.

263

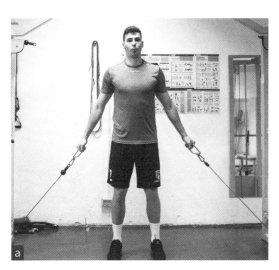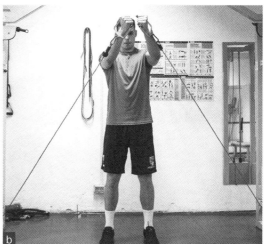

Dual-cable front raise.

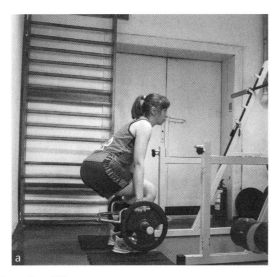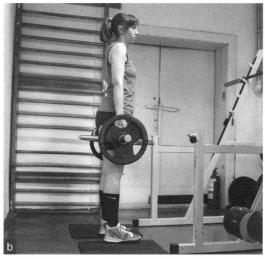

Hex-bar deadlift.

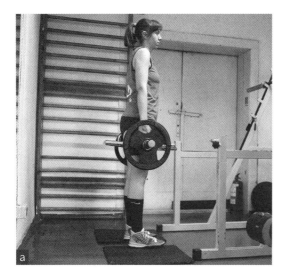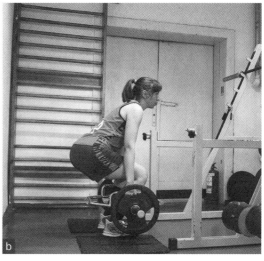

Hex-bar squat.

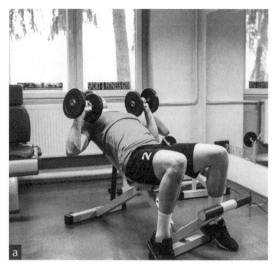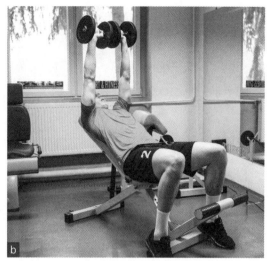

Incline dumbbell press.

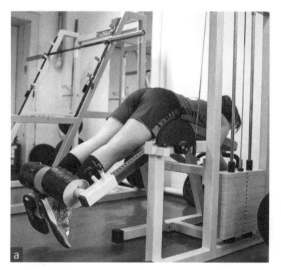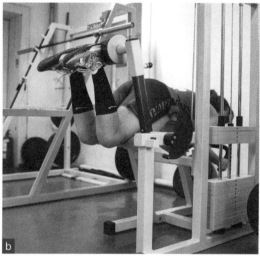

Leg curl.

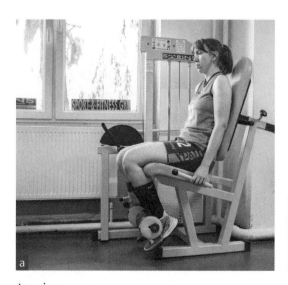

Leg extension.

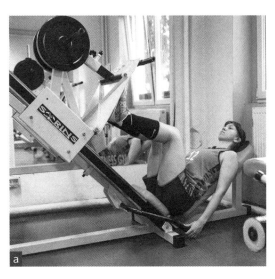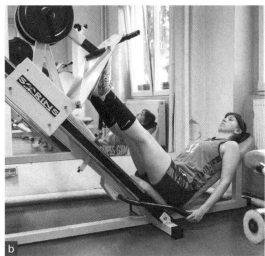

Leg press.

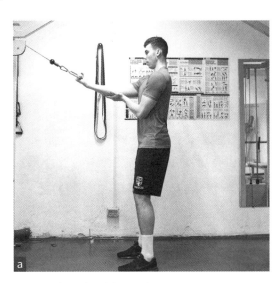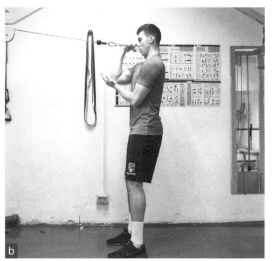

One-arm overhead cable curl.

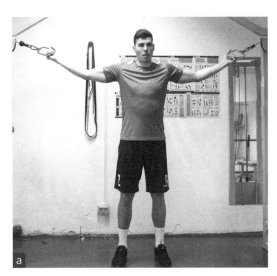

Overhead cable curl.

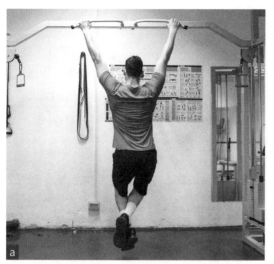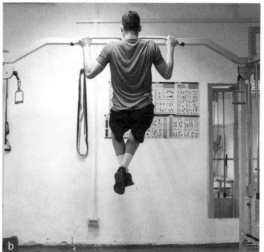

Pull-up.

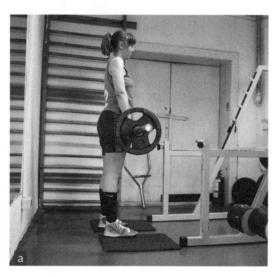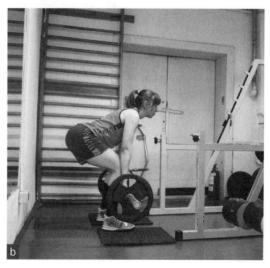

Romanian deadlift.

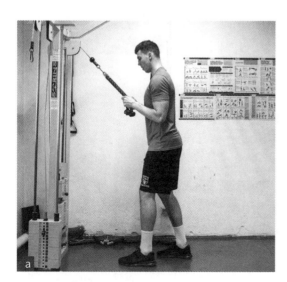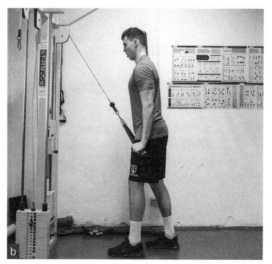

Rope triceps extension.

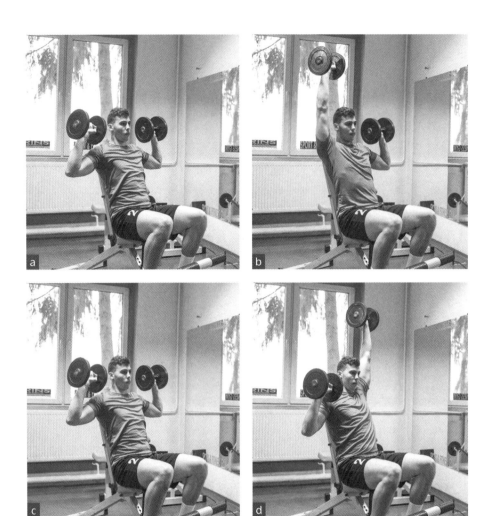

Seated alternating dumbbell presses.

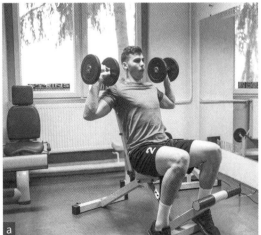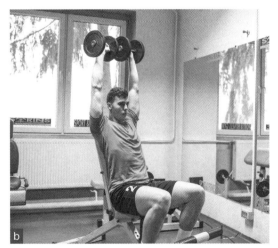

Seated overhead press.

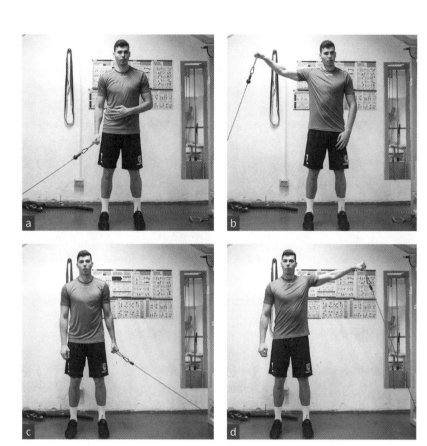

Single-arm cable lateral raise.

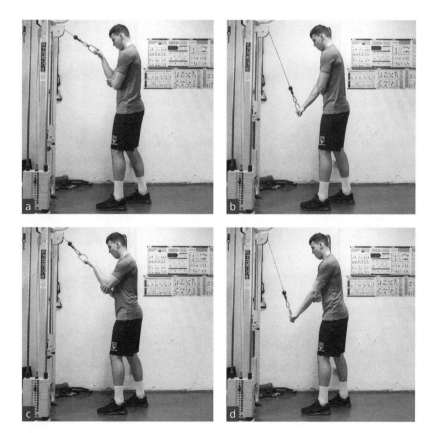

Single-arm cable triceps extension.

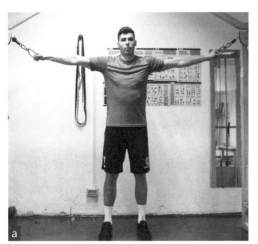 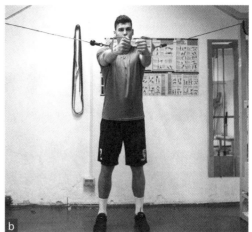

Standing cable chest fly.

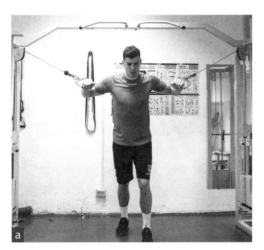 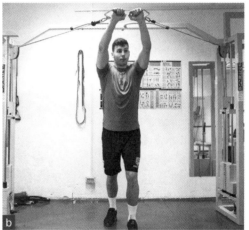

Standing cable chest press.

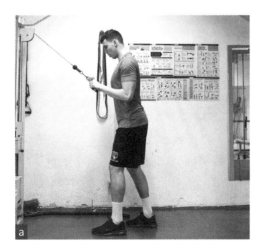 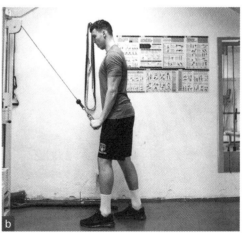

Standing cable EZ-bar triceps extension.

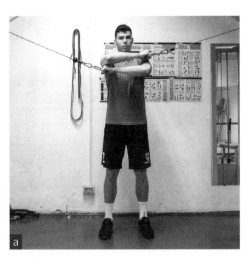 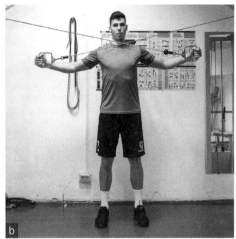

Standing cable rear deltoid fly.

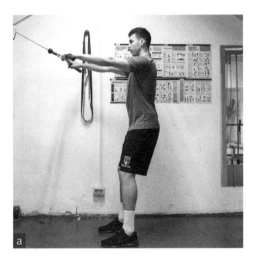 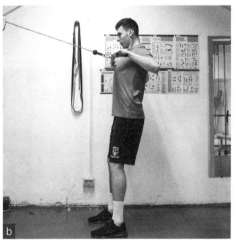

Standing cable row.

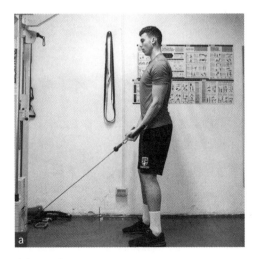 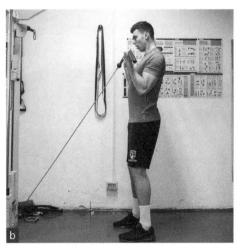

Standing cable curl.

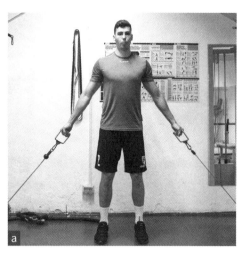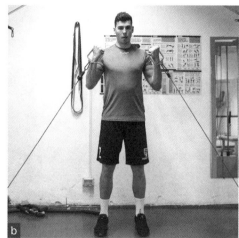

Standing double cable curl.

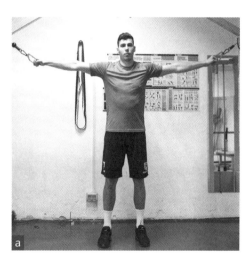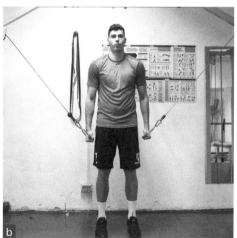

Standing double cable pull-down.

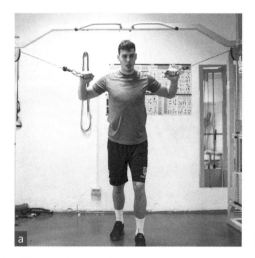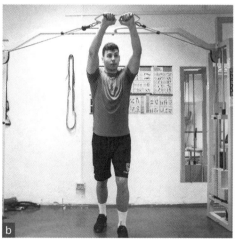

Standing incline cable chest press.

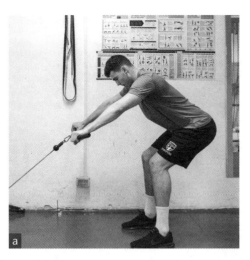
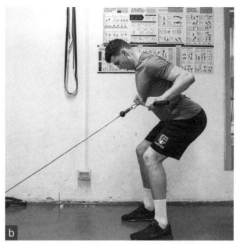

Standing low cable row.

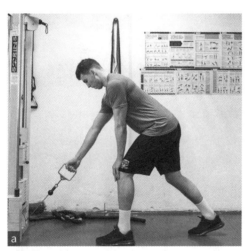
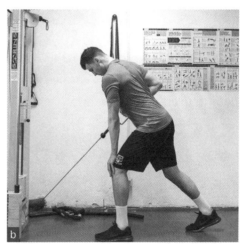
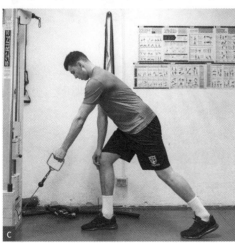
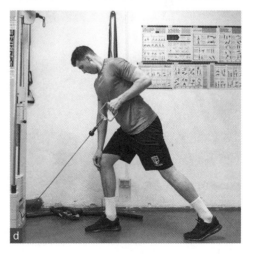

Standing one-arm cable row.

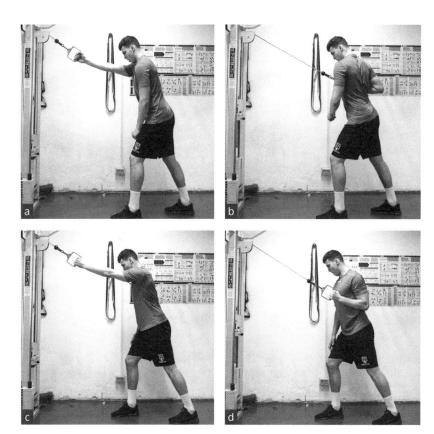

Standing one-arm overhead cable row.

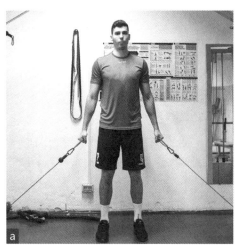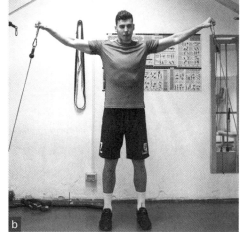

Standing two-arm cable lateral raise.

274

Glossary

accelerate—The ability to increase frequency of running or rate of a motion.

acceleration—The ability to increase movement action or velocity in a minimum amount of time.

acceleration–deceleration coupling—The ability to slow down quickly after running with maximum velocity.

actin—Thin filament; a protein involved in muscle contraction.

adaptation—Positive changes in the functions of the body because of training.

adenosine triphosphate (ATP)—A complex high-energy phosphate compound formed with the energy released from food and stored in muscle cells. It allows for the release of energy when its phosphate bonds are broken.

aerobic endurance—The ability to exercise at moderate intensity for an extended period.

aerobic energy system—See oxidative anergy system.

agility—The ability of a player to quickly change direction (cut) during the game. It is a highly desirable quality in most team sports, particularly on offense and for playmakers. Agility is clearly enhanced by, and strongly dependent on, a player's level of maximum strength.

agonist muscles—Muscles contracting to perform a physical action.

alactic endurance—The capacity of an athlete to repeat short-duration (5-12 sec) maximum-intensity activities or drills and to tolerate the fatigue induced by such activities.

alactic energy system—See phosphagen energy system.

anaerobic—In the absence of oxygen.

anaerobic energy system—See glycolytic energy system.

antagonist muscles—Muscles relaxing during a motion or return of the movement to the original position.

anatomical age—Numerical assessment of a child's physical growth in relation to chronological age.

biological age—An indication of age based on sexual maturation.

biomotor (motor) abilities—The physical abilities used in a sport, such as agility, flexibility, speed, strength, and endurance.

carbohydrate—A basic foodstuff, it is a compound composed of carbon, hydrogen, and oxygen.

clean—Lifting a weight from the floor to the chest.

concentric contraction—The shortening of a muscle during contraction.

connective tissue—Ligaments and tendons that connect the muscles to the bones to perform an athletic action

crossbridge—Projections around the myosin filament that latch onto the binding site on actin, initiating a muscle contraction.

detraining—A reversal of adaptation to exercise caused by a longer duration of inactivity.

eccentric contraction—Muscle contraction during which the muscle lengthens.

endurance—The capacity to perform work for an extended period.

energy—The capacity to perform work.

energy system—Metabolic system involving a series of chemical reactions, which form waste products and manufacture ATP.

ergogenesis—The proportions, expressed in percentages, of the three energy systems that supply energy for a given sport.

extension—Stretching a joint, when the two parts of a joint move away from each other.

fast-twitch (FT) muscle fiber—A muscle fiber characterized by fast contraction time beneficial to speed, power, and agility activities.

fatigue—A state of discomfort and decreased efficiency resulting from training.

flexibility—The range of motion of a joint.

flexion—A bending movement around a joint that decreases the angle of two body parts.

glycogen—A storage form of carbohydrate that is found in the skeletal muscle and liver.

glycolytic energy system—Energy system, also known as lactic energy system, that provides energy through the breakdown of glucose without the presence of oxygen. It supplies energy for 20 to 90 seconds. Often it is associated with a high level of fatigue.

hypertrophy—An increase in the size of the muscles because of a strength-training program.

intensity—The qualitative aspect of work performed during training, such as speed, agility, power, and maximum strength (MxS).

intermuscular coordination—The ability to synchronize all muscles of a kinetic chain (movement).

intramuscular coordination—The capacity to voluntarily recruit as many motor units as possible in an athletic action.

lactate—A salt formed from lactic acid (must be eliminated from the system before an athlete can return to maximum efficiency).

lactic endurance—The ability to perform medium-duration work lasting 30 to 90 seconds.

lactic energy system—See glycolytic energy system.

macrocycle—A training plan of a 4- to 6-week duration.

maturation—Progress toward adulthood.

maximal aerobic power—Maximum rate at which oxygen can be used during intense exercises.

maximum strength (MxS)—The highest force an athlete can lift or overcome during one maximal contraction. See also one-repetition maximum (1RM).

metabolite—Any substance produced by a metabolic reaction (chemical reactions occurring during sporting athletic activities).

microcycle—A training plan for one week.

model or **modeling**—A training system that models, mimics, the specifics of athletic actions during a game/competition. Modeling a competition or game readies an athlete for the future contest.

movement time—The capacity of an athlete to quickly move a limb or parts of the body as fast as possible in the desired direction.

multilateral development—The development of all abilities of an athlete as required by the selected sport or position played.

muscular endurance—The ability of a muscle to repeatedly exert force against resistance.

muscular strength—The capacity of an athlete to perform work or overcome a resistance.

myosin—Thick filament; a protein involved in muscular contraction.

myotatic stretch reflex—A muscle contraction in response to the stretching within a muscle.

neuromuscular training—A type of training that involves athletes performing exercises (e.g., agility and quickness exercises) at a very high intensity (90%-95%), which taxes the neuromuscular system.

obese—An overweight person or excessive fat accumulation that can present a risk to health.

one-repetition maximum (1RM)—See maximum strength (MxS).

overtraining—A decrement of performance caused by overwork.

overuse injuries—A muscle, ligament, or joint trauma, or injury, caused by exaggerated, repetitive, specific training.

overweight—See obese.

oxidative (aerobic) energy system—The primary source of ATP during low-intensity, long-duration physical activity, this system utilizes carbohydrate, fat, and sometimes (but rarely) protein to resynthesize ATP in the presence of oxygen and make energy available for activity.

oxygen debt (oxygen deficit)—The anaerobic contribution to the total energy cost of an activity.

periodization—A systematic sequencing of training phases during a training plan. This concept is also valid for planning the development of physical abilities, such as strength, speed, agility, and endurance.

phosphagen—A group of compounds; it collectively refers to ATP (adenosine triphosphate) and CP (creatine phosphate).

phosphagen (alactic, ATP-CP) energy system—An anaerobic (without the presence of oxygen) energy system that provides energy for a short term (<12 sec).

physiology—A branch of the science of biology, the study of living organs and the whole human body, during physical activity.

plyometric training—Drills using an explosive, reactive type of exercises. It is often called jump training.

power—Unit of work expressed per unit of time (power = work/time). It is often considered a factor of intensity. Also, it is the scientific term that refers to work where speed and strength are the main contributors.

power endurance—Athletes' capacity to apply, nonstop, a power action for a long time.

prime movers—Muscles performing the main technical skills. See also agonist muscles.

preparatory phase—The first phase of an annual training plan, where the scope is to ready an athlete for competitions.

reaction time—The time it takes the neuromuscular system to respond to a stimulus (athletic action).

recovery (exercise recovery)—A pause between bouts of training that replenishes energy.

repetition—A sporting action, sprint, drill, or weight training, that is repeated several times during training.

rest interval—The pause, in minutes or seconds, taken during speed, agility, strength, and endurance training.

set—The total number of repetitions an athlete performs before taking a rest interval (pause).

slow-twitch (ST) muscle fiber—A muscle fiber characterized by slow contraction time, low anaerobic capacity, and high aerobic capacity, all making the fiber suited for low power output activities.

speed—The ability to cover a given distance in the shortest time period (run, swim, etc.).

speed endurance—The ability of an athlete to maintain a high level of speed for a longer period. For instance, in a 100-meter race, the ability to maintain a high velocity in the last 20 meters depends on the level of speed endurance. In team sports, it also refers to the ability to repeat many sprints at high velocity.

step loading method—A training method where the load is increased in steps, usually one week.

stop-and-go drills—Exercises in which athletes accelerate to maximum velocity, decelerate to a stationary stop, and again accelerate in another direction.

strength—The force generated by muscle contractions.

stretch-shortening cycle (SSC)—A physiological manifestation in which muscle fibers contract concentrically (shorten) or eccentrically (lengthen) during many power-based sport activities, such as plyometric exercises.

supercompensation—Also known as general adaptation syndrome, it refers to the body's response to stressors and how it adapts to them.

training—The process of executing repetitive, progressive exercises or work that improves the potential to achieve optimum performance. For athletes, it means using long-term programs that condition the body and mind for the specific challenges of competition and lead to excellence in performance.

training demand—A summation of all the factors used in training or game situations.

volume—The amount of work during all aspects of training and sporting contests.

References

Afonzo, J., J. Olivares-Jabalera, and R. Andrade. 2021. Time to move from mandatory stretching? We need to differentiate "Can I?" from "Do I have to?" *Frontiers in Physiology*. https://www.frontiersin.org/articles/10.3389/fphys.2021.714166/full

Alaranta, H., H. Hurri, M. Heliovaara, A. Soukka, and R. Harju. 1994. Flexibility of the spine: Normative values of goniometric and tape measurements. *Scand. J. Rehab. Med.* 26:147-54.

American Heart Association. 2018. Recommendations for Physical Activity in Kids Infographic. https://www.heart.org/en/healthy-living/fitness/fitness-basics/aha-recs-for-physical-activity-in-kids-infographic.

Aoyagi, M.W., A.B. Cohen, A. Poczwardowski, J.N. Metzler, and T. Statler. 2018. Models of performance excellence: Four approaches to sport psychology consulting, *J. Sport Psychol. in Action* 9(2): 94-110. .

Avalos, M, P. Hellard, and J.C. Chatard. 2003. Modeling the training–performance relationships using a mixed model in elite swimmers. *Med Sci. Sports Exerc.* 35(5): 838-46.

Bacil, E.D.A, O. Mazzardo, Jr., C.R. Rech, R.F. Legnani, and W. de Campos. 2015. Physical activity and biological maturation: A systematic review. *Rev. Paul. Pedriatr.* 33(1): 114-21.

Baker, J. 2003. Early specialization in youth: A requirement for adult expertise. *High Ability Studies*, 14(1): 85-94.

Bangsbo, J., M. Mohr, and I.P. Krustrup. 2006. Physical and metabolic demand of training and match-play in elite football players. *J. Sports Sc.* 24(7): 665-74.

Bangsbo, J., F.M. Iaia, and P. Krustrup. 2007. Metabolic response and fatigue in soccer. *Int. J. Sports Physiol. Perform.* 2(2): 111-27.

Behm, D.G., A.D. Faigebaum., B. Falk, and P. Klentrou. 2008. Canadian Society for Exercise Physiology position paper: Resistance training in children and adolescence. *Appl. Physiol. Nutr. Metab.* 33(3): 547-61.

Behm, D.G., J.D. Young., and J.D. Whitten. 2017. Effectiveness of traditional strength vs. power training on muscle strength, power, and speed in youth: A systematic review and meta-analysis. *Front. Physiol.* 8: 423.

Behringer, M.A, A. Vom Heede., M. Mathews., and J. Mester. 2011. Effects of strength training on motor performance skills in children and adolescence: A meta-analysis. *Pediatr. Exerc. Sci.* 23: 186-206.

Beliard, S, M. Chauvreau, T. Moscatiello, F. Cros, F. Ecarnot, and F. Becker. 2015. Compression garments and exercise: No influence of pressure applied. *J. Sports Sci. Med.* 14(1): 75-83.

Bell, R.D., L. DiStefano, N.K. Pandya, and T.A. McGuine. 2019. The public health consequences of sports specialization. *J. Athl. Train.* 54(10): 1013-20.

Benton, D., A. Maconie, and C. Williams. 2007. The influence of the glycaemic load of breakfast on the behaviour of children in school. *Physiol . Behav.* 92(4): 717-24.

Blackhurst, N.R., J.C. Peterson, V.W. Herzog, and E.P Zimmerman. 2015. A comparison of static stretching versus combined static and ballistic stretching in active knee range of motion. *Internet J. Allied Health Sci. Pract.* 10: 20.

Boisseau, N., M.Vermorel, M. Rance, P. Duché, and P. Patureau-Mirand. 2007. Protein requirements in male adolescent soccer players. *Eur. J. Appl. Physiol.* 100(1): 27-33.

Bompa, T.O. 2006. *Total training for coaching team sports: A Self-Help Guide.* Toronto: Sport Books.

Bompa, T.O. 1993. *Periodization of strength: The new wave in strength training.* Toronto: Veritas.

Bompa T. and G.G. Haff. 2009. *Periodization: Theory and methodology of training.* Champaign, IL: Human Kinetics.

Bompa, T.O. and C. Francis. 1995. Force-time analysis of Canadian sprinters. Unpublished data. Toronto: York University.

Bompa, T.O. and M. Carrera. 2015. *Conditioning young athletes.* Champaign, IL: Human Kinetics.

Bompa T.O. and C. Buzzichelli. 2021. *Periodization of strength training for sports.* Champaign, IL: Human Kinetics.

Bowman, S.A., S.L. Gortmaker, C.B. Ebbeling, M.A. Pereira, and D.S. Ludwig. 2004. Effects of fast-food consumption on energy intake and diet quality among children in a national household survey. *Pediatrics* 113(1): 112-18.

Branta, C.F. 2010. Sport specialization. *J Phys. Educ. Rec. Dance* 81(8): 19-28.

Bray, G.A., S.J. Nielsen, and B.M. Popkin. 2004. Consumption of high-fructose corn syrup in beverages may play a role in the epidemic of obesity. *Am. J. Clin. Nutr.* 79(4): 537-43.

Brenner, J.S. and the Council of Sports Medicine and Fitness. 2016. Sports specialization and intensive training in young athletes. *Pediatrics*, 138(3): 2016-2148.

Cain, D.J., J. Difiori, and N. Mafulli. 2006. Physical injuries in children and youth sports: Reason for concern? *Br. J. Sport Med.* 40:749-760.

Cain, D.J. and N. Maffulli. 2005. Epidemiology of children's individual sports injuries. *Med. Sports Sci.* 48: 1-7.

Canadian Hockey Association. 1993. Ottawa, Ontario.

Capranica, L. and M.L. Millard-Stafford. 2011. Youth sport specialization: How to manage competition and training? *Int. J. Sports Physiol. Perform.* 6(4): 572-579.

Carling, C, J. Bloomfield, L. Nelsen, and T. Reilly. 2008. The role of motion analysis in elite soccer: Contemporary performance measurement techniques and work rate data. *Sports Med.* 38(10): 839-862.

Cattelan M, C. Varin, and D. Firth. 2013. Dynamic Bradley-Terry modelling of sports tournaments. *J. R. Stat. Soc.* Series C 62(1): 135-150.

Centers for Nutrition Disease Control and Prevention (CDC). 2015. 24/7: Saving Lives, Protecting People. Guidelines & Recommendations. Last reviewed November 27, 2017. https://www.cdc.gov/cdctv/emergencypreparednessandresponse/cdc-24-7-transcript.html

Clark, K.P. and P.G Weyand. 2014. Are running speeds maximized with simple-spring stance mechanics? *J. Appl. Physiol.* 117(6): 604-615.

Clarkson P.M. and M.J. Hubal. 2002. Exercise-induced muscle damage in humans. *Am. J. Phys. Med. Rehabil.* 81(Suppl 11): S52-69.

Colomer, C.M.E., D.B. Payne, M., Mooney, A. McKune, and B.G. Serpell. 2020. Performance analysis in rugby union: A critical systematic review. *Sports Med.* 6(1): 4.

Colyer S.L., R. Nagahara, Y. Takai, and A.I.T. Salo. 2018. How sprinters accelerate beyond the velocity plateau of soccer players: Waveform analysis of ground reaction forces. *Scand. J. Med. Sci. Sports.* 28(12): 2527-35.

Crane, J. and V. Temple. 2015. A systematic review of dropout from organized sport among children and youth. *Eur Phy Educ Rev.* 21(1): 114-131. https://doi.org/10.1177%2F1356336X14555294

Cushion, C. 2007. Modelling the complexity of the coaching process. *Int J. Sports Sci. Coach.* 2(4): 395-401.

Cyrenne, P. 2009. Modelling professional sports leagues: An industrial organization approach. *Rev. Ind. Org.* 34: 193-215.

Dahab, K., and T. McCambridge. 2009. Strength training in children and adolescence: Raising the bar for young athletes? *Sports Health* 1(3): 223-26.

Daniels, S,R., D.K. Arnett, R.H. Eckel, H. Robert, S.S. Gidding, S. Samuel, L.L. Hayman, S. Kumanika, L.L. Shiriki, T.N. Robinson, B.J.

Scott, S. St. Jeor, and C.L. Williams. 2002. Overweight in children and adolescents: Pathophysiology, consequences, prevention, and treatment. *J. Am. Med. Assoc.* 288(14): 1728-32.

Dasuri, K., L. Zhang, and J.N. Keller. 2013. Oxidative stress, neurodegeneration, and the balance of protein degradation and protein synthesis. *Free Radic. Biol. Med.* 62: 170-85.

Dolci, F., H.H. Hart, A.E. Kilding, P. Chivers, and B. Piggott. 2020. Physical and energy demand of soccer: A brief review. *Strength and Cond J.* 42(3): 70-77.

Dorn T. W, AG., Schache , M G Pandy. 2012. Muscular strategy shift in human running: Dependence of running speed and angle muscle performance. *J Exp Biol.* June 1; 215(Pt 13): 1944-56.

Dorn T.W., A.G Schache, M. G. Pandy. 2012. What muscles are moving us while we run? Updated: Dec 8 2019. *J Exp Biol.* 215: 1944-56.

Douglas A., K. Johnston, M.A. Rotondi, V.K. Jamnik, and A.C. Macpherson. 2019. On-ice measures of external load in relation to match output in elite female ice hockey. *Sports* 7(7): 173.

Duarte, R., B. Escofier, M. Rumpf, and J. Wiemeyer. 2016. Modeling and simulation of sport games, sport movement and adaptation to training. Report from *Dagstuhl* Seminar 5(9):38-56.

Duffey, K.J., and B.M. Popkin. 2008. High fructose corn syrup. Is this what's for dinner? *Am. J. Clin. Nutr.* 88: 1722S-1732S.

Eime, R.M., J.A. Young, J.T. Harvey, M.J. Charity, and W.R. Payne. 2013. A systematic review of the psychological and social benefits of participation in sports for children and adolescence: Informing development of a conceptual model of health through sport. *Int J Behav Nutr Phys Act.* https://doi.org/10.1186/1479-5868-10-98.

Ekblom, B. 1986. Applied physiology of soccer. *Sports Med.* 3(1):50-60.

Ekstrand, J. 2021. UEFA Medical Committee Annual Report. https://editorial.uefa.com/resources/0275-151e15e03052-f1013331ca02-1000/uefaannualreport202021_englr_1_.pdf.

Eliassen, W., A.H. Saeterbakken, and R. van den Tillart. 2018. Comparison of bilateral and unilateral kinematics and muscle activation. *Int. J. Sports Phys. Ther.* 13(5): 871-81.

Engel, F.A., C. Stockinger, A. Woll, and B. Sperlich. 2016. "Effects of compression garments on performance and recovery in endurance athletes." In *Compression garments in sports: Athletic performance and recovery*, edited by F. Engel and B. Sperlich, 33-61. Switzerland: Springer International Publishing.

Enoka, R.M. 2015. *Neuromechanics of human movement.* 5th ed. Champaign, IL: Human Kinetics.

Erčulj, F. 1997. Comparison of various criteria of playing performance in basketball. *Kinesiology* 29 (10): 45-51.

Fabricant, P.D., N. Lokomkin, D. Sugimoto, F.A. Tepolt, A. Straccioloni, and M.S. Kocher. 2016. Youth sports specialization and musculoskeletal injuries: A systematic review of the literature. *Phys. Sportsmed.* 44(3): 257-62.

Faigenbaum A.D., W.J. Kraemer, C.J. Blimkie, J. Jeffreys, L.J. Micheli, M. Nikta, and T.W. Rowland. 2009. Youth resistance training: Updated position statement paper from the National Strength and Conditioning association. *J. Strength Cond. R J. Strength Cond. Res.* 23(5 Suppl): S60-79.

Fair, R. 2017. The steep economics cost of contact sports injuries. PBS News Hour. Last modified October 20, 2017. https://www.pbs.org/newshour/economy/making-sense/the-steep-economic-cost-of-contact-sports-injuries.

Feeley, B.T, J. Agel, and R.F. LaPrade. 2016.When is too early for single sport specialization? *Am. J. Sports Med.* 44 (1): 234-41.

Fox, E. 1984. *Sports physiology.* 2nd ed. New York: Saunders College.

Gidding S., B. Dennison, L. Birch, S. Daniels, M. Gilman, A. Lichtenstein, R.T. Rattay, J. Steinberger, N. Stetter, and L. Van Horn. 2005. American Heart Association scientific statement: Dietary recommendations for children and adolescents. A guide for practitioners: Consensus statement from the American Heart Association. *Circulation* 112: 2061-75.

Granacher, U. and R Borde. 2017. Effects of sport-specific training during the early stages of long-term athlete development on physical fitness, body composition, cognitive, and academic performances. *Front. Physiol.* 8: 810.

Gustavsson, H, J.D. DeFreese, and D.J. Madigan. 2017. Athlete burnout: Review and Recommendations. *Curr. Opin. Psychol.* 16: 109-13.

Halberg, N., M. Henriksen, N. Söderhamn, B. Stallknecht, T. Ploug, P. Schjerling, and F. Dela. 2005. Effect of intermittent fasting and refeeding on insulin action in healthy men. *J. Appl. Physiol.* 99: 2128-2136.

Harre, D. 1982. *Trainingslehre (Learn About Training).* Berlin: Sportverlag. Health Day News, Oct. 10, 2019.

HealthDay News. 2019. *World Mental Health Day.* Oct. 10, 2019

Heitner, D. 2015. SportsMoney: Sports industry to reach $73.5 billion by 2019. *Forbes,* October 19, 2015.

Hemner, S.R., A. Seth, and S.L. Delp. 2010. Muscle contribution to propulsion and support during running. *J. Biomech.* 43(14): 2709-16.

Hensley, L. 2019. If you stop exercising here is how quickly you'll lose strength. *Global News.* July 20, 2019. https://globalnews.ca/news/5653575/how-long-does-it-take-to-lose-muscle-mass/

Herbert, R.D. and M. Gabriel. 2002. Effects of stretching before and after exercising on muscle soreness and risk of injury: A systematic review. *Br. Med. J.* 325:468-70.

Holt, N.C. and C. Neely. 2011. Positive youth development through sport: A review. *Ibero-American Journal of Exercise and Sports Psychology* 6(2):299-316.

Horníková H., E. Zemková. 2021. Relationship between physical factors and change of direction speed in team sports. Appl Sci. 11(2): 665. https://doi.org/10.3390/app11020655

Horsfield, I. 2015. Arsenal plot £45m bid for Manchester United and Chelsea target Isco. May 13, 2015. https://www.express.co.uk/sport/football/576966/Arsenal-preparing-45m-bid-Manchester-United-Chelsea-Isco

Horsfield, J. 2015. Football coaching manual. London, United Kingdom.

Huxley, A.F. and R. Niedergerke. 1954. Structural changes in muscle during contraction; interference microscopy of living muscle fibers. *Nature.* 173 (4412):971-3.

Ingraham, S.J. 2003. The role of flexibility in injury prevention and athletic performance: Have we stretched the truth? *Minnesota Med.* 86(5): 58-61.

Janssen, I. and A.G. LeBlanc. 2010. Systematic review of health benefits of physical activity and fitness in school-aged children and youth. *Int. J. Behav. Nutr. Phys. Act.* 7(40): 1-16. doi:10,1201/b 18227-14

Jayanthi, N.A., E.G. Post, T.C. Laury, and P.D. Fabricant. 2019. Health consequences of youth sports specialization. *Athl. Train* 54(10): 1040-49.

Johns Hopkins Medicine. 2022. Sports safety. Position paper. The John Hopkins University.

Karli, U., A. Guvenc, A. Aslan, T. Hazir., and C. Acikada. 2007. Influence of Ramadan fasting on anaerobic performance and recovery following short time high intensity exercise. *J. Sports Sci. Med.* 6(4): 490-97.

Kavey, R.E., S.R. Daniels, R.M Lauer, D.L. Atkins, L.L. Hayman, and K. Taubert. 2003. American Heart Association guidelines for primary prevention of atherosclerotic cardiovascular disease beginning in childhood. *Circulation* 107(11): 1562-1566.

Kimmons, J.C., J. Seymour, M. Serdula, and H.M. Blanck. 2009. Fruit and vegetable intake among adolescents and adults in the United States: Percentage meeting individualised recommendations. *Medscape J. Med.* 11(1): 26.

References

Kohl, H.W. III and H.D. Cook, eds. 2013. *Educating the student body: Taking physical activity and physical education to school.* Washington, D.C.: National Academic Press.

Krasilshchikov, O. 2014. Multilateral training: Re-examining the concept practically. *Malaysian J of Sports Science and Recreation.* 10(1): 1-15.

Krissansen, G. 2007. Emerging health properties of whey protein and their clinical implementations. *J. Am. Coll. Nutr.* 26 (6):7135-7235.

Kumar, C.K.K. and S. Chakrabarty. 2010. A comparative study of static stretching versus ballistic stretching on the flexibility of the hamstring muscles of athletes. *Br. J. Sports Med.* 44: i16.

Laffaye, G. and P. Wagner. 2013. Eccentric rate of force development determines jumping performance. *Computer methods in Biomechanics and biomechanical engineering* 16(1): 82-83.

Law, B, P. Post, and P. McCullagh. 2017. Modeling in sport and performance. *Psychology.* https://doi.org/10.1093/acrefore/9780190236557.013.159

Lim, S., J.M. Zoellner, J.M. Lee, B.A. Burt, A.M. Sandretto, W. Sohn, A.I. Ismail, and J.M. Lepkowski. 2009. Obesity and sugar-sweetened beverages in African-American preschool children: A longitudinal study. *Obesity* 17(6):1262-68.

LoDolce, M.E., J.L. Harris, and M.B. Schwartz. 2013. Sugar as part of a balanced breakfast? What cereal advertisements teach children about healthy eating. *J. Health Commun.* 18(11): 1293-1309.

Luc, T., I. Mujika, and T. Busso. 2009. Computer simulations assessing the potential performance benefit of a final increase in training during pre-event taper. *J. Strength Cond. Res.* 23(6): 1729-36.

Manchado C., J. Pers, F. Navarro., A. Han., E. Sung., and P. Platen. 2013. Time-motion analysis in women's team handball: Importance of aerobic performance. *J. Hum. Sport Exerc.* 8(2): 376-390.

McCambridge, T.M., and P.R. Striker. 2008. Strength training by children and adolescence. American Academy of Pediatrics Council and Fitness. *Pediatrics* 121(4): 835-40.

McArdle W.D., E.I Katch, and V.L. Katch. 2007. *Exercise physiology: Energy, nutrition, & human performance.* 6th Ed. Baltimore: Lippincott Williams & Wilkins.

McInnis, S.E., C.J. Jones., and M.J. McKenna. 1995. The physiological load on basketball players during competition. *J. Sports Sci.* 13: 387-97.

Merkel, D.L. 2013. Youth sport: Positive and negative impact on young athletes. *J. Sports Med.* 4: 152-260.

Mero A., P.V. Komi, and R.I. Gregor. Biomechanics of sprint running. *Sports Med.* 13: 376-92.

Meyers R.W., S. Moeskops, J.I. Oliver, M.G. Hughes, J.B. Cronin, and R.S. Lloyd. 2019. Lower-limb stiffness and maximal sprint speed in 11-16 year-old boys. *J Str Cond Research* 33(7): 1987-1995.

Miller P.E., R.A. McKinnon, S.M. Krebs-Smith, A.F. Subar, J. Chriqui, L. Kahle, and J. Reedy. 2013. Sugar-sweetened beverage consumption in the U.S.: Novel assessment methodology. *Am. J. Prev. Med.* 45(4): 416-21.

Morgan, R.E. 2013. Does consumption of high-fructose corn syrup beverages cause obesity in children? *Pediatr. Obes.* 8(4): 249-54.

Morin, J.B., P. Gimenez, P. Edouard, and P.J. Arnal. 2015. Sprint acceleration mechanics: The major role of hamstrings in horizontal force production. *Front. Physiol.* 6: 404.

Mostafavifar, A.M., T.M. Best, and G.D. Myer. 2013. Early sport specialisation, does it lead to long-term problems? *Br. J. Sports Med.* 47(17):1060-61.

Mota, G.R, M.A. de Moura Simim, I. A. dos Santos, J.E. Sasaki, and M. Marocolo. 2020. Effects of wearing compression stockings of exercises performance and associated indicators; a systematic review. *J. Sports Med.* 11: 29-42. https://doi.org/10.2147%2FOAJSM.S198809

Murphy, J.R., D.C. Button., A. Chaouachi., and D.G. Behm. 2014. Prepubescent males are less susceptible to neuromuscular fatigue following resistance exercises. *Eu. J. Appl. Physiol.* 114: 825-35.

Murray, J.F. 2018. The ten biggest issues seen in private practice. Sports psychology and clinical psychology. https://johnfmurray.com/news-events/sports-psychology-article-the-10-biggest-issues-seen-in-private-practice/

Naumovski, E. 2001. "Formulating a model for talent identification, development, and selection in women basketball." MA thesis, Toronto: York University.

Nettle, H. and E. Sprogis. 2011. Pediatric exercise: Truth and/or consequences. *Sports Med. Arthrosc. Rev.* 19(1): 75-80.

Nicklas, T.A., C. Reger, L. Myers, and C. O'Neil. 2000. Breakfast consumption with and without vitamin-mineral supplement use favorably impact daily nutrient intake of ninth-grade students. *J. Adolesc. Health.* 27: 314-21.

O'Dea, J.A. 2003. Why do kids eat healthful food? Perceived benefits of and barriers to healthful eating and physical activity among children and adolescents. *J. Am. Diet. Assoc.* 103(4): 497-501.

Ogden, C.L., K.M Flegal, M.D. Carroll, and C.L. Johnson. 2002. Prevalence and trends in overweight among US children and adolescents, 1999-2000. *J. Am. Med. Assoc.* 288 (14):1728-32.

Pain, M.T. and A. Hibbs. 2007. Sprint starts and the minimum auditory reaction time. *J. Sports. Sci.* 25(1): 79-86.

Pandy, M.G., A.K.M. Lai, A.G. Sache, Y. Chung Lin. How muscles maximize performance in accelerated sprinting. *Scand J Med & Sci in Sport.* 16 Jul. 2021.

Passer, W. 2012. Children in sports: Participation motives and psychological stress. *Quest* 33 (2): 231-44.

Pasulka, J., N. Jayanthi, A. McCann, L.R. Dugas, and C. LaBella. 2017. Specialization patterns across various youth sports and relationship to injury risk. *Phys Sportsmed.* 45(3): 344-352.

Paul, D.J, T.J. Gabbett, and G.P. Nassir. 2016. Analysis in team sports: Testing, training, and factors affecting performance. *Sports Med.* 46, 421-42.

Peirce, N., C. Lester, A. Seth, and P. Turner. 2018. The role of physical activity and sport in mental health. https://www.fsem.ac.uk/position_statement/the-role-of-physical-activity-and-sport-in-mental-health/

Perroni F, G.P. Emereziani, F. Pentene, M.C. Gollotta, L, Guidetti, and C. Baldari. 2019. Energy cost and energy sources of an elite female soccer player to repeated sprint ability test: A case study. *The Open Sports Sciences Journal* 12: 10-16.

Post, E.G., S.M. Trigsted, J.W. Riekena, T.A. McGuine, M.A. Brooks, and D.R. Bell. 2017. The association of sport specialization and volume with injury history in youth athletes. *Am. J. Sports Med.* 45(6): 1405-12.

Powers, S.K. and E.T. Howley. 2008. *Exercise physiology: Theory and application to fitness and performance.* 7th ed. New York: McGraw-Hill.

Pozzi, F., H.A. Plummer, E. Shanley, C.A. Thigpen, C. Bauer, M.L. Wilson, and L.A. Michener. 2020. Preseason shoulder range of motion screening and in-season risk of shoulder and elbow injuries in overhead athletes. *British Journal of Sports Medicine.* 54 (17): 1019-27.

Radnor, J.M., R.S. Lloyd., and J.L. Oliver. 2017. Individual response to different forms of resistance training in school-age boys. *J. Strength Cond. Res.* 31: 787-97.

Raedeke, T. and A.L. Smith. 2004. Coping pressures and athlete burnout. *Journal of Sports and Exercise Psychology* 26: 4.

Rader, R.K., K.B. Mullen, R. Sterkel, R.C. Strunk, and J.M. Garbutt. 2014. Opportunities to reduce children's excessive consumption of calories from beverages. *Clin. Pediatr.* 53: 1047-54.

Ratel, S. 2011. High-intensity and resistance training and elite young athletes. *Med. Sport Sci.* 56:84-96.

Rivier M.L., L. Louit., A. Strokosh, and L.B. Seitz. 2017. Variable resistance training promotes greater strength and power adaptation than traditional resistance training in elite youth rugby players. *J. Strength Cond. Res.* 31: 947-55.

Richards, J.D., A. Chohan, and R. Erande. 2013. *Tidy's physiotherapy.* 15th ed. Edinburg: Elsevier.

Rumpf, M.C., J.B. Cronin, I.N. Mohamad, S. Mohamad, J.L. Oliver, and M.G. Hughes. 2015. The effect of resisted sprint training on maximum sprint kinetics and kinematics in youth. *Euro L Sport Sci.* 15(5): 374-381.

Sebastian, R.S., C. Wilkinson Enns, and J.D. Goldman. 2009. US adolescents and MyPyramid: Association between fast-food consumption and lower likelihood of meeting recommendations. *J. Am. Dietic Assoc.* 109: 226-35.

Sasaki, K. and P.R. Neptune. 2006. Differences in muscle function during walking and running at the same speed. *J. Biomech.* 39(11): 2005-13.

Seitz, B.L., A. Reyes, T.T. Tran, E.S de Villarreal, and G.G Haff. 2014. Increase in lower body strength transfer positively to sprint performance: A systematic review with meta-analysis. *Sports Med.* 44(12): 1693-702.

Sharma, K.D. and P. Hirtz. 1991. The relationship between coordination quality and biological age. *Med. Sport* 31: 3-4.

Sonoda, T., Y. Tashiro, Y. Suzuki, Y. Kajiwara, H. Zeidan, Y. Yokota, M. Kawagoe, Y. Nakayama, T. Bito, K. Shimoura, M. Tatsumi, K. Nakai, Y. Nishida, S. Yoshimi, T. Aoyama. 2018. Relationships between agility and lower limb muscle strength. targeting university badminton players. *J Phys Ther Sci.* 30(2): 320-323.

Squire, J.M. Muscle contraction: Sliding filament theory, sarcomere dynamics and the two Huxleys. *Glob Cardiol Sci Pract.* June 30, 2016 (2): e201611. http://dx.doi.org/10.21542/gcsp.2016.11.

Stanford Children's Health (Children's Orthopedics and Sport Medicine Center). 2019. Position paper.

Stead, R. and M. Neville. 2010. The impact of physical education and sport on education outcomes: A review of literature. Position paper. Institute of Youth Sport. Loughborough University.

Steinbach Chiropractic Clinic. 2018. Position paper. Complete concussion management.

Struzik, A., K. Karamanidis, A. Lorimer, J.W.L. Keogh, and J. Gajewski. 2021. Application of leg, and joint stiffness in running performance: A literature overview. *Appl Bionics Biomech.* 2021: 9914278.

Taylor, M.J.D. and R. Beneke. 2012. Spring mass characteristics of the fastest men on Earth. *Int. J. Sports Med.* 33(8): 667-70.

Thomson, R.L. and J.D. Buckley. 2011. Protein hydrolysates and tissue repair. *Nutr. Res. Rev.* 24: 191-97.

Thorpe, R.T., G. Atkinson, B. Drust, and W. Gregson. 2017. Monitoring fatigue status in elite team sports athletes: Implications for practice. *Int. J. Sports Physiol. Perform.* 12: S227-34.

Tomkinson, G. 2013. "Global Changes in Cardiovascular Endurance of Children and Youth Since 1964: Systematic Analysis of 25 Million Fitness Test Results from 28 Countries" (presentation: American Heart Association's Scientific Sessions, Dallas, TX, November 16-20, 2013).

Tonnessen E, T. Hangen, and S.A. Shalfawi. 2013. Reaction time of elite sprinters in athletic world championships. *J. Strength Cond. Res.* 27(4): 885-92.

Trappe, S., M. Harber, A. Creer, 0P. Gallagher, S. Slivka, K. Minchev and D. Whitsett. 2006. Single muscle fiber adaptation with marathon training. *J Appl Physiol.* 101:721-27.

Trauth, J., J. Sheffer., S. Hasenjager, and C. Taxis. 2019. Synthetic control of protein degradation during cell proliferation and developmental processes. *ACS Omega.* 4(2): 2766-78.

Turner, A.N. and I. Jeffreys. 2010. The stretch-shortening cycle: Proposed mechanisms and methods for enhancement. *J. Strength Cond Res.* 17: 60-67.

Turner, N.J. and S.F. Badylak. 2012. Regeneration of skeletal muscle. *Cell Tissue Res.* 347(3) 759-74.

Udofa, A.B., L.J. Ryan, K. Clark, and P. Weyand. June 14-18, 2017. "Ground Reaction Forces During Track Events: A Motion Based Assessment Method." (presentation: 35th Conference of the International Society of Biomechanics in Sport, Cologne, Germany, June 14-18, 2017).

University of Wisconsin Health. 2016. Dynamic stretching vs. static stretching. University of Wisconsin School of Medicine and Public Health. https://www.uwhealth.org/news/dynamic-stretching-versus-static-stretching.

U.S. Department of Agriculture. Food and Nutrition Service. 2022. Child nutrition programs. https://www.fns.usda.gov/cn

Urbach, A.C. 2001. "An analysis of the energy demand in the sport of basketball." MA thesis, Toronto: York University.

Valovich McLeod, T.C., L.C. Decoster, K.J. Loud, L.J. Michell, J.T. Parker, M.A. Sandrey, and C. White. 2011. National Athletic Trainers' Association Position Statement: Prevention of Pediatric Overuse Injuries. *J. Athl.* Train 46(2): 206-20.

Van Someren, K.A. 2006. The physiology of anaerobic endurance training. In *The Physiology of Training,* edited by G. White, 85-115. London, UK: Elsevier.

Vanelli, M., B. Iovane, A. Bernardini, G. Chiari, M.K. Errico, C. Gelmetti, M. Corchia, A. Ruggerini, E. Volta, and S. Rossetti,. 2005. Breakfast habits of 1,202 northern Italian children admitted to a summer sport school. *Acta Biomed.* 76(2): 79-85.

Weyand, P.G., D.B. Sternlight, M.J. Bellizzi, and S. Wright. 2000. Faster top running speeds are achieved with greater ground force not more rapid leg movement. *J. Appl. Physiol.* 89:1991-99.

Weyand, P.G., R.F. Sandell, D.N.L. Prime, M.W. Bundle. 01 April, 2010. The biological limits to running speed are imposed from the ground up. J Appl Physiol 108 (4): 950-961.

Wiersma, L.D. 2020. Risks and benefits of youth sport specialization. *Pediatr. Exerc. Sci.* 12(1): 13-22.

Zoladz, J.A., D. Semic, B. Zawadowska, J. Majerczak, J. Karasinski, L. Kolodziewski, K. Duda, and W.M. Kilarski. 2005. Capillary density and capillary-to-fibre ratio in vastus lateralis muscle on untrained and trained men. *Folia Histochem. Cytabiol.* 43:11-17.

Index

Note: The italicized *f* and *t* following page numbers refer to figures and tables, respectively.

A

acceleration, 121-122, 154
acceleration–deceleration coupling, 136
Achilles tendon, 111-112, 111*f*, 121
actin, 96, 108
adaptation. *See also* anatomical adaptation training
  in agility training, 157
  endurance and, 164, 165, 167, 168
  microcycle planning and, 64
  in modeling of training, 82
  in multilateral development, 20
  neural, 107, 110
  nutrition considerations and, 60
  plateaus in, 115-116
  specialization and, 18, 23
  in strength training, 106
  to training loads, 27, 29
addictive disorders, 5
aerobic capacity, 20, 165, 166
aerobic endurance, 23, 37, 67, 71, 164, 166-168
aerobic energy system. *See* oxidative energy system
age categorizations, 25-27, 25*t*
agility. *See also* flexibility
  assessment of, 98, 100, 101*t*
  building foundations for, 16, 35
  components of, 67, 153
  energy systems and, 65
  guidelines for training, 155-157
  maximum strength and, 11, 37, 38, 96, 158
  modeling training for, 86
  multilateral development of, 20
  periodization of, 112, 113*t*, 157-158, 158*t*, 159*t*
  pitfalls of contemporary training for, 95
  power in relation to, 154
  in simulation training, 85
  strength training and, 105
  variety of training and, 24
agility ladders, 155
agonist muscles, 24, 104
alactic endurance, 164-165
alactic energy system. *See* phosphagen energy system
alternating bent-over rows, 233
alternating cable front raises, 261
alternating dumbbell chest presses, 233
alternating dumbbell curls to presses, 234

American football
  ergogenesis of, 68*t*, 75-76
  injury statistics related to, 8
  position-specific characteristics in, 72
American Heart Association, 17, 42
anaerobic capacity, 20, 165
anaerobic endurance, 37, 167-168
anaerobic energy system. *See* glycolytic energy system
analysis phase of game modeling, 82, 84*t*
anatomical adaptation (AA) training, 97, 113-114, 114*t*, 115*t*, 127-129
anatomical age, 25-26, 25*t*
anger, 5, 12
antagonist muscles, 24, 104, 133
anticipation practice, 138
anxiety, 4, 5, 11, 88
application phase of game modeling, 82, 84*t*
arch exercise, 206, 235
arousal activities, 88
athletic development
  agility training and, 158
  endurance training and, 172
  flexibility and, 32-34, 159-161
  multilateral training program for, 20
  nutrition considerations and, 45, 52*t*
  optimization of, 16
  stages of, 31-38, 32*t*
athletic formation stage (U15)
  agility training for, 158, 159*t*
  anatomical adaptation training and, 113-114
  endurance training for, 172, 173*t*
  exercises for use in, 190-205
  flexibility training for, 161, 161*t*
  nutrition considerations, 52, 52*t*, 55
  scope of training during, 34-35
  speed training for, 148*t*, 149
  strength training for, 126-127, 126*t*
ATP-CP energy system. *See* phosphagen energy system
audiovisual training, 140-141

B

back extensions, 183, 190, 206, 215, 224, 231
back squats, 235
barbell back squats, 235
barbell bench presses, 245
barbell calf raises, 236

barbell front squats, 236, 262
barbell Romanian deadlifts, 237
baseball
  ergogenesis of, 68*t*, 74
  injury statistics related to, 8
  position-specific endurance in, 171
basketball
  ergogenesis of, 68*t*, 74-75
  injury statistics related to, 8
  position-specific characteristics in, 72, 73*t*
  strength and power training in, 106
  time–motion analysis of, 73
behind the neck lat pull-downs, 237
bench presses
  close-grip flat, 240
  dumbbell, 190-192, 241
  flat, 241, 259
  incline, 245, 261, 265
  with legs up, 190, 192
  in science-based strength training, 98, 100, 100*t*
bent-over rows, 233, 238
biceps curl to overhead press, 238
biological age, 26-27
biomotor abilities. *See* motor abilities
bodyweight squats, 183
bounding exercises, 37, 119, 128, 158
box squats, 184, 193
breakfast, 46-51, 49*t*
burnout, 12, 15, 18, 21, 24

C

cable chest presses, 257, 270, 272
cable curls, 257, 266, 271-272
cable fly, 270, 271
cable front raises, 261, 264
cable lateral raises, 258, 269, 274
cable overhead presses, 258
cable pull-downs, 263, 272
cable rows, 204, 239, 258-259, 263, 271, 273-274
cable triceps extensions, 262, 269, 270
calf presses, 98-100, 100*t*, 111, 117-119, 190, 206, 224, 240
calf raises, 236
carbohydrates, 41-43, 52-56
cardiorespiratory system, 3, 20, 32-35, 113, 163, 171
center of gravity (COG), 124, 133, 142, 156
central nervous system (CNS), 86-87, 105, 135, 139, 155, 157, 165

About the Authors

Tudor O. Bompa, PhD, revolutionized Western training methods when he introduced his groundbreaking theory of periodization in his native Romania in 1963. He has personally trained 11 Olympic medalists (including 4 gold medalists) and has served as a consultant to coaches and athletes worldwide.

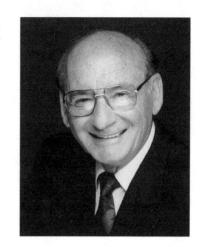

Bompa's books on training methods, including *Periodization: Theory and Methodology of Training* and *Periodization of Strength Training for Sports*, have been translated into 19 languages and used in more than 180 countries for training athletes and for educating and certifying coaches. Bompa has been invited to speak about training in 46 countries and has been awarded certificates of honor and appreciation from such prestigious organizations as the Ministry of Culture of Argentina, the Australian Sports Council, the Spanish Olympic Committee, the National Strength and Conditioning Association (2014 Alvin Roy Award for Career Achievement), and the International Olympic Committee.

A member of the Canadian Olympic Association and the Romanian National Council of Sports, Bompa is a professor emeritus of York University, where he began teaching training theories in 1981. In 2017, Bompa was awarded the honorary title of *doctor honoris causa* by the Polytechnic University of Timisoara.

Sorin O. Sarandan, PhD, is an assistant lecturer at Polytechnic University of Timisoara in Romania. He has worked as a conditioning coach since 2003 and currently serves as a conditioning coach at Sorin Sport & Fitness as well as the Municipal Sports Club in Timisoara. Sarandan has a master's degree in sport management from West University of Timisoara and a PhD in mechanical engineering from Polytechnic University of Timisoara. He served as the conditioning coach for fencer Bodo Benjamin when he won the national title in men's foil in 2021 and 2022. He was also the strength coach to Biea Flavius, winner of the International Boxing Association's Intercontinental Super Welterweight title. He has also coauthored a number of articles in journals, including *Mechanics of Advanced Materials and Structures*, *Materials Today: Proceeding*, and *IOP Science*.

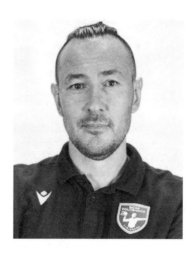

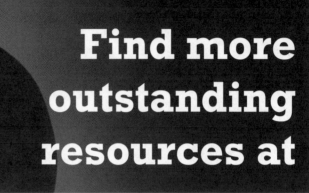
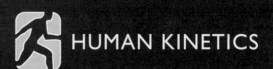

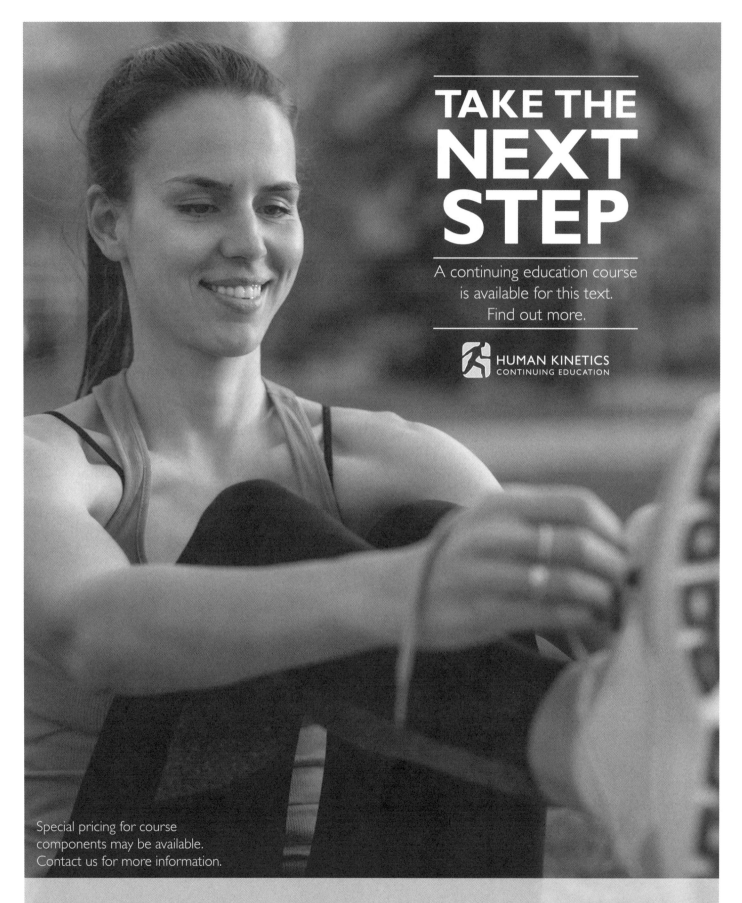